Enlightened Immunity

Enlightened Immunity

Mexico's Experiments with Disease Prevention in the Age of Reason

Paul F. Ramírez

STANFORD UNIVERSITY PRESS
STANFORD, CALIFORNIA

Stanford University Press
Stanford, California

Printed in the United States of America on acid-free, archival-quality paper

Library of Congress Cataloging-in-Publication Data

Names: Ramírez, Paul F., author.
Title: Enlightened immunity :
Mexico's experiments with disease prevention in the Age of Reason /
Paul F. Ramírez.
Description: Stanford, California : Stanford University Press, 2018. |
Includes bibliographical references and index.
Identifiers: LCCN 2017057766 (print) | LCCN 2017059181 (ebook) |
ISBN 9781503605800 (electronic) | ISBN 9781503604339 (cloth : alk. paper)
Subjects: LCSH: Public health—Mexico—History—18th century. | Public health—Mexico—History—19th century. | Epidemics—Mexico—History—18th century. | Epidemics—Mexico—History—19th century. | Vaccination—Mexico—History—18th century. | Vaccination—Mexico—History—19th century.
Classification: LCC RA451 (ebook) |
LCC RA451 .R36 2018 (print) |
DDC 362.10972—dc23
LC record available at https://lccn.loc.gov/2017057766

Typeset by BookMatters in Sabon LT Pro 10/12

Contents

Maps, Figures, and Tables

MAPS

FIGURES

TABLES

Preface

The seeds of this book began germinating on the campus of the University of California, Berkeley, in the fall of 2006. The occasion was a symposium on Bolívar and the Bolivarian revolution in Venezuela, in which anthropologist Charles Briggs and physician Clara Mantini-Briggs presented research on Misión Barrio Adentro, a revolutionary healthcare program developed on the Cuban model. Interviews with barrio residents showed how experiences in clinics had modified the relationship between Venezuela's citizens and the Bolivarian state. That the manner in which citizens were recognized in healthcare initiatives might shape the provision of care brought me back to the socially distinct settings of colonial Mexico, where efforts to introduce immunizations and other measures of disease control at the end of the eighteenth century dovetailed with intermittent programs to acculturate rural *pueblo de indios*. I hoped to understand the role of politics and culture in a field that seemed enamored with frameworks of biopolitics, medicalization, and medical hybridity.

As in Venezuela, the relationship of the Bourbon state to subjects and tributaries in Mexico was in flux. In these years of scientific discovery and debate, the manner in which immunization would be introduced and used looked as uncertain as the political scene in the wider Atlantic world. These are times when the future seems to offer possibilities that the socioeconomic structure might not ultimately allow. Revolutions in medicine, like other kinds, have a way of doubling back, returning, revolving. But the *contingent* moment, to use the technical term, with its anticipation that things might be otherwise, holds out the promise of insights about technology, citizenship, and ways of knowing that can inform other humanities disciplines, the human sciences, and the way we think about the politics of health care and immunity today. How are new medical techniques and measures designed and implemented? What insights and sensibilities do ordinary people contribute to the process? *Enlightened Immunity* attempts an answer. The book explores the ways that heterogeneous communities and cultures are made visible across fragmented regions, the different forms in which medicines, practitioners, and preventive paradigms reach them, and the mediation of subjects and their knowledge, following the Colombian communication studies scholar Jesús Martín-Barbero, through performances, protests, processions, and ritual.

In the course of completing it, I have incurred numerous personal and professional debts. The financial support of the University of California's Chancellor's Fund, the University of California Institute for Mexico and the United States (UC MEXUS), the Mabelle McLeod Lewis Memorial Fund, and the Muriel McKevitt Sonne Chair made possible extended research trips to archives and libraries. The Dana and David Dornsife Fellowship at the Huntington Library, San Marino, California, facilitated a research leave in 2012–2013 to revise the manuscript. The Alice Kaplan Institute for the Humanities at Northwestern University contributed financial support for publication.

The patient labor of the archivists and librarians at the repositories listed in the notes made available most of the sources on which this book is based. The staff of the Archivo General Municipal de Puebla and the Archivo General del Estado de Oaxaca; Berenise Bravo Rubio and Marco Antonio Pérez Iturbe at the Archivo Histórico del Arzobispado de México; Martha Whittaker at the Sutro Library at California State; Walter Brem and Theresa Salazar at the Bancroft Library; and Hortensia Calvo and David Dressing in the Latin American Library at Tulane also endured my questions and requests and shared their knowledge of the sources and history.

In Berkeley, colleagues and friends who commented on drafts and advised on the conceptualization of the project include Victor Goldgel Carballo, Steve Gross, Bea Gurwitz, Sarah Hines, John Kelleher, Larissa Kelly, Dan Lee, Brian Madigan, Sean McEnroe, Rob Nelson, Kinga Novak, Matt O'Hara, Abena Osseo-Asare, Sylvia Sellers-Garcia, Chris Shaw, and Sarah Wells. Linda Lewin and Mark Healey supplied scholarly and professional guidance early on and again at the end. The theoretical vision of William Hanks is apparent in several chapters. Margaret Chowning endured messy first chapters, refined arguments along the way, and remains an admired mentor, colleague, and friend. Bill Taylor's work on peasant politics and religion first drew me to the historical profession. I have often returned to his publications and teachings in search of good questions, or when the answer seemed to come too quickly.

In Mexico City, Miruna Achim, Claudia Agostoni, Adriana Rodríguez Delgado, Javier Salinas Sáenz, and Zeb Tortorici encouraged this work and provided food, *café*, or shelter. Brian Connaughton always inspires with his insights into religion and public discourse. Linda Arnold's determined indexing of Mexican archives has benefited numerous researchers, including me. From Seville, José Hernández Palomo came through in a critical moment.

At Washington University in Saint Louis, Jean Allman, Daniel Bornstein, Maggie Garb, Christine Johnson, Ahmet Karamustafa, Steve Miles, Tim Parsons, Mark Pegg, and Yuko Miki took an interest and welcomed me. Billy Acree, historian in disposition if not in name, merits special mention. At the Huntington Library I developed some of the book's themes in conversations with Lily Geismer, Claire Gherini, Brian Klopotek, Cynthia Nazarian, Michele Navakas, Katie Paugh, Jason Sharples, and Derek Burdette, who kindly shared his work on Mexican confraternities from afar. At Notre Dame, Karen Graubart, Alex Martin, Jaime Pensado, and Evan Ragland graciously advised a visitor. At Northwestern, for several years my institutional home, Ken Alder, Mariana Cracium, Brodie Fischer, Paul Gillingham, Sean Hanretta, Laura Hein, Daniel Immerwahr, Camilo Leslie, Melissa Macauley, Michelle Molina, Daniel Stolz, Helen Tilley, and Keith Woodhouse supported and encouraged me and the project in the final stages.

Research on rumors and flight into "regions of refuge" was first presented at the 2009 meeting of the American Society of Ethnohistory, at the invitation of Martha Few and with helpful comments from Mary Karasch and Noble David Cook. Jennifer Hughes made possible a lively symposium on "Epidemics and History" at the University of California, Riverside. Other portions of the book were developed in presentations at the Katz Center for Mexican Studies at the University of Chicago, the Klopsteg Lecture Series in the Science in Human Culture Program at Northwestern, and Yale's School of Medicine, in a workshop convened by Mariola Espinosa. I learned much on this last occasion from Diego Armus, Pablo Gómez, Gilberto Hochman, Adrián López-Denis, Steven Palmer, Julia Rodriguez, Gabriela Soto Laveaga, and Adam Warren. Early on, Adam shared unpublished work from his pioneering study of medicine and population management in Peru. I am grateful for his friendship and advice.

Amy Smith Bell, Peg Duthie, Roger Gathman, Margo Irvin, Nora Spiegel, and the two anonymous reviewers for Stanford University Press guided this volume to completion, with maps provided by Bill Nelson. Material in the second and third chapters appeared previously as "Enlightened Publics for Public Health: Assessing Disease in Colonial Mexico," *Endeavour* 37:1 (March 2013): 3–12, and "'Like Herod's Massacre': Quarantines, Bourbon Reform, and Popular Protest in Oaxaca's Smallpox Epidemic, 1796–1797," *The Americas* 69:2 (October 2012): 203–235.

More a part of it than they know, this book is for my parents, Crescencio and Laura, and grandparents, Juana, Leoncio, Mary Jo, and Russell, whose patience for works in progress is unsurpassed.

Enlightened Immunity

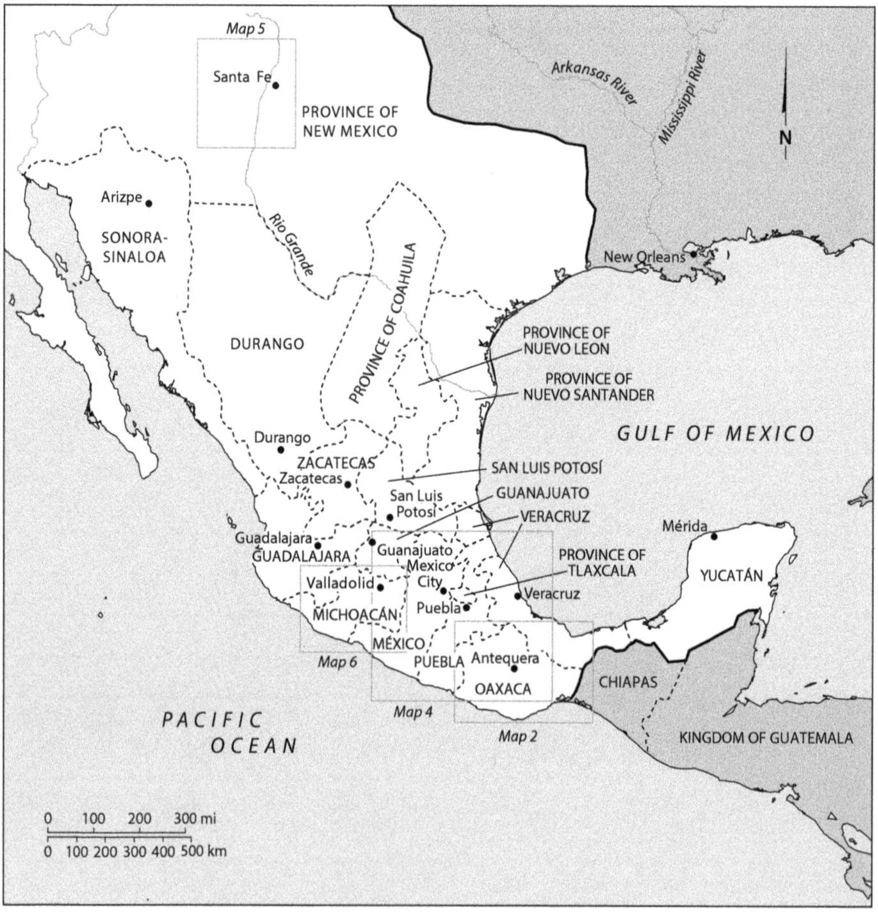

Map 1. Viceroyalty of New Spain.

Introduction

Minerva's Children

Looking back on his time in the plantation society of the Caribbean, things must have seemed simpler. A graduate of the prestigious University of Montpellier, Esteban Morel (1744–1795) served a tour of duty in the French Caribbean as court physician for the French and Spanish Bourbons. On the island of Guadeloupe, he certified surgeons and apothecaries in military hospitals, visited pharmacies to inspect medications and prescriptions, and oversaw some eight thousand inoculations among the island's enslaved workers and slave owners, observing outcomes and instructing others to inject smallpox fluid from one body to the next. Departing on a *peregrinaje* (pilgrimage), as he called it, he sought out additional healing experience in the climates of Venezuela, Cuba, and New Orleans (and looked after interests in the mining centers of Guanajuato and Real de Catorce) before he settled in Mexico City in 1778.[1]

In the cosmopolitan capital of the viceroyalty of New Spain, Morel found a welcoming cultural scene and a population besieged by smallpox. It was a time when vapors from desiccated lakes, sudden drops in temperature, and suspicious odors prompted persons of means to visit a physician or barber-surgeon for preemptive bleeding and sparked bonfires and pungent fumigations with sulfur. Documents from the period are stained where drops of vinegar landed for disinfection, the acrid material of the paper the remnants of a time when disease was sensed in the nose. Morel noticed the ways that residents came together to pray for divine intercession, filing out into the streets to plead with saints to intercede.

He agitated for a different approach. The inoculation technique that he had practiced on the island Guadeloupe was still largely unknown in colonial Mexico. Hopeful to prevent a full-blown epidemic, city officials and the viceroy supported Morel's proposal to initiate trials. A public advertisement announced the availability of inoculation for residents aged three and up under the supervision of Dr. Morel, "trained and expert in the matter." Meanwhile, in a clinic set up in a partitioned room in his own home, Morel—eager to demonstrate inoculation's effectiveness on Indian bodies—conducted experimental trials on six *indios* and *indias* between the ages of three and ten. The children were injected with live smallpox following a preparatory period of several days and segregated to contain the infection.[2] Along with eight Spanish children who were inoculated in their homes, these were the first recorded trials in Mexico City.

Morel documented the outcomes in a treatise on inoculation that he submitted to the city council for publication. In a prefatory letter he thanked the municipal authorities for their support but reminded them that the beds designated for inoculation in the convent hospital of San Hipólito lay empty. The few inoculations carried out in private homes or in Morel's makeshift clinic had been successful, but in one week ten patients who were being prepared for the procedure perished from smallpox. Now rumors swirled about amputations and deaths. As the tide of public opinion turned, the city council declined to publish Morel's treatise and sidelined inoculation measures in favor of a renewed focus on atmospheric conditions and sanitation. The treatise languished as an unrealized vision in the city council's files.

In possession of considerable training and practical experience, Morel had navigated an interconnected Atlantic world. Yet the medical learning he brought, developed on the estates of the Caribbean and further refined on children in Mexico City, ran aground in the streets and homes of New Spain's upper classes. Why, in light of such vigorous efforts? Morel suggested one possibility in the treatise, a litany of responses to the most common moral, medical, and theological objections. On its first page Morel conjured a tableaux for the frontispiece, in which a figure of Minerva, goddess of wisdom and medicine's muse, would appear with shield in the portico of the capital's municipal building, with smallpox victims arrayed in the dark shadows below to represent the misery, death, and deformity caused by smallpox. To the right, in the same light bathing the goddess, a group of joyful children playing with toys or in the hands of the inoculator, indicated the procedure's complete safety.[3] An icon of the Enlightenment, Minerva became patron and protector, who would guide the population out of the darkness of pestilence and misery and into the light of reason, health, and immunity.

Although he failed to introduce inoculation, Morel correctly anticipated opposition and predicted that the rhythms of emergencies would dictate the pace of reform. More than orders, instructions, and missives arriving from the Spanish metropolis, he thought that acceptance of a medical novelty depended especially on the degree to which the population perceived the severity of the disease it was to remedy. Recent studies of enlightened absolutism and reform in Spanish America and Europe have confirmed Morel's prediction, destabilizing the *absolutist* nature of the Bourbon state. In the aftermath of these revisions, projects look more precarious than seamless, translated and initiated by colonial actors, according to factors, connections, and patterns that have their own cadences and logic.[4] We are left looking to other phenomena—the tastes of merchants, the flow of information in urban centers, the salient effects of microbes on the body—for convincing explanations for change.

In 1794, in an atmosphere of paranoia about the French Revolution, Morel was swept up in the reaction. He died in a cell of the Mexican Inquisition while awaiting trial on the charge of deism, months before inoculations commenced en masse in villages and towns in New Spain. He had been prescient in another respect: when the time came to promote and adopt new techniques, the path would be paved by a host of celestial and terrestrial mediators and agents. In an age when ships and newspapers throughout the Atlantic bore the name of the goddess of medicine, many more emblematic Minervas—patrons across the viceroyalty—would mediate cultures, knowledge, and public health programs. The people, rituals, and routines responsible for this transition in Mexico have remained in the shadows. *Enlightened Immunity* attempts to bring them to light.

DISEASED POPULATIONS

When Morel arrived in Mexico City, judges, city officials, physicians, architects, and the police were in the midst of a program of urban reform that had begun to transform the city center. Cities teemed with human waste, piles of refuse, and filthy drinking water, and other obstacles to good health. Among those who indicted Mexico City's dismal sanitary record was the talented lawyer and *oidor* (royal judge) Baltasar Ladrón de Guevara (1725–1804), whose 1788 *discurso* (essay) evoked a city redolent of putrid odors. Guevara believed that the pathological effects of poor atmospheric conditions might be countered by the methods of enlightened administration, informed by principles of rational order, or *policía*. Guevara had in mind efficient municipal planning: clean air, clear sight lines, regularity in public spaces (down to the size and shape of lettering on homes and businesses), and especially the suppression of transgressions by individuals and groups. Public health suffered owing to *desórdenes* (disorders) that consisted not only of violations of the municipal code but also exemptions and special privileges that undermined its spirit. Frequently, regulations were simply not enforced.

The result was repeated abuse, including the resale of articles of clothing previously worn by infected residents, ineffective cleaning of the city's aqueducts, decomposing meat passing through poorly controlled entrances, and lice and the stench of urine brought into public spaces by swine, which contaminated the air and facilitated the spread of epidemics. The ad hoc conglomeration of barrios further deprived the city of rational beauty and salubrious air, of symmetrical and rectilinear street grids that, in Guevara's view, had been the hallmark of the "enlightened" sixteenth-century monarchs, Charles V and Philip II. The proximate remedy was ventilation, more trees for shade and clean air for residents strolling through the Alameda, and aromatic plants such as chamomile, jasmine, peppermint, rosemary, rue, thyme, watercress, "and others that embalm the atmosphere and facilitate healthy and pleasant respiration with their emanations."[5] As in such European cities as Madrid, Paris, and Venice—which served as ideals of rational planning—cleanliness and regularity in Mexico City's appearance would bespeak the calm, health, and good order within.

Penned at the height of the Bourbon monarchy's interest in enlightened administration and healthy human populations, Guevara's essay articulated itself around the defining axis of happiness and liberty, which derived from the ability to live within the constraints established by a clean, ordered urbs. The contemporary interest in *policía*—indicated by regulations on burial practices, the use of public spaces, and ceremonial life—has been construed as a manifestation of anxiety among the upper classes: poorly masked and frequently contested measures to control plebeians, who were viewed as inherently disorderly in their living habits and associations.[6] Vagrants, beggars, pilgrims arriving for feast-day celebrations, and the lower classes in general were most often and easily targeted by reformers, and modern historians have readily seen them as victims of a regime of discipline under the rhetoric of the Enlightenment.

It is a selective reading that edits out systematic criticisms aimed at the social elite, who behaved in ways prejudicial to the common good and were not above reproach. If the physical environment was so potentially deleterious to human health when not managed with a rational hand, private actors were accessories in this tale of negligence, carelessness, and self-interest. They were the *manos poderosas* (powerful or favored persons; literally "hands") cited in streams of petitions received by the General Indian Court (Juzgado General de Indios) from indigenous villages (*repúblicas de indios*) beginning in the seventeenth century. In seeking out viceregal protection, communities accused justices and administrators, Spanish ranchers, parish priests, and Indian governors of usurping land, rigging elections, extracting excessive tribute, and submitting villagers to a variety of onerous labor exactions. These abuses inflicted harm on the petitioners, the king's most humble and deserving subjects (as they stressed), and offended the authority of the royal person.[7]

Enlightened diagnosticians in pursuit of social reform referred to these and other discursive and legal traditions. Guevara looked nostalgically to the rectilinear grids of the sixteenth-century "golden age" of Spanish American urban planning. The long-serving archbishop of Mexico, Alonso Núñez de Haro y Peralta (tenure from 1772 to 1800), a major figure in urban and public health reforms, found historical justification in the patristic era of the early Catholic Church. In the 1779 smallpox outbreak, when he ordered victims buried in new *camposantos* (cemeteries) rather than overcrowded churches, he announced that "the ancient discipline of the [Church] Fathers" must be restored "as current circumstances permit" to maintain the decorum of the church building, to achieve indispensable public health (*salud pública*), and to compel uniform cooperation.[8] The reformist narrative presented an image of old, sound habits of thought, behavior, and speech that had been undermined by inertia and neglect. New restraints and regulations were a restoration rather than an innovation.

In fact, steps by residents and officials to introduce rational planning and protect the populace from disease were already entangled in conversations about health, population, and industry taking place across the Atlantic and deep in the agricultural countryside. The Swiss physician Samuel-Auguste Tissot announced a troubling demographic trend in the first lines of his widely read 1761 advice manual on health and medicine: "It is an unyielding fact known to all and shown by census registers that the number of inhabitants of Europe has declined. This depopulation has many causes, and I would be pleased if I could remedy one of the principal ones, which is the poor method employed in the curing of diseases."[9] Tissot's work was published in six Spanish editions over the century, and the supposed demographic fact of Europe's population decline worried ministers of absolutist states at a time when a healthy workforce was indispensable to agriculture and industry.

The Spanish statesman Pedro Rodríguez, Count of Campomanes, was so concerned by reports that he fully endorsed inoculation, still controversial in the Spanish world, in his influential 1774 essay. "The Indies suffer even greater devastation from smallpox" than Europe, he observed, and "we are indolent in view of such repeated devastation, which we could easily stem."[10] If there were doubts about the means to achieve it, monarchs agreed that healthy populations were the responsibility of enlightened states. New Spain's reformist viceroy, the Conde de Revillagigedo (tenure from 1789 to 1794), advised his successor that few matters were as worthy of a ruler's attention as prevention of epidemic illness. "If in governing New Spain the necessary precautions for public health had always been taken," he reasoned, "we would not have seen frequent epidemics, to which is and should be attributed in great part the depopulated state of the provinces of these kingdoms."[11] In Lima, the city's creole (of Spanish descent born in the Americas) physicians positioned themselves at the center of this debate, as the antidote to decline through applications of "useful knowledge."[12]

Although inoculation remained mostly unknown, the Bourbon notion of the state as guarantor of healthy populations moved ahead in New Spain, the source of nearly half of Spain's mineral wealth and the most populous and wealthiest of its colonies.[13] Indian tributaries, some 90 percent of the population and a vital source of revenue, participated in economies centered on regional and provincial capitals, where they were separated from the royal treasury by layers of intermediaries who controlled trade and tribute. In an arrangement known as the *repartimiento de comercio* (a system of monopoly trade), district governors, sometimes in partnership with merchants and parish priests, distributed merchandise and animals or advanced cash on woven goods or future crops to villagers. To regalist ministers, the practice invited abuse, consolidated the power of these individuals in the countryside at the expense of royal officials, and undermined competition and economic progress.[14]

A vast reorganization of administration was proposed to integrate populations into the economic realm of Spain and eliminate these inefficiencies. Beginning in the middle of the century, the mendicant orders were removed from *doctrinas,* or "protoparishes" of Indian subjects (many were still administered by the Augustinian, Dominican, and Franciscan orders), which were placed under the authority of diocesan priests. With the appointment of regalist or reform-minded bishops to posts at the top of the ecclesiastical hierarchy in the Americas, vast territories were implicitly attached more firmly to royal control.[15] The secularization of parishes accelerated in the wake of Spain's defeat at the hands of the English in the Seven Years' War, when reformers under Charles III (1759–1788) sought to diminish the privileges and social influence of corporate communities, especially those of the Catholic Church.[16]

The intent was to transition from the traditional partnership between monarchy and the church, in which priests and district governors were powerful mediators between Indian communities and colonial authority, to one in which governance was centralized and rule-bound.[17] José de Gálvez (1720–1787) epitomized this modernizing spirit. As minister of state, he instituted new French-style intendancies designed to temper the influence of semi-independent creole administrators, whose payment for posts and vast social networks motivated them to turn a profit rather than serve the Crown. Promulgated in 1786, the new royal ordinance

(Real Ordenanza de Intendentes) transformed provincial capitals into administrative centers under the rule of salaried intendants who were assisted in the countryside by subdelegates.[18] The decades-long movement to secularize parishes, standardize fees and feast days, and introduce Spanish-language instruction to indigenous pueblos encountered opposition from both priests and parishioners.[19] But in commerce, administration, and education, the ideology of enlightened governance made a mark on the countryside.

Less often considered within this movement is the emphasis on administering healthy populations. On April 15, 1785, José de Gálvez wrote to the viceroy of New Spain—at the time, his brother—to inform him of the king's wishes to protect his American subjects from infectious disease. Administrators in New Spain were to enact a program for disease management that had recently been followed to good effect in Louisiana. Sick persons, conceived as sources of contagion, were to be isolated in a chapel or rural building, distant and downwind from populations to avoid contamination of healthy persons. Gálvez assured his brother that these measures posed minimal risk to Spain's American vassals ("el ningún riesgo que de su ejecución puede resultarles [sus vasallos de América]"). When Bernardo de Gálvez (1746–1786), former governor of Louisiana and Cuba, succeeded his father as viceroy of New Spain months later, he declined to issue the *bando* that his uncle had ordered; instead he left the mandate to prelates and secular administrators to enact. He apparently thought this route more effective and was overwhelmed in any case by the devastating famine that he faced in his brief term as viceroy. Bernardo de Gálvez died after just a year in office, at the age of forty, perhaps himself a victim of rampant disease.[20]

The program enacted the idea that disease spread by communication with infected persons, which meant infirmaries at a distance from nucleated settlements, rapid separation of infected victims, and limited contact with patients. Adapted from a 1784 medical treatise by the Spanish surgeon Francisco Gil (whose anticontagion measures had reportedly been tested in the royal monastery of San Lorenzo, on the island of Mallorca, and in Spanish-governed Louisiana), it temporarily resolved the debate over inoculation by rejecting it as too dangerous, in favor of quarantines and *cordons sanitaires* around infected communities. An extract of Gil's treatise circulated to parish priests and royal governors in 1788, with orders to follow its instructions in the event of an outbreak.[21] Resembling in its specifics measures enacted in medieval England and Italy to contain plague and other contagious diseases, the program was novel in its universal implementation, in the incorporation of medical opinion about infection by proximity (as opposed to miasma), and in its vision of governance in which public utility necessitated restrictions on movement, even when potentially harmful to commercial interests.[22] Thus it bore the features of the moment: uniformity through fixed rules, to be enforced without preference ("sin distinción") of caste, class, or gender.

Disease management had become one of the means to a productive state and a measure of Spain's modernity. Inspired in part by European models of statecraft and sanitation, public health initiatives evolved in tandem with bureaucratic restructuring of the countryside and signaled the most comprehensive plan of defense against disease yet. The program was characterized as a restraint on arbitrary private interest (and corporate exemptions) to restore the "liberties" of Spanish subjects to be productive contributors to the Spanish state. Defending American pueblos from the ravages of infectious disease—whose consequences went beyond mortality to include the debilitation of producers and consumers, social unrest, and flight from devastated villages to cities that filled with destitute and starving masses—would, it was thought, allow Spain to participate on more equal footing with France and Britain for territory, trade, and oceanic supremacy.[23] Administrators on the ground were motivated to eliminate *desórdenes* well beyond the cities in which antiepidemic and sanitary measures had usually been applied before.

As a result, by the time a ship armed with Edward Jenner's smallpox vaccine reached the port of Veracruz in 1804, communities across colonial Mexico had years of experience with modernizing health initiatives. Officially known as the Real Expedición Filantrópica de la Vacuna (Royal Philanthropic Vaccination Expedition), the undertaking has long been recognized as the start of mass vaccinations in Mexico. Twenty-two children along with nurses, caretakers, and physicians set sail from La Coruña, Spain, in November 1803 to transport vaccine to subjects across the four continents of Spain's empire. Following stops in the Canary Islands, Puerto Rico, Caracas, and Cuba, teams moved across Mexico by horse carriage and by foot to transfer vaccine to children, to train practitioners and administrators, and to establish vaccination juntas in district seats and capital cities to coordinate future efforts. It was an unprecedented achievement, but its story, in which communities struggled to make immunized populations a reality, is inseparable from a deeper history of reforms in managing disease.

Enlightened Immunity locates the vulnerabilities of late colonial public health projects, as evident in expressions of confusion, contradiction, and contestation. One paradox had to do with the role assigned to the Catholic Church, traditionally a pillar of viceregal power whose members were at once sympathetic to the reforming spirit and part of an institution under threat. José de Gálvez, viceroys, magistrates, and local authorities in New Spain all turned instinctively to parish priests when they sought to implement reforms. Guevara signaled their authority when he contrasted the esteem in which the lower classes held the viceroy and Mexico's archbishop; while the former was shown little consideration in public, the prelate received extraordinary demonstrations of respect. In Guevara's words: "Once the plebeians (who make up without doubt four-fifths of the crowds in this city) see him at a distance, even if in his carriage, they make ready, halt, and even kneel, devoutly removing their hats to receive his blessing, and remain several minutes directing their gaze at him and by their demeanor show the most humble and blind deference."[24] Such displays elicited grudging respect from Guevara, who reasoned that the clergy must be involved in instituting reforms, by persuading parents from the pulpit and in the confessional, for instance, to teach modesty and public cleanliness to their children. Plenty of prelates were ardent reformers; it remained to ensure that such a potential force for progress not become an obstacle to change. The role of priests in public life would be constrained, as some hoped, or else more rational public health practices would penetrate within colonial society. According to Guevara, both would not prevail.

DISTANT ENCOUNTERS: THE WIDOWS OF GUICHICOBI

In January 1796 communities of salt workers, fishermen, and farmers on the Isthmus of Tehuantepec, the narrow landmass that connects the heartland of Mexico to Chiapas and Guatemala, were tasked with enforcing the new anticontagion regime as smallpox spread into New Spain. Not only were parents there asked to relinquish their infected children to isolation, villagers were recruited to assist by providing care and patrolling roads. In San Juan Guichicobi, two widows who had volunteered to minister to the sick children in the infirmary on the outskirts of the village approached Joseph Mariano, the friar overseeing preparations, about an apparent oversight. In halting Spanish they asked, "Father, if a child cries during day or night and wants to feed, who will call its mother to give it milk? We no longer have it." Lifting their *huipiles* (cotton blouses) to illustrate their point, they bared their breasts, which looked to the friar like the slack pouches used to transport *pulque* (agave liquor) or the sagging buttocks of a corpse. Mariano reassured the women that he knew how to make a milk substitute from wine, beetles (*cochinita de humedad*), and *atole* (a corn drink) with butter, to which they allegedly replied, in their native Mixe, "Who knows if that is true?"[25]

Contemporary medical understandings of infectious disease, distilled in a program of prevention and treatment by Bourbon reformers, affected some of the poorest producers and tributaries at the end of the colonial period. Viceregal orders prohibiting villagers from interacting with contagious members of the community targeted susceptible children especially but somehow failed to address nursing infants or the provision of milk (to say nothing of milk substitutes). The question posed by the widows, expressing commonsense anxieties about sustenance and the dangers of the new infirmary, along with the friar's response, alluded to material conditions in which the livestock that might provide an alternate source of milk were scarce, as were other resources to sustain villagers under quarantine. In effect, the exchange between the bilingual widows and their pastor was part of a combined effort to improvise a solution, to make viable a modernizing scheme developed for places that were more hypothetical than real.

The significance of the encounter in San Juan Guichicobi depends as well on what the historical literature on medical reform in Spanish America has trained us to see. Even if economic activity brought producers, merchants, and carriers on the Isthmus into regular contact with other ethnicities, classes, towns, and regions, it was a place viewed by administrators (and by Mexicans and travelers since) as remote in linguistic, cultural, and geographic senses. Because of an accident of geography, with Tehuantepec in the immediate path of contagion, many villagers nevertheless had early and immediate experience with experiments in disease prevention, and they responded to measures that depended for success on communal cooperation. Villagers there and elsewhere would soon express an opinion about the sanitary and quarantine measures in which they were involved. These laypeople appear awkwardly in a literature that has tended to emphasize critical publics for Enlightenment learning as masculine, urban, creole, and literate. *Enlightened Immunity,* the first full-length study of the inception and reception of public health programs in Mexico during this eventful period in the history of medicine, seeks to revisit and reconsider the ways they fit in the picture.

Seeing through the haze of the intervening centuries is a tricky proposition. In the last decades of the nineteenth century, germ theory and modern immunology, backed by modernizing states and informal empires, helped justify unsavory medical campaigns throughout Latin America. Under the influence of critical theory (from Foucault's history of "biopower" to the feminist questioning of patriarchal structures), the modern developments once hailed by historians of medicine look rather regressive in retrospect, compelling us to understand the ways in which ordinary people experienced the state and medical power as untrustworthy, disciplining, or intrusive. Examples for Latin America abound. In the name of public health and progress, social workers, psychiatrists, medical doctors, and the police regulated and reformed some of the poorest citizens of Mexico.[26] Favelas and tenements in port cities were razed, emptied, and fumigated, and their sick isolated in sanatoriums. In 1901, when yellow fever threatened the economy of the United States, sanitarians and engineers from the occupying government teamed up with Cuban health officers to implement invasive sanitation measures on the island, including a mosquito eradication campaign that ruined supplies of drinking water.[27]

The spread of immunization, so emblematic of advances in scientific health care, took place in campaigns that were no less heavy handed. In 1904 a forced immunization drive in Rio de Janeiro coincided with an assault on tenements, under the auspices of an urban renewal and beautification project, and precipitated a major riot that forced the government to rescind a compulsory vaccination article in the health code.[28] Though many submitted willingly, more than a few of those immigrants and working poor who dared resist elsewhere were vaccinated at gunpoint or under threat of corporal punishment. Multiplied, examples would seem to illustrate the rise of what the anthropologist James Scott has called the "high modernism" of twentieth-century totalitarian states. He traces the impulse to impose rationalism and order on populations through control of environments, bodies, and health to the eighteenth century, when governments across Europe acquired the desire and capacity to engineer ambitious human-improvement programs in a "broadening and deepening" of old objectives of statecraft related to productivity and human health.[29]

With their utopian ends and tendency to regard local knowledge and experience in reductive or dismissive ways, the reforms in health pursued by Bourbon ministers, prelates, intendants, priests, district governors, and physicians in Spanish America seem to invite similar assessments. The Bourbon monarchy generally sought to restrict the flexibility characteristic of their Hapsburg predecessors, after all, and to that end promulgated reformist programs that were less tolerant of regional variations and customs. Occasionally these schemes were put into practice violently. A study of the neighboring kingdom of Guatemala turns up examples of intimidating shows of force and "militarized spaces" in inoculation campaigns during the mid-1790s, including the erection of pillars to whip intransigent subjects, which gave way to a medicalized society with the arrival of Jennerian vaccine.[30] Research on subsequent vaccination campaigns highlights both symbolic and physical violence, as when a smallpox outbreak in Guatemala's western highlands moved the creole physician (and future president) Cirilio Flores to impose quarantine on Quetzaltenango in April 1815. Following attacks by Indian residents on the quarantine house to liberate its patients, the priest in Tejutla, fearing a general riot, demanded an end to invasive house inspections and coercive vaccinations. Sixty armed men were nevertheless stationed around the plaza during Easter week to ensure compliance. In historian Greg Grandin's interpretation of these incidents, they are symptomatic of a trend toward state meddling in "nearly every aspect of community life" in the pre-Independence years, and prefigured the liberal state's interventions in a 1837 cholera outbreak, when it sought to incorporate Indians as modern, hygienic, educated, ladino (non-Indian) citizens.[31] Honed in medical campaigns, elite paternalism in regard to Indians apparently found ever-greater expression in an era of heightened nationalism and liberalism.

The Mexican case offers striking if not surprising similarities having to do especially with the way acculturating discourses and projects acquired focus through medical practice. In a 1780 smallpox outbreak, one priest in rural Oaxaca pronounced that "all of the Indians, generally speaking [*generaliter locuendo*], have such horror and fear of the hospitals that it is not possible to persuade them to go there to be healed, because they respond that they die."[32] Such commentaries on Indian nature were among the more innocuous tropes propagated during epidemics. Often these gave way to blanket condemnations of superstition, stubbornness, or timidity; violent campaigns against *temascales* (sweat baths) and other rural healing practices involving alcohol or herbal treatments; and occasionally even whippings or incarceration of villagers who contravened orders for quarantine to seek out markets or tend their fields. At the same time, the Mexican context suggests a meaningful contrast. Administrators invoked and cautiously monitored public opinion, aware of the considerable dangers of popular discontent. Assaults on local healing practices by medical officials or priests might turn villages into states of siege, but communal flight and protest remained viable options long after teams of vaccinators first arrived in the countryside. Documented violence is exceptional, in other words, perhaps because violence was an expensive and ultimately ineffective way to manage public health if prevention was to "work" in any sense.

And there were undoubtedly successes in disease management, no less significant for being modest. Hundreds of registers in archives in Mexico and Spain document the names, ages, and caste status of children vaccinated by priests, district governors, physicians, and local healers, a feat sustained, with starts and stops, through years of insurgency. These sources present a puzzle that has not been sufficiently explored in the literature on medicine and health care in Latin America. Why, with little prior experience and so many reasons for suspicion, did parents allow their children to be immunized in the first place? Medicine was still firmly in the ancien régime: therapeutics remained ineffective, controlled tests were few, and the population was overwhelmingly rural and illiterate. Even today, with the benefit of historical perspective, studies in peer-reviewed journals, and far higher literacy rates, immunization can be controversial. Why did peasants voluntarily participate two hundred years ago, when so much conspired against it? How did certain schemes to improve the human condition *succeed*?

The introduction of preventive techniques forms a pivotal chapter in the history of medicine and public health, yet the historical literature on Mexico offers few sustained descriptions of how campaigns operated on the ground, much less explanations for why parents assented to epidemic measures or immunization technologies when they did. More nuanced understandings of the mechanisms of rule, the mediating role of local knowledge, the nature of medical and scientific technologies, and the scope of debate in colonial cities, towns, and villages would help to crossfertilize histories of medicine. The ways in which natural philosophers, physicians, and administrators addressed different publics across regions or invoked their learning is an especially obscure topic, perhaps because Mexico's geographically fragmented public sphere has discouraged the pursuit of these connections.[33] Broadening the chronological and methodological approach might help to situate disease and public health within a fuller political and socioreligious context.

Instead, the imperial crisis brought about by the Napoleonic invasion of Spain and the king's abdication of the throne in 1808, so transformative of Spanish America, has marked a rupture for historians interested in the origins of modern modes of sociability, a moment when questions of representation and critique moved to the fore. The political crisis ushered in not only a decade of economic catastrophe, disease, famine, and warfare, but also critical experiments in Atlantic republicanism and self-rule. Studies of political representation and culture in Spanish America emphasize new reading and publishing practices, maintaining an imperiously urban and literary focus on a "geography of modernity" that is almost perfectly coextensive with places of print and literacy, above all Mexico City—at the time second only to Madrid in publishing.[34] In histories of medicine and public health, this emphasis is reinforced by the fact that publication and correspondence about scientific matters took place in urban centers, where the handful of institutions that promoted, produced, or divulged "modern" medical practice and scientific methods were based.[35]

Some of the most compelling research on late colonial Spanish America has challenged the assumption that people acquired information about their world or engaged in politics primarily through print and political literature. Studies have taken issue with the "public sphere" model as developed by the German social theorist Jürgen Habermas, which emphasized what appear retrospectively as the most modern modes of communication, to the exclusion of other ways of sharing and shaping information, such as pasquinades and rumors.[36] The historian of science

Jorge Cañizares-Esguerra stands out for questioning both the primacy of textual analysis and the embrace of Europe (and specifically France) as the core of the Enlightenment universe: creole intellectuals in Mexico City spilled much ink refuting European works that disparaged the populations of the New World as physically, culturally, or intellectually inferior and elaborated an "aggressively modern" historical project that, in certain respects, was not literary at all. By examining ancient Mesoamerican monuments and ruins, glyphs, and Mexican antiquities, these creole writers illustrated the superiority and antiquity of the New World while showcasing the critical capacities of Americans. Though the protagonists are similar—clergy, students, and intellectuals in a cosmopolitan center oriented toward the Atlantic world—the political pamphlets in studies of high politics are secondary, drastically altering the picture of Enlightenment knowledge.

With the shift to this side of the Atlantic and a more eclectic documentary base, barriers of class, gender, and geography have yet to be crossed. Histories of science that move to deemphasize national boundaries and narratives of progress tend to highlight the accomplishments and identities of those creole classes that most actively fueled Iberian expansion in the early modern world and eventually formed the political backbone of the new Latin American nations. It remains difficult to shake the notion that a critical "willingness to question authority," taken as a fundamental characteristic of the "radical modernity" of Spanish America, was for the most part limited to elite, literate, Spanish circles.[37] The construal of the modern critical mind's genesis at the upper echelons is largely a result of the objects of study—history writing, scientific investigation, political philosophy, and national identity.

If the major problems in need of consideration are a matter of perspective and definition, how are the dominant "practices and ideas" defined, and by whom? By restricting these to questions of nationalism, the decline of empire, class identity, and the significance of Mesoamerican artifacts and civilization for modern polities, the opinions and concerns of many ordinary people—peasants, artisans, weavers, and others who were not trained scientists, technicians, inventors, natural historians, collectors, or functionaries—have been inadvertently marginalized. Most laypeople in New Spain did not, strictly speaking, consume technical scientific studies in Mexico City's literary journals as part of a reading public, or contribute in writing to its production by way of debate, experimentation, or collection, although whether they contributed otherwise is another matter. They were peripheral insofar as most lived beyond centers of publication and were infrequently involved in industry and major problems of statecraft. In sum, the historiography has made clear, on one hand, that Mexico in the eighteenth century was enlightened in unique ways; on the other hand, it has generally not considered how various parts of society fit into the whole. That the lower classes were excluded or forsaken is often assumed, rather than demonstrated.

Disease presented society with another sort of crisis of equal or greater concern to people than the political, historiographical, or absolutist ones.[38] From the beginning of Spanish rule in the Americas, contagious disease was a constant wherever European friars and settlers traveled to gather converts to Christianity.[39] These "virgin soil" epidemics, caused by pathogens and vectors against which indigenous populations lacked immunological defenses, were particularly destructive in their physiological, social, and cultural effects. In acute infections of measles or smallpox, chronic diseases such as typhoid or dysentery, and tropical and semitropical ones such as malaria, microbes wreaked havoc on human bodies and communities. Preceded or accompanied by drought, famine, or warfare, disease outbreaks might weaken or depopulate communities to the point of total collapse and exacerbate subsistence crises, which had grave implications for the Europeans who depended on these ailing communities for food.[40]

For the "mature" colony of Mexico, spanning the eighteenth and early nineteenth centuries, studies of demographic impact, timing, and regional variation show that the effects of disease on human migration, land tenure systems, and sanitary reforms remained considerable.[41] Cycles of settlement along the northern frontiers of New Spain even recapitulated some of the early demographic, epidemiological, and immunological patterns. In the mid-eighteenth century a Jesuit priest in the Pimería Alta, in Sonora, observed that a great scourge of measles had decimated fully half the Indian population of the *cabecera* (head town) of Tubutama—but also, miraculously, brought into the mission residents of outlying settlements, apparently for subsistence and baptism.[42] Although not all contemporaries invoked the hand of God to explain such episodes, it is rare to read sources from the period without finding some trace of famines, acute infections, anxieties about health, and physical disease.

When epidemics struck, intellectuals, bureaucrats, physicians, merchants, priests, and village leaders converged to cope with heightened mortality, pursue explanations, and restore stability. Bureaucrats and physicians arrived as urban emissaries in barrios and outlying Indian pueblos to heal, diagnose, and report, sometimes leaving behind rich documentary trails.[43] Not only officials and medical practitioners, but also pamphlets, microbes, plant remedies, and instruments moved across the Atlantic and between cities and their hinterlands; eventually Jenner's cowpox vaccine followed these itineraries into provincial capitals and beyond. One such traveling object, the pastoral letter (*carta pastoral*), like the sermon, aimed to inculcate proper Catholic practice, orient the faithful toward God and the Catholic monarch, and define what it meant to be a good Catholic. One such *carta* issued by the bishop of Oaxaca to priests and parishioners in his diocese conveyed news of the arrival of the vaccinating expedition from Spain. Exhorting parents and grandparents to adopt vaccination for the young, Jenner's vaccine was presented as divinely ordained and a gift from King Charles IV (1789–1804), who had previously provided schools for Castilian language instruction and improvements in industry, agriculture, and the arts. Now the king sought to secure the health of his vassals at great cost, "to protect you from the contagious illness of smallpox." As copies traveled to parishes throughout the countryside, the *carta* linked the Spanish capital of Antequera to auditors in the parishes of Oaxaca, where portions were read or paraphrased; mediated between literate and oral cultures; made present the monarch in virtual interaction with his American subjects; conveyed Jenner's experiments in England to vaccinators and parents in rural Mexico; and finally, as the bishop surely intended, aligned the celestial realm with the terrestrial, where the vaccine was to be used.

This ecclesiastical genre makes rare appearances in histories of disease and preventive medicine. Rather than assume that the announcement fell on deaf ears, following such an intermediating object across geographic divisions discloses another dimension of the way preventive techniques and programs were communicated, interpreted, and occasionally adopted. Applying this same hermeneutic to more traditional sources, such as instructional pamphlets and periodicals, we can discern some of the features of and reasons for practice. While some were dismissive of the lower classes, others believed that medical science might accord with popular views and earnestly tried to close a perceived educational and cultural gap. The authors of a simple instruction (*método sencillo*), published to treat fevers and pulmonary illnesses afflicting residents of Mexico City in the early Republic, employed "a simple language," they wrote, avoiding "the technical terms of the art [of healing]" in order to "place science within the reach of those who do not understand it."[44] Such vernacular productions and scientific transpositions had their beginnings in the colonial past, when attempts to teach people best practices in healing or the latest fashions in medical science required translations in the dual sense: knowledge physically relocated, and converted into other media, forms, and systems. Though Bourbon reformers complained of the number of intermediaries that stood between Spain and its tributaries, in colonial Mexico, where even saints performed indispensable mediating roles for towns and villages, preventive medicine would have remained a utopian dream without these intermediary links.[45]

The story told in this book is as much about false starts and minor victories as the "conquest" of a particular disease. At the nexus of *pueblos de indios,* the Catholic Church, and urban institutions and media, it takes its cue from studies of the Enlightenment that insist that other ways of apprehending the world made possible the production of knowledge.[46] Not only were these epistemologies, or modes of knowing, compatible with textual learning; literacy is imperfectly understood without these dimensions. Scholarship on the French case proves illustrative. In the years preceding the French Revolution, the monarchy and Parisian police devoted considerable resources to gauging rumors uttered by popular classes, because speech conveyed newsworthy—and potentially dangerous—information and criticism. If not public opinion in the Habermasian sense, this style of speaking warrants serious consideration because it shaped perceptions and attitudes (and was taken seriously by authorities as an expression of popular mood).[47] In the following century, residents of rural France are said to have lived in an "auditory landscape," in which, following a revolutionary campaign to desacralize bell ringing, the practice once again communicated messages and news from a national sphere beyond the village. Bells became "a prerequisite of modernity," according to historian Alain Corbin, "in a society increasingly subject to haste but as yet without any other means of transmitting information simultaneously."[48] The same scholar has documented a "perceptual revolution" in the olfactory register, beginning perhaps with the vinegar used in France's battle with miasmic putrefaction. Vinegar reflected a relationship between chemical science and broader cultural practice; while communities of experts weighed, measured, and classified harmful exhalations in the atmosphere to quantify disease, society became more attuned to foul odors in everyday life. "We have lost sight of that connection," Corbin observes, "because we operate with a history of science that favors the discovery of scientific truth and neglects the history of scientific error."[49] Focusing on reading publics alone obscures the multiple forms of social criticism, perception, and practice that were not strictly literary but that made a difference in the adaptation, elaboration, and experience of enlightened knowledge.

Whether they intended a playful meaning, by baring their breasts the widows of Guichicobi communicated what they knew and feared about complications resulting from the separation of unweaned children from their mothers. To understand this exchange and the binaries (clergy / laity, male / female, urban / rural, European / Indian, scientific literacy / folk orality) that structure it, we need a sense of the endogenous knowledge and rituals that conditioned external forces and policies. Whatever his thoughts about their rusticity, the friar reported their words and actions, suggesting one way that embodied, multilingual exchanges produced effects beyond local settings. Other villagers critical of government policies did not hesitate to raise matters that urban bureaucrats and physicians had not sufficiently considered when formulating public health policies and occasionally ventured "to express their interests in loud, coarse, and, yes, abrasive ways."[50] In this manner authorities were compelled to come to terms with what laypeople knew about disease and health, and what they reckoned the important questions to be.

Disease prevention, like any scheme to conquer or convert, was a matter of what anthropologist Marshall Sahlins called "distant encounters": unpredictable meetings of communities with agents of state-sanctioned policies and practices. Tracking these encounters, we will see more clearly the restraints on critique in a compound public sphere fractured by class, gender, generation, geography, and caste, as well as restraints on the authority of scientific reason.[51] The world contracts in curious ways when infection travels, according to the living logic of microbes instead of the paper logic of colonial Mexico's cordoned administrative units. The resulting encounters put into relief the conflictual and unpredictable structure in which global policies and technologies and notions of public happiness acquired relevance (as menaces or benefits) for "consumers" and "producers" beyond those who ordinarily read scientific journals or followed intellectual debates in societies or periodicals. These laypeople—agriculturalists, artisans, day laborers, the urban underclass—were not mere spectators of the encroachment of state policy on intimate and communal spheres of life but participants in it. They felt these developments in powerful ways, and it is fairly inconceivable that they would not have had something to say.

ORGANIZATION OF THE BOOK

Enlightened Immunity situates the eighteenth- and early nineteenth-century transition in medical techniques, theories, and policies within a backstory of epidemic management in colonial Mexico. The organization is a methodological nod to the epistemologies and habits through which people viewed their world, their environment, and their health. Individual chapters in Part I ("Contagion") examine the complex of rituals and practices—religious, political, and medical—to which communities turned to resolve disease emergencies and address public health reforms. Part II ("Immunization") is a case study of the rituals, debates, and complications surrounding the introduction of preventive techniques in Mexico.

Most scholars agree that the *peste* that struck the Valley of Mexico from 1736 to 1739 was an outbreak of typhus. The epidemic decimated cities and wiped entire villages off the map.[52] Preceding the outbreak, the louse-borne bacillus that causes it would have been invading human settlements and larger cities from the countryside, where months of failed harvests (occasioned by droughts and hailstorms) had destroyed the grains on which their hosts fed. Contemporaries did not perceive the microbial culprit, or the virus that spread smallpox across the viceroyalty in 1779 or 1796, which required sufficient numbers of immunologically vulnerable human hosts to survive. Nor were they likely to identify the coughs and sneezes that spread pneumonia or pleurisy, what contemporaries called "dolores de costado," following another viceregal-wide famine around 1784.

Instead, residents of colonial Mexico turned to saints, herbal remedies, and *cordons sanitaires* to combat these disease outbreaks. The epidemic of 1737 in Mexico City, documented by an eyewitness and promoter of the cult of the Virgin of Guadalupe, provides a point of departure for a deeper history of public pageantry in cities and towns, when appeals to saints transformed urban centers into thoroughfares of statues and devotees. Chapter 1 examines how these dramas were regularly sponsored by corporate bodies and actively solicited by laypeople well into the eighteenth century, when administrators aggressively pursued sanitation and hygiene campaigns alongside divine succor.

Publishing practices in the Atlantic world inspired physicians, natural philosophers, clerics, and others conversant in learning about climatic conditions, sanitation, and the sciences of anatomy, botany, chemistry, and statistics to forge connections with one another and with communities in need to improve medical care in New Spain. Chapter 2 examines this process beginning in 1768, when the rise of a scientific periodical press offered a novel means to collect and disseminate learning about health care, natural remedies, and scientific developments. Reproducing a conceit of colonial healing manuals, the print culture of the Enlightenment went further to shape a repository of vernacular knowledge from correspondents in cities, towns, and villages. Some even hoped that this venue might induct a broader swathe of women, Indians, and mixed-race *castas* into scientific and medical practice.

The government's anticontagion measures occasioned novel experiments in disease management with the arrival of another epidemic of smallpox at the end of the eighteenth century. Chapter 3 draws on judicial inquiries, administrative correspondence, and legal briefs and petitions filed by guilds, villages, religious orders, and administrators to reconstruct the complaints of agriculturalists, artisans, merchants, priests, and local governors as communities wrestled with disease and royal policies. Following months of social unrest in the intendancy of Oaxaca, the viceregal government confirmed the technological shift already under way in rural villages by endorsing inoculation. Colonial Mexico's mediated social structure, oriented toward commerce, production, and revenue, gave a platform to the voices of many more rural actors aggrieved by the official measures. Their concerns form the core of the chapter.

These experiences tilled the landscape for Jenner's smallpox vaccine. Part II examines the ways in which the new technology traveled, through multiple media, communities, and personnel, and years of insurgency. Today, vaccinations against deadly diseases are often genetically engineered in labs, to simulate one portion of a virus to stand in for the real thing. The early modern approach was at once simpler and more complex. It involved introducing into otherwise healthy, nonimmune persons a live version of the virus against which it was meant to protect. In the earliest practice, human smallpox was often simply injected into the skin, which produced a mild case of smallpox. Known as inoculation, or variolation, the procedure triggered the formation of antibodies that conferred protection against a deadlier case. The term "vaccine" derives from inoculation's replacement: the Spanish word *vacuna* referred to the bovine variety of smallpox virus, or cowpox, injected from an infected cow (*vaca*) into a person. The infection similarly produced antibodies to protect against the human virus, but with lower risk of death, and without the possibility that it might spark an outbreak of smallpox. Whether drawing on a reservoir of smallpox or cowpox, the organic material was often transmitted from person to person, by transferring the fluid from the mature pustule on the arm of an immunized person (the "arm to arm" method).

Today the public health principle behind this method of prevention is called herd immunity, which refers to the way that the protection of enough individuals against disease works to defend an entire community. Early modern views on the mechanism were more diffuse, with considerable disagreement about how the procedure worked, who was capable of practice, and its value and safety.[53] Drawing on the insights of historians of science, who note that novel technologies must be "domesticated" before they work, as well as previously unavailable archival records of immunization campaigns in Mexico, this section of the book situates the twice-told tale of the Royal Vaccination Expedition against immunization's promotion and practice over decades.[54] Moving thematically and chronologically, the chapters show how ceremonial routines, colonial healers, and political rituals brought laypeople into contact with foreign medical matter and techniques and fulfilled, however imperfectly, vaccination's radical potential.[55]

Chapter 4 traces the domestication of the technique in medical treatises, sermons, pastoral letters, legal briefs, and public ceremonies, as physicians, bishops, and ministers aimed to convince governments, parents, and other caretakers of its value. These colonial genres and rituals, along with gifts of coins and cookies to parents and children, rendered preventive medicine viable and sacred for diverse publics in New Spain. These ceremonies did not last, however, and in the chaotic decade of insurgency (1810–1820)—a time of acute warfare, infection, and famine—the ability of a shattered government to sustain programs of disease prevention was overwhelmed by a perennial shortage of funds. Chapter 5 considers the types of skill and expertise involved in the propagation of vaccine in these years. Priests, female healers, Spanish administrators and Indian governors, as well as barbers and surgeonsm helped coordinate vaccinations in campaigns that adhered to the dictates of disease outbreaks and warfare as often as those of medical professionals. The final chapter returns to the experience of medical reform in *pueblos de indios,* where rumors and political action mediated the arrival of urban practitioners, Atlantic technologies, and Enlightenment convictions. This process allowed parents and Indian officials to assess and interpret these medical interventions, discern efficacy, and occasionally shape more acceptable campaigns.

The Royal Vaccination Expedition has from its inception been a source of considerable national pride and contention, which requires an additional note. Upon the triumphant return of its director, the Spanish surgeon Francisco Xavier de Balmis (1753–1819), to Spain after circumambulating the globe, readers of a special edition of the *Gazeta de Madrid* learned not only of the feats of the team throughout Spanish America, "and even including the gentiles and neophytes of the Pimería Alta" (on New Spain's northwestern frontier), but of the fact that Balmis had introduced vaccine in Macao and Canton, China, which not even the English had managed in multiple attempts. In case the irony was lost on readers, the article stressed that though the English nation had discovered and publicized vaccine, it was the Spanish who were consummating its use.[56] This national myth making was no less evident in the counternarrative being written in Mexico City, where a special issue of the viceroyalty's newspaper, the *Gazeta de México,* announced the successful vaccination of several orphans in the capital's foundling home—months in advance of the expedition's arrival. This feat had been made possible with vaccine fluid acquired from Havana via the *ayuntamiento* (city council) of Veracruz, thanks to the viceroy's patronage and the patriotic efforts of creole physicians.[57] When the Spanish surgeon José Salvany arrived in the capital of Lima, Peru, as head of the South American branch of the expedition, creole councilmen and physicians there were even less inclined to credit him with success or follow his lead.[58] (For their part, both Balmis and Salvany later cast aspersions on the quality and viability of these early American vaccinations.)

Full-throated claims in print to the glory bestowed on nations and people by a modern public health program attune us to the considerable stakes of this history, which frequently exacerbated elite rivalries by pitting the paternalism of peninsular physicians, natural philosophers, and authorities against the "patriotic science" (in Cañizares-Esguerra's phrase) of creoles. Discussion of these conflicts has been mostly relegated to chapter notes in this book because they have been well studied elsewhere and because they were often less salient to the actors whose views are highlighted.[59] Instead, these chapters pursue realities of disease, quarantine, and vaccination that have been less fully documented, including matters of ritual, technology, genre, accessibility, and emotion, which no less shaped this late movement to improve the health of New Spain's populations.

In Mexico smallpox was declared eradicated by President Miguel Alemán Valdés in 1952, following more than 150 years of work by physicians, nurses, priests, administrators, and medical brigades to introduce vaccine in the countryside. By then, medical practice and ideas about disease and immunity had changed dramatically, but preventive medicine still depended on familiar political routines and stoked the fear and anxiety of parents and children. Today, conversations about the possible hazards of immunization—from autism to multiple sclerosis to infant death syndrome—proliferate in even the most "developed" nations. In the United States, where the polemics have been especially virulent and vaccination rates comparatively low, citizens reluctant to vaccinate their schoolaged children can make use of personal belief exemptions (PBEs) to opt out.[60]

With a far more complex immunization schedule—vaccines for measles, mumps, rubella, diphtheria, tetanus, chickenpox, and pertussis—and more literate and informed citizenries, we have scarcely stopped debating imperatives of public good, divine will, and human liberty, and what peasants in colonial Mexico might have called *manos poderosas* in the form of politically influential chemical and pharmaceutical industries, seemingly poised to compromise public health and the natural health of our bodies.[61] The logic of this skepticism merits serious consideration. In considering the patrons, benefactors, healers, and translators who worked as mediators across different communities and cultures in colonial Mexico, there may be lessons for us in the history recounted in this book.

PART I

Contagion

CHAPTER I

Devotions of Affliction

The Dramaturgy of Colonial Epidemics

> The God of the Hebrews hath met with us: let us go, we pray thee, three days' journey into the desert, and sacrifice unto the LORD our God; lest he fall upon us with pestilence, or with the sword.
>
> —Exodus 5:3 (King James)

In 1563 the Council of Trent reaffirmed the importance of images of Christ, the Virgin Mary, and the saints as the means by which the faithful might direct appropriate honor, adoration, and veneration: against Protestant "iconoclasm," sacred images were deemed to be reminders of God's miracles and other gifts of mercy.[1] Trent bestowed legitimacy on a culture of sacred images that came to flourish in colonial Mexico, where groups of all social backgrounds crossed the fine line drawn between appropriate honor for the prototype, and superstitious attention to the image. In rural areas saints in sculpted form became guardians of households and benefactors of corporate villages, regularly invoked as intercessors between humans and God.[2] Saint images evolved a special role during emergencies, when people entreated them to govern justly, behave virtuously, and to look on the suffering with mercy because this, according to prayer booklets for devotion, was their nature. These celestial patrons became the intermediaries of first and last resort for the resolution of disease crisis.

As the French historian Fernand Braudel wrote in his magisterial study of the early modern world, epidemics were of central importance throughout the course of civilization. Human societies lingered in a biological ancien régime prior to advances in public health and natural science in the nineteenth century, he wrote, and "wherever he lived, man could only count on a short expectation of life, with a few extra years in the case of the rich."[3] Those with the means to escape a city or town besieged by pestilence often did, while those left behind diagnosed, healed, blamed, prayed, atoned, and supplicated. This is the dramaturgy of an epidemic: the typical ways that people perceive, manage, negotiate, and finally assess an outbreak, once its moment has passed.[4]

The eighteenth century has been taken as a watershed moment in the typical pattern of response. In Europe, some governments appear to have moved away from religious assessments of emergencies, in which theological explanations reigned, to impassive "modern" modes of relief that were based on natural, physical, and scientific explanations.[5] A similar story has been suggested for Mexico, where studious interest in the natural order became fashionable and insights from empirical study were applied to remediate and resolve earthquakes, famines, and contagious disease outbreaks.[6] Were the religious processions that reigned perhaps incompatible with medical theories rooted in the body and environment? Studies of devotional images in Mexico have shown how important they were in managing sickness and restoring health, but lack of attention to public devotions has made it difficult to subject this supposed shift in civic response to closer scrutiny at the level of the city, barrio, neighborhood, or town.[7]

This chapter considers the special role of devotional images in the dramaturgy of Mexican epidemics through years of reform. Mexico City, the largest urban center in the Americas at the time, was administratively, economically, and demographically preeminent in New Spain. With its high population density, fragmented administration, and frequent communication with the countryside, the city was also a common locus of disease outbreaks. At the end of 1736, royal, ecclesiastical, and municipal authorities noted increasing reports of *matlazahuatl*, most likely typhus, from the city's barrios. The official response addressed food, clothing, beverages, and the environment as well as the relationship of celestial healers to the ailing population. Despite efforts to mitigate the damage, the epidemic was the most severe to ravage the Valley of Mexico in living memory. In its aftermath the *ayuntamiento* (city council) commissioned Cayetano Cabrera y Quintero (a creole poet and cleric) to commemorate the Virgin of Guadalupe's role and election as patron of Mexico City.[8] Finally published after years of delays and paper shortages, the five-hundred-page *Escudo de armas de México*, ostensibly about Guadalupe, the capital's "shield of arms," documented much more: dozens of saint images, miracles, cures, and acts of thanksgiving and mutual aid enlisted by officials and laity alike in their prolonged battle with contagion.[9]

Read in combination with official correspondence, meeting minutes, decrees, and the government's newspaper, Cabrera's chronicle offers unique testimony to the paternalistic impulses of the capital's elite, along with the spell cast by devotional images in colonial Mexico. The reader is led through hospitals, churches, and streets of the capital and introduced to a world of baroque ceremony in which ritual measures help to contain corrupted vapors and consecrate pestilential thoroughfares. This universe is at once familiar and unsettling to the modern reader, insofar as communal relief efforts and civic duty mix easily with celestial intervention (figure 1.1). Cabrera's vision highlights Mexico City's streets and shrines, and especially the transient ephemera of public rituals: the *posas* (improvised open-air altars) that appeared during religious and civic processions, the decorations adorning doorways and façades, and the sculptures and saintly attire transformed for the occasion by devotees.[10] A focus on the city's northern sector, the processional region that centers on the main plaza and extends to the shrine of Guadalupe, on the hill of Tepeyac, allows us to trawl through the rich network of religious associations, barrios, and other communities here and to see local struggles to cope with critical illness. Here, Spanish viceroys made ceremonial entrances, devotees of Guadalupe converged on her shrine, residents of the indigenous *parcialidad* (sector) of Santiago Tlatelolco worshipped in and around their famous Franciscan church, and the Jesuits concentrated many of their buildings and educational activities.

There were significant changes and continuities in these typical behaviors and responses through years of urban reform. In the last decades of the eighteenth century, administrators preoccupied with disease and its effects, social disorder, and scarce revenues were more willing than ever to impose a vision of rational urban planning and sanitation, with measures to ensure that the atmosphere would not be corrupted by noxious particles from exposed cadavers, refuse, and animals. According to the historian Pamela Voekel, reforms in the use of public space, including mortuary rituals and burial practices, were supported by a rising middle sector in Mexico City and in the Atlantic port of Veracruz, whose enlightened sensibilities led them to avoid the ostentatious privileges associated with burial in churches in favor of a more restrained laying to rest.[11] How did public devotions fare in this environment of urban rationalism? Reports from the official gazette and municipal records of emergency management from Mexico City, along with Guadalajara, seat of the second *audiencia* (royal court), and Puebla, a center of textile production known for its piety, provide a counterpoint of devotional life in cities, towns, and settlements across the viceroyalty.

The *matlazahuatl* crisis of 1737 is in some ways an obligatory starting point for this history because it both preceded the period of most intense urban and public health reforms, providing a benchmark for change, and

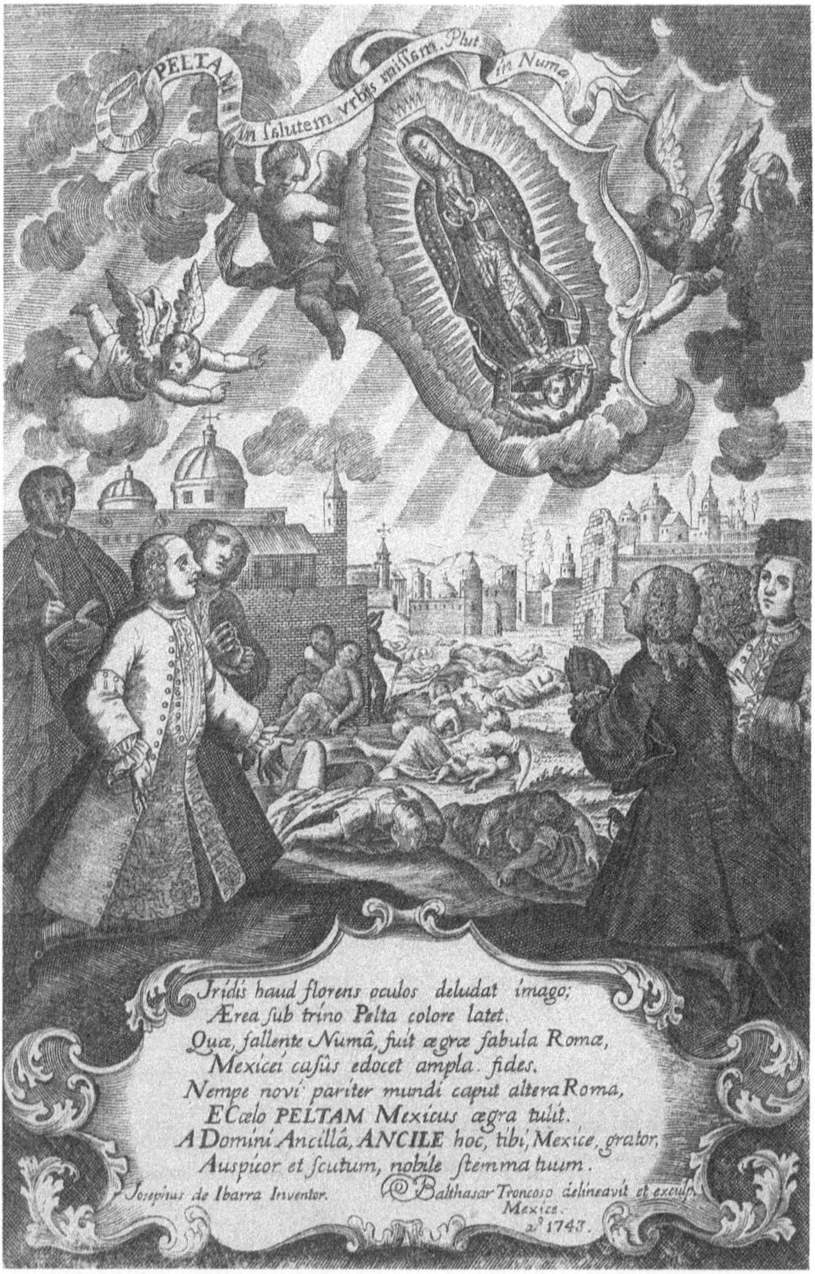
PELTAM in ſalutem urbis miſſam. Plut in Numa.
Jridis haud florens oculos deludat imago;
Ærea ſub trino Pelta colore latet.
Quæ, fallente Numâ, fuit ægræ fabula Romæ,
Mexicei caſûs edocet ampla. fides.
Nempe novi pariter mundi caput altera Roma,
E Cœlo PELTAM Mexicus ægra tulit.
A Domini Ancillâ, ANCILE hoc, tibi, Mexice, grator,
Auspicor et ſcutum, nobile ſtemma tuum.
Josephus de Ibarra Inventor.
Balthasar Troncoso delineavit et excuſ.
Mexice.
a.º 1743.

Figure 1.1 Guadalupe intercedes on behalf of Mexico City. This 1743 engraving illustrates Cayetano Cabrera y Quintero's chronicle of the 1737 epidemic.

SOURCE: Cabrera y Quintero, *Escudo de armas de México*.

served future generations as a point of reference against which new outbreaks were measured. Like Cabrera's chronicle, an exceptional record of fleeting dimensions of life, the city's public spaces overflowed with melting wax, clouds of smoke and vapor, and people and saints in motion. Residents hungry for signs of animation in a saint looked to its transformed dress and saw meaningful reflections of their own predicament projected back. The epidemic yielded renovations of all kind, including the renewal of self, as people prepared for the afterlife; reconstructions of chapels; and the burgeoning fame of Guadalupe and other sacred images like Nuestra Señora de la Bala (Our Lady of the Bullet), whose devotees took the statue in the church adjoining the pesthouse of San Lázaro to the cathedral for a devotional act, "healing, if not Mexico City of its fever, then the chill that its cult has caught."[12] Within this baroque culture of epidemic control, distinct devotions ebbed and flowed in popularity according to local patterns that resist a single narrative. Nevertheless, it too underwent a crisis; this chapter tells the story of how it might be reborn, in recognizable form, in an environment that some desperately wanted to be clean, modern, and enlightened.

MANAGING UNCERTAINTY

In November 1736 the first case of *matlazahuatl* fever was discovered in a textile workshop in Tacuba, on the outskirts of Mexico City. By the new year, *matlazahuatl* had reached the city center, and more than a thousand patients lay sick in the capital's hospitals. They presented with headache and high fever, swelling of the face, and delirium. Blood flowing from the nose and rotting fingers and toes produced an unbearable stench. By the fourth or fifth day, the less fortunate, their skin covered with eruptions, perished from their illness.[13] Statistics compiled by Cabrera from registers totaled 40,157 deaths in a population still shy of 100,000, with 9,787 interred in the cathedral and the city's main chapels, and another 13,721 in the Royal Indian Hospital and the city's predominantly Indian parishes.

Cabrera's chronicle drops readers into one of the largest urban centers in the early modern world, with its attendant mess: its streets muddy, unpaved, poorly lit, and littered with trash and excrement. The fetid conditions of Mexico City, like its great opulence, were the result of wealth flowing in from mining sectors and productive agricultural regions of New Spain. European administrators, merchants, professionals, and traders settled in the capital for reasons of comfort, culture, and access to the productive regions, typically in the *traza*, the central sector originally marked off for Spanish colonists. The majority of the city's churches, cathedral, convents, and monasteries were located here, but observers noted as well more modest huts, crowded tenements, and dilapidated building. In these lived Indians from outlying barrios as well as Africans and *castas* of mixed ancestry, who mingled in the opulent city center as peons, artisans, domestic servants, water carriers, porters, street vendors, and unskilled workers on public works projects.[14] Both in the Spanish *traza* and the Indian-only *parcialidades* and barrios beyond, a large floating and intransigent population transgressed physical and administrative boundaries, spawning repeated complaints about social mixing.[15]

As officials pursued explanations for disease and other disorders, they repeatedly sought to reinforce the boundaries that were undermined in urban economies, spaces of diversion, public worship, and domestic life. Rising rates of infection spurred urgent sanitation campaigns by the municipal government and the Protomedicato, the tribunal of medical officials. Because officials suspected that filth and disease were being transmitted through public spaces, some of the first measures sanctioned by the city council included the elimination of dangerous materials from streets. This meant removing rotting corpses and infected clothing and relocating the living, the urban poor. Decrees ordering improved sanitation and regulation of public activity came in quick succession. On January 24 the council agreed that to ameliorate putrefaction and its effects, the chapter heads of each district should place votive candles in their homes, reflecting a constant concern with illumination as an antidote to corrupted airs. Juan Antonio de Vizarrón (1658–1747), the archbishop of Mexico (who served as viceroy as well for the duration of the epidemic), was petitioned to prohibit transport of the deceased through streets, a practice that was expected to increase with the number of funerals. The following day, the city council approved financial assistance of 20 pesos daily to hospitals serving Indian residents in the barrios of El Hornillo and San Sebastián Atzacoalco.[16] On January 28 the archbishop's legal adviser mandated, under penalty of excommunication, that nothing be sold or traded in portals, plazas, or other public places during celebrations.[17] Medical and spiritual aid was provided at six pharmacies run by religious societies (and sponsored by the city council with the collaboration of the Protomedicato) in the barrios of San Pablo y San Pedro, Empedradillo, and Jesús Nazareno, which dispensed fixed-price medications totaling more than 35,000 pesos. No less central to these efforts, the infected were segregated in lazarettos founded to serve the barrios of San Juan de la Penitencia and Atzacoalco.[18]

Cabrera observed that in general infection concentrated in Indian barrios, in the cramped *chozas* (huts) of poorer residents, as well as in textile workshops, places "where either voluntarily, or forced like meek sheep, those Indians worked to weave clothes."[19] When considering the high incidence of sickness among these populations, physicians identified four causes, in accordance with humoral views of the body: the abuse of *aguardiente* (brandy liquor) and pulque; inadequate nourishment, attributed to excessive expenditures on alcohol (rather than low wages), whose consumption constricted capillaries and obstructed blood circulation; the overheating of bodies at work followed by nights on the cold floors of huts, which similarly constricted blood vessels, especially during the winter months of the epidemic; and drinking cold water while perspiring and overheated, with the same physiological effect. Of these Cabrera informed readers that use and abuse of *aguardiente* was the principal cause, as indicated by the barrel of *aguardiente* found in the Tacuba textile workshop.[20] In these ways the perception of disease incubating in the living and working conditions of the poor opposed the city center to its Indian periphery, as one historian has noted, where piles of garbage, packs of stray animals, and "corrupt odors" were perceived as the origin of infestation and were "considered sufficient to explain why epidemics 'arrived from outside' or originated in those places."[21]

Citing the living conditions, supposedly lax morals, and weak physical constitution of impoverished communities of *indios*, municipal, ecclesiastical, and medical officials who explained the epidemic did not see the lice or fleas on rats that likely propagated bacterial infection to residents and workers in the *obraje*. Textile workshops stored raw materials arriving from beyond the city, and the crowded conditions made them ideal sites to incubate the rickettsia microbe and spread infection throughout Mexico City. Without a theory of germs, officials instead rekindled ongoing debates about the role of intoxicating beverages in the proliferation of human and social ills. A decree of February 16, 1736—months before the epidemic struck—banned an array of beverages, including *aguardientes* of cactus, cane, and honey, *mistelas* (adulterated brandies), wines, *tepaches* (a fermented drink mixed with brown sugar or pineapple), mezcal (distilled agave), and others whose consumption undermined "good customs." These produced drunkenness and other excesses, including robberies, homicides, sacrileges, disorders in production and trade, and unspeakable sins, "with the shameful ruin of servants, slaves, and officials, and what is more, of many high-class persons of distinction, who indulge in similar excesses."[22]

Months later, on June 6, 1737, Archbishop Vizarrón, in coordination with the city council, issued an outright ban on alcohol consumption in the city. He informed the Crown that the Protomedicato, summoned to reflect on the "general, pestilential illness," had deemed the principal cause "excess in consumption of beverages," in which Indians especially indulged, drinking until they were falling-down drunk. The experts thought "that because there were so many producers of false *aguardientes* and *mistelas*, distilled with mixtures and dangerous additives to give them strength on the cheap, Indians filled up continuously on these harmful liquors and contracted a corruption of their blood that was causing their deaths."[23] Citing medical opinion, and the barrel of pulque in Tacuba, the ban deemed intoxicating beverages the source of harm to public health (*común salud*) and specifically the herbs, roots, and other ingredients used to adulterate brandy.[24] Unlike other attempts to regulate production and consumption, it introduced no provision to mitigate the effects on royal income.[25]

Alcohol abuse allowed medical experts and the ruling elite to explain the excessive mortality and morbidity witnessed in indigenous barrios in culturally familiar terms and to suggest policies to address it. Since the beginning of Spanish rule, the overconsumption of alcoholic beverages had been repeatedly cited as a cause of moral decay and illness among indigenous populations. In their response to King Philip II's survey of the Americas the notables of Chimalhuacan-Atenco named the "great vice of drunken binges" as the reason for their community's general decline.[26] Alcohol appeared in the reports of priests and government officials in connection with a slew of social ills, "sweeping statements of excessive drinking and general indictments of pulque and *tepache*," whose wide availability in Mexico became "the cause of virtually all sins and social problems, including idolatry, rebellion, poverty, illness, violent crimes, infidelity, and incest."[27] Within living memory the 1692 riot in Mexico City's plaza, which compelled authorities to temporarily resettle Indians in barrios at the city's periphery, had been officially blamed on alcohol consumption.[28]

The *matlazahuatl* epidemic sharpened the medical edges of this diagnostic tool. Whereas the first (1736) ban on alcohol made no distinction of class or ethnicity when singling out those who abused prohibited beverages ("irrespective of the person's *calidad*"), and furthermore said little about the physical harms they caused, by the end the authorities were fully persuaded that high Indian mortality was bound up with this group's excessive consumption of doctored pulque and *aguardientes*.[29] Explanations for disease, illness, and death recycled discriminatory discourses rooted in the cultural schema of colonial life, and in the process confirmed the moral suspicions of New Spain's ruling classes.

The government's attempts to control alcohol consumption in 1737 came too late to have an effect. Indigenous communities were not, in any case, patiently awaiting diagnosis. Instead, they turned to herbs, purges, bleedings, and a host of celestial advocates for succor. In its final issue of the year, the *Gazeta de México*, the government's official paper, reported that many devout and miraculous images, "until then not seen, even in the most urgent necessities experienced by the city," had been carried in procession that year.[30]

PESTILENTIAL DEVOTIONS

Desperate times called for devotional measures. In his report to Spain, Archbishop Vizarrón wondered how the epidemic had persisted so long, given months of sustained efforts to thwart it. Besides the six infirmaries established for Indians, the pharmacies treating the poor for free, the four physicians assigned to barrios to heal the sick in their homes, and the constant ministrations of priests and physicians, he noted more than a dozen official processions and public acts of devotion. In his words: "Beyond these human measures, spiritual aid has been solicited from divine providence, with prayers, novenas, and rogations to God, His Holy Mother, and the saints, special advocates [*abogados*] of this city and people, seeking to calm His most justified wrath with processions and public penance."[31]

These acts, with their complicated protocols, had origins in medieval and early modern Europe. Especially in times of pestilence, flooding, and earthquakes, images in sacred precincts were turned to as celestial patrons, to mediate between populations, nature, and the unpredictable ire of an omnipotent God. In *rogativas*, or penitential acts, communities characteristically made a vow (*voto*) to an intercessor in exchange for relief, after which households sent members to the saint's procession to honor the contract. As William Christian has noted, certain shrines and images around Madrid acquired reputations for medical aid in an age when the bleeding and poultices offered by popular and professional healers were out of the reach of most people. "At these shrines the fee was reasonable," he observes, "it could be paid in kind, it was payable only if the cure was successful, and it was generally set by the patient."[32]

Marian shrines and devotions found nutritive soil in the pestilential ecology of the Indies. In the first century of Spanish rule, Mesoamerican populations were devastated by repeated epidemics of measles, influenza, and smallpox. In combination with evangelical efforts, in which friars promoted religious images to attract Amerindians to Christianity, this demographic reality encouraged a devotional model in which small statues of Mary and Christ were venerated as repositories of divine presence. One of these, the wooden statue of Our Lady of Remedios—placed in her chapel on the hill of Totoltepec after she reportedly intervened for the Spanish in battles against Aztec warriors in 1520—made the first of many recorded visits to downtown Mexico City in 1576, during an outbreak of what Nahuatl-speakers called *cocolixtli* ("great sickness"), shortly after the city council was designated caretaker of the shrine.

A firsthand account comes from Spanish surgeon Alonso López de Hinojosos (c. 1535–1597), who at the time was employed at the Royal Indian Hospital in the *parcialidad* of San José. Hinojosos recalled that the viceroy dispatched him and a team of governors and a translator to the barrio of Santa María, to investigate the mounting numbers of deceased. Finding a hundred sick in one day, the city's astrologers and physicians, called by the viceroy, identified the summer season, dry climate, and extreme swings in temperature as the cause. Hinojosos was appointed to perform anatomies in the hospital alongside Francisco Hernández, the king's physician and first *protomédico* (medical official) of the Indies (Hernández was experimenting with the herbs that would bring him fame in Europe). The dissections reportedly uncovered a poison in the body that produced rib cages stretched by enlarged livers, abscessed and enlarged gall bladders, urine thick and red with blood, and maddening, feverish thirst. When herbal treatments failed, physicians realized that they were witnessing neither the effects of a celestial conjunction of stars, as astrologers thought, nor corruption of the elements, but the will of God.[33] Interrupting an episcopal review, the archbishop returned to Mexico City, apportioned funds for priests to provide food, medicine, and other care to the indigenous population, entrusted the important *parcialidad* of Santiago Tlatelolco to the Jesuits, and ordered prayers, supplications, and sacrificial masses in the city's churches "for the health of humankind."

The great *cocolixtli* epidemic, as Hinojosos's account makes clear, was critical for afflicted communities, medical practice, and the social order. Losses among indigenous and African population left mines and estates everywhere without a workforce and moved panicked administrators to employ local herbal remedies and activate prayerful rhythms to call on celestial aid. Hinojosos described the ceremonious arrival downtown of the statue of Remedios, "an image of great veneration and devotion that resides in a chapel two leagues from this city on its main altar." At the end of a *novenario* (novena), or nine-day prayer cycle, during which "masses and prayers were said continuously for her to plead with her precious Son for the health and common good of these kingdoms," the diminutive statue was returned, "accompanied by the viceroy, the archbishop, religious orders, clergymen, and many from throughout the city."[34]

Instances of pestilential pageantry in the following years helped forge and reinforce relationships with advocates in other towns and villages. The *Zodíaco mariano* (a compendium of marvels associated with Marian images drafted in the seventeenth century) recounts how, in 1648, the *cabildo* (city council) of the provincial capital of Mérida secured permission from the head of the Franciscan order to bring the sculpted image of the Virgin of Izamal to town during an especially punishing epidemic. It was carried some forty miles on the shoulders of Spaniards and Indians, over protests from Izamal's indigenous community, who kept the friar hostage to ensure the return of their image. In Mérida healthy and sick residents alike processed it through the streets and lavished on it precious jewels and gifts in the Franciscan convent church. (For her role the Virgin was later elected patron of the city.)[35] Devotees of the Virgin of Zapopan, a league outside Guadalajara, processed with the statue to the cathedral for a *novenario* in 1663, during an outbreak of *sarampión* (measles) and smallpox. Called by the bishop to testify to the Virgin's role, the city's physicians confirmed "that since the moment the sovereign image entered the city they had noticed such improvement that of numerous dangerously sick only two remained at risk of death."[36] The same source suggests how some viewed these images and acts in sanitary terms: in 1686, with the city of Guatemala overcome by epidemic, the sculpted image of Nuestra Señora de la Merced (Our Lady of Mercy) was removed from her convent church in procession "to purify the air by way of the streets of the city."[37] By the eighteenth century, extra-urban statues like Remedios and Zapopan made regular visits to city cathedrals and churches, often over the protests of the Indian caretakers of their shrines.[38]

These were the patterns of response featured in the *Gazeta de México* when the paper began reporting devotional acts for an end to the epidemic in Mexico City. In the first three months of 1737 the city council sponsored seventeen processions and *novenarios*, a remarkable commitment in light of the observation that its European counterparts often fled in epidemics, leaving residents to cope on their own.[39] Many of these were jointly sponsored by the city council, viceroy-archbishop, lay religious sodalities, local communities, and religious orders, and were structured to reflect the hierarchies of urban life. Cabrera's chronicle depicts several in poetic detail. On December 14, 1736, for instance, the city council reminded the viceroy of favors the capital had acquired from the Virgin of Loreto in the epidemics of 1727 and 1734. "That which in the present urgency seemed most to the liking of the Lady of the City [Loreto]," Cabrera reflected, "was a devout *novenario*, or nine day Deprecation."[40] Because the image was housed in the church adjoining the Jesuits' College of San Gregorio, two blocks north of the city center, a committee on festivals convened to coordinate the event notified the head of the Society of Jesus.[41] With the cooperation of the custodians of San Gregorio and the permission of its rector, the *novenario* began on December 17 and concluded on Christmas Day. So many among the devout took refuge at Loreto's shrine that it seemed Mexico had relocated to a new home; they went "not only owing to the stimulus of devotion, but by order of physicians," who, like the healers in plague-stricken Rome depicted in the histories of Herodian, advised "that by means of the fresher air that blows there and the plentiful *laureles* [laurel trees] they would be protected against contagion."

The act concluded without sign of the epidemic's retreat. While city councilmen considered other measures, certain devout residents, in

Cabrera's reporting, insisted on taking out the "remedy of Loreto" once more, hoping to steer her toward the main plaza. Because the cathedral was claimed for Remedios at the time, they resolved to bring her to the Casa Profesa, the Jesuit school on the west side of the *traza*, two blocks away, "where, making a further deprecation to her, she would incline her mercy to our requests, purifying on the way there and back the vapors that were infesting Mexico City."[42] The chaplain of the monastery of Santa Inés donated three hundred wax candles for the clergy who would participate and the same number of printed invitations, distributed to notables before the event. As usual, announcements were posted in public places. Some, Cabrera remarked, including residents of Santiago Tlatelolco and San Juan, hardly needed to be invited. "As the afflicted Indians of the city," desperate for relief, "they came more out of necessity than by invitation."[43]

On January 20, 1737, the procession congregated in the afternoon, headed south and east past several convents, and paused for a *posada* (shelter) in the cathedral before arriving at the Jesuit school at eight o'clock in the evening, where members keeping vigil received Loreto's statue.[44] It traversed at most eight city blocks in five and a half hours, suggesting the immense scale and deliberate pace of the event. In procession were many notables, among them the city's corregidor (royal governor) with Loreto's banner; the cathedral clergy, with distinguished priest don Juan Joseph de la Mota carrying the processional cape; city councilmen in the lead; and enough of the populace that, when exiting the wide plaza of San Gregorio College, participants funneled into the narrower streets well after the statue's departure. The *posada* at the cathedral delayed the procession further: accompanied by organ music and singing, Loreto was brought to the main altar, placed in the gallery, and worshipped, at which point Loreto and Remedios and their faithful might have passed one another in the magnificent interior of the church.[45]

Cabrera depicted the procession through the heart of downtown by an elaborate metaphor. Like the string of beads used in praying the *rosario* (rosary), the traditional Catholic devotion to Mary, the faithful made up a human rosary, the beads of which were many, "and of various colors," Cabrera noted, "who either pressed together by the tensed string of fear, or more plausibly, strung along on the gold thread of fervent devotion, made up indistinguishably this Rosario." The faithful were "white and black; men who count, and alongside them others who do not; men of the country, and from abroad; small and large, ecclesiastic and secular; in short all as one, and strung together under one Cross in one Rosary with lights in their hands."[46] The gazette confirmed (with less flourish) this impression of mass participation, reporting that "the number who went out in procession [*alumbrando*] was greater than those who watched it."[47]

In subsequent days the faithful and sick filled the church of the Casa Profesa to confess and be consoled (*desahogarse*). The archbishop and three of the city's principal guilds donated some 100 and 1,350 pesos for wax candles, respectively.[48] After considerable donations of wax and money, there was silver enough in the coffers by the end to renovate the chapel under the college's rector. On December 10, 1737, the new chapel premiered to less than critical acclaim; some complained that the brighter light cast strong shadows that detracted from Loreto's beautiful face.[49]

The other most prominent Marian advocations in the city, Remedios and Guadalupe, received similar regal treatment. Their *novenarios* were coordinated so that one followed the other in ten-day segments, apparently to ensure that devotees might pay respects to all. The effect was a neat escalation to Guadalupe, whose devotion was attaining unprecedented popularity in Mexico City, as signaled in the providential end toward which Cabrera's narrative arcs: the salvation of the entire capital by her mercy. Features of Guadalupe's devotion included a strong association with floods, including a visit to the cathedral during an inundation from 1629 to 1634, in a city whose inhabitants were constantly attuned to of the ebb and flow of water. Since then, she had been physically fixed at Tepeyac, which created challenges in 1737. When city councilmen proposed that the populace accompany Guadalupe to the cathedral once other *novenarios* concluded, Archbishop Vizarrón cited Guadalupe's natural immobility and countered that, if it was not possible, in light of precedent, to take Guadalupe from her sanctuary in procession, then she should be supplicated there.[50]

On Wednesday, January 30, residents left their dwellings and "crowded into nearby hills, plazas, flats and roads, the causeway and other roads becoming cordons of people, restless villages [*poblados movedizos*], linking Mexico City to Guadalupe, and uniting the city with its environs." The devout were reportedly drawn by "her fame and experience preserving against contagion, and the good smell of the place." Miraculously, in Cabrera's telling, few died during those propitious days or henceforth (excepting the occasional careless accident at the shrine). "Contagion dispersed from Guadalupe's precinct; it encircled the circumference but did not enter."[51] Like medieval shrines and tombs, which acquired a "force field" within which the saint's power to heal was most pronounced, Tepeyac had become a sanctuary in another sense—a place of refuge, somehow immune from the vapors infesting the city, where the faithful might take shelter from contagious disease.[52]

When city councilmen appealed to Rome and the Congregation of Rites in the following years, irrefutable evidence of Guadalupe's role in bringing about the end of the epidemic would enhance their case for confirmation as patron. In Cabrera's chronicle, commissioned for this purpose, the purity of the Tepeyac shrine prevails over all others. Nevertheless, even with growing popularity, residents did not simply rely on Guadalupe, or on special protectors against the plague, in a unified gesture of supplication. Within the city was a messier constellation of communities and devotional images. On February 16, 1737, the specialist Saint Roche was one of seven devotions for which Mexico City's *ayuntamiento* approved acts of deprecation, along with the Blood of Christ, Saint Joseph, Saint Sebastian (another plague saint), Saint Rosalia, Saint Raphael, and Saint Christopher.[53] Fort their part the devout came together in neighborhoods, churches, and around dozens of images. Cabrera's chronicle confirms that local preferences as much as choreographed pan-urban events drove the activities of urban communities, who acted on relationships with their own patrons to bring relief.

URBAN VILLAGES IN MOTION

In referring to *poblados movedizos* in his description of Guadalupe's procession, Cabrera acknowledged the many parishes, neighborhoods, and barrios in which residents associated and identified. Following the elaborate Loreto procession back to its beginnings in the sector north of the city, and zooming in on neighborhoods there, it is possible to imagine the concerns and activities of the students and devotional groups associated with the Jesuits at the time of the epidemic, alongside other communities in rituals of penance, supplication, and thanksgiving. Though recently embroiled in controversy over remittances of the tithe owed the Crown from their vast cattle estates, the Jesuits remained respected healers and educators who oversaw no fewer than three schools in Mexico City: the Casa Profesa, the Colegio de San Pedro y San Pablo (a merger of several colleges intended primarily for Spaniards and mestizo residents), and San Gregorio College, established in 1588 for the instruction of the sons of Nahua nobles.[54]

Among the associations affiliated with San Gregorio College was the Good Death Society (Congregación de la Buena Muerte), founded in 1710 to provide financial support and spiritual benefits to members.[55] The devastating impact of the epidemic appears in the group's register for 1737: names struck through or marked with crosses on the page reveal the group struggling to fill vacant offices and maintain organizational stability.[56] Its stricken Indian members came from the adjoining districts and barrios of Las Salinas, San Pablo, San Sebastián Atzacoalco, and Santiago Tlatelolco. Members served the community by providing alms to the poor, attended to Our Lady of Sorrows and the Blessed Sacrament (the devotion of the Eucharist or sacred host), and labored around Loreto's image in the church adjoining San Gregorio.[57] Atzacoalco's patron, San Sebastián, was also protector against pestilence, whose feast day, January 20, marked the beginning of Loreto's procession. Perhaps its members were among the faithful who, as Cabrera reported, "persisted in taking out the remedy of Loreto" and pressed for that significant date as an appropriate compromise when adjusting to the schedule for Remedios.[58] Buena Muerte members, residents of Atzacoalco, and others who lived or labored in Loreto's charismatic presence might have hoped for special grace in their battles against contagion when she appeared for days at the center of citywide devotion. Given their pursuit of a good death, perhaps they found mercy in that feared moment of *agonía.*

Accompanying Loreto to the Casa Profesa, devotees with candles, incense, and bells sought to purify "the vapors that infested Mexico," cutting through the pestiferous air by means of light, prayer, and image. The descriptions portray a mixture of the miraculous and the miasmatic, invoking the sensory, tactile, and visual dimensions of healing, what one anthropologists has called the "ritual sentience" that produces a new awareness of the environment.[59] It is a reminder that, in the structured opposition between purity and pollution, medicine and religion shared similar impulses. With the blood, sores, and other bodily evidence of sickness all around, and the most noxious elements of early modern cities—inadequately disposed garbage and sewage and the remains of human cadavers—physicians, laypeople, and clerics behaved as though contagion could be seen and smelled, like the smoke from fires, incense, and gunpowder that were used as countermeasures. Allowing that Cabrera's depictions were exaggerated to demonstrate a "Christian commonwealth," they reflect features of healing in a Catholic society, which required a cleansed conscience in preparation for the afterlife and the familiar, comforting presence of holy men and beloved saints.[60] During the epidemic, mortuary rituals involving saintly figures, the consecrated host, oil, candlelight, and fragrant incense wafting from the censer and boat of the priest opposed dirt and rot. Priests with access to holy oil, the viaticum, and the expiating power of confession toiled regularly in infested barrios, lower-class huts, and *obrajes* throughout the city. Pastors of the Veracruz parish made trips to three infected textile workshops and several barrios to administer the rite of extreme unction to victims past hope for recovery. The work reportedly exhausted the clergy laboring in the church and hospital of Saint Catherine, where they "nearly lived with the sick."[61]

In the Indian parish of San José, Franciscan priests drew dangerously close to the dying and dead to confess or administer sacraments, "holding the sacred viaticum in one hand, and in the other a vessel to collect the blood that appeared as discharge in nearly all of the sick, and which impeded, at the moment when it was in greatest demand, the aid of the confessions they administered."[62] Pastors from this parish joined forces with those in Veracruz to administer sacraments to the sick in the charitable hospital for parishioners of San José.[63] Jesuit priests and mendicants from the nearby Discalced Carmelite convent were singled out for their zealous administration of sacraments and other remedies: in "continuous movement" for nearly nine months, "they performed in this district alone up to 11,000 *estaciones* [rogations or prayers] and 24,000 *óleos* [anointings] and confessions."[64] Sebastián Atzacoalco, the Indian barrio adjacent to San Gregorio College, found its clergy so fatigued that its parish called on members of the neighboring Jesuit colleges to help with confessions of the sick. Meanwhile, Atzacoalco's parishioners performed a *novenario* to San Sebastián, special plague protector, and while out in procession brought him to individual homes in the barrio to comfort the afflicted.[65]

Like activities at shrines, the attentive ministrations of priests, healers, and lay devout in procession formed nodes of ritual activity intended to restore the integrity of sick bodies, souls, and infected spaces.[66] While some of the city's physicians recommended that individuals stay home rather than participate in religious processions that "heated up" the air in the city center and mixed healthy with sick, others were exploring the salubrious effects of the clean air in and around shrines.[67] The record of processions indicates that the physicians who prescribed isolation were mostly ignored. Residents followed in the footsteps of Athanasius Kircher, German Jesuit and polymath, whose vision of a subterranean world of rivers and fire influenced efforts by natural scientists to expel dirt from urban centers; in this universe regular movement was a guarantor of good health.[68]

The activities that drew the most sustained attention in Cabrera's chronicle came during an incident in the Indian *parcialidad* of Santiago Tlatelolco, where casualties had overwhelmed its parish. In response, on Shrove Tuesday in 1737 (March 5), residents carried out in procession a statue of their patron Saint James, the conquering "Moor Slayer," dressed as a flagellant.[69] Cabrera wrote admiringly of the predominately indigenous district (of *indios mexicanos*), with its wide plazas, innumerable small houses, and magnificent domed parish church, which was designed by Juan de Torquemada for the Franciscan convent and dedicated to Santiago, "patron of the Spains."[70] On Shrove Tuesday members of the city council and numerous residents crowded into the neighborhood to venerate the miraculous sculpture of Saint Anthony, one of several images housed on the left of the main chapel. After mass a procession was conducted around the cloister of the convent, with Saint Anthony escorted by his confraternity and also "by the bizarre statue of Santiago." As Cabrera described it,

...in this procession of blood, in which many went as humiliates and penitents, many who saw the image were mortified [as well], for the image of the Holy Apostle [Santiago]—which by virtue of its sculpture and aptitude [ordinarily] mounts a horse, confronts and attacks, raises his sword and arm, and is dressed and armed as a knight—on this occasion had been dressed as a penitent, giving him the vague appearance of doing more to punish rather than assist. Dressed as he was in a purple tunic, wearing a crown of thorns that reached his eyes, mounted on his vigorous beast, and brandishing a penitential whip instead of a sword, he resembled that other Celestial Knight [Jesus Christ].

Modern readers of this passage wade through double meanings and complicated turns of phrase before seeing that the faithful had improvised with unexpected and, to Cabrera's eyes, distasteful modifications to the dress and behaviors of their saint. The episode caused Cabrera to remark on the "devout sincerity of the Indians, who always do as they see done." He offered this explanation in justification of their actions: "They had seen other images, respectable and devout, in the dress and adornments of penitence, and so to go out in the streets with theirs, without concern that it was of another aptitude, and on horseback, they dressed Santiago in the same way." If this imitation reflected mere simplicity, as he thought, then it should be celebrated; if indecent, then corrected.[71]

Displays of penitential enthusiasm were familiar responses to natural or manmade disasters. Epidemics and drought in Barcelona, Mexico City, and Seville frequently witnessed flagellants take to the streets to counter disease or bring rains as members of confraternities.[72] At Tlatelolco the conquering knight had been transformed and incorporated into the procession, a transformation aided by the sculpted form of processional images that "were meant to engage and provoke the viewer" and "were among the most illusionistic sculptures ever made."[73] Dressed as Christ, Santiago became one more flagellant, vividly spilling blood with and on behalf of his devotees, a reminder of the ease with which an imagined ontological boundary between deity and human was transgressed.[74] It was the blood spilled in these events that especially drew the attention of contemporary observers.[75] Cabrera compared "this procession of blood" to the equally condemnable practice of the city's physicians, who bled their patients all over the capital in a desperate bid to improve their condition or, in his view, to extract as much income as possible, bleeding them twice. The physician "torments the patient in a thousand ways, presses him and nearly breaks his limbs, cutting him and squeezing blood from various parts, pretending that he removes the problem, and though [the patient] may appear to recover from the treatment, it is no more than a lie and punishment for their sins." For good reason, Cabrera observed, *indios* refused to see these physicians again.[76]

Though not identical to medical bleeding, the spilling of blood by flagellants implied, in the broadest sense, blood as the material sign of sin and atonement, and of sickness of the humors in the body.[77] Patron, patronym, and brother, the saint takes up his own whip when the afflicted community repents; Santiago's refashioning is theirs, their suffering his. But too much blood spilled by patients or by flagellants offended the cleric's sensibilities. For Cabrera, Santiago Tlatelolco, with its magnificent church and images, bore monumental witness to Mexico's celebrated past, but its residents, who by his admission were in greatest need, actively sought relief in expiatory rituals and multiple devotional images. As the epidemic continued, some residents took a miraculous crucifix in the church, the Santo Cristo del Milagro, in procession to Guadalupe's sanctuary, which Cabrera approvingly documented. They sang praises, made supplications along the way, did penance, and when they returned heard a sermon on the danger posed by the pestilence and the need to ask forgiveness and mend their ways.[78]

Relief came in many modes, even within Tlatelolco. Much like peasants in early modern Spain, "flexible and open to new options," residents of Mexico City apparently sought protection in "a host of small changes and rearrangements" in the configuration of relations between humans and intercessory saints.[79] These might interact with and even stand in for a barrio, village, or city, calling to mind Emile Durkheim's discussion of sacred objects as containers harboring society's feelings, shared emotions, and moral obligations.[80] Cabrera rejected any such symbiosis in the flagellant procession, but it was happening throughout the city. Sculptures of Santiago, San Antonio, San Sebastián, Loreto, Remedios, and Guadalupe were "shields of arms," in Cabrera's organizing metaphor, which possessed figurative and transformative properties to assume a share of the epidemic's burden. On April 28, 1737, the day after Guadalupe's swearing in as patron, the Cristo Renovado, a miraculously restored crucifix in the care of the Discalced Carmelites, was mobilized for yet another *novenario* in the cathedral. A long miraculous history held that it had restored itself, cured the blind and crippled, and in 1697 saved Mexico City from illness, demonstrating its capacity to protect against contagion.[81] Declining reports of death around this time indicated that it had intervened once more, and April 28 was deemed the official end of the epidemic, adding another wrinkle to the biography of this crucifix.[82]

Eventually commemorated in large-scale paintings commissioned by notables and merchants, the prints and statues transformed and restored at the time no less confirmed the investment of the faithful in these mediators. Not just a story of social control and isolation, the process from crisis to recovery invited broader participation from residents that was neither simply coordinated by patriarchs nor necessarily out of step with the government's response. The poor were undoubtedly subjected to the authority and policies of city officials in these months. Yet secular, religious, and medical authorities achieved limited results in controlling alcohol consumption, and isolation in lazarettos was only ever part of a multifaceted effort to provide relief. Instead of yielding, communities intensified their efforts with new processions, drawing on saints more powerful or familiar with disease, or increasing the workload of familiar figures, transformed for the diseased occasion. From the perspective of lay urban communities, it was a more complex and accessible way of placing blame and restoring health than the fixation on alcoholic beverages. Little wonder these images were so frequently touched up in the aftermath.

PRODUCING ENLIGHTENED MIRACLES

When he departed New Spain in 1794, the Conde de Revillagigedo, seen by historians as one of the most effective viceroys of colonial Mexico, left instructions for his successor that reviewed his achievements on behalf of public health. He highlighted the advancement of medical practice, including new *cátedras* (professorships or chairs) of anatomy and physiology in Mexico City's general hospital; the botanical expedition of Martín de Sessé; improved sanitation; the establishment of public cemeteries at a safe distance from cities; lazarettos to contain infectious patients during two outbreaks of smallpox (which he credited for the avoidance of full-blown epidemics); and other efforts to introduce *policía* in the capital, such that livestock no longer roamed the streets, carts regularly collected waste, and physicians saw that the furnishings and clothing of the sick did not circulate in flea markets for resale. While the personal cleanliness of the lowest classes (*clase ínfima de la plebe*) left much to be desired, a recent directive sought to eliminate the rampant disorders associated with *temascales* and other baths, generally used by Indians "since the time of their heathenism." When it came to managing disease, with its implications of civilization, acculturation, and enlightenment, Revillagigedo had reasons to be optimistic.[83]

Conspicuously missing was any mention of miraculous images, suggesting the distance traversed from the 1737 *matlazahuatl* epidemic. Evidently new confidence in their ability to locate and control sources of infection had changed the ways people spoke and conceived of public health. A wave of administrators, perhaps including many more upwardly mobile professionals who fashioned themselves *sensatos* (enlightened or rational people), achieved dramatic reforms in urban hygiene, planning, and upkeep in the second half of the century.[84] By the time of

Revillagigedo's rule, it has been argued, the populace was undergoing sustained reeducation in matters ranging from burial practices to eating, drinking, bathing, urinating, defecating, and the use of public space, including devotional processions and other public displays of worship.[85] In this view, processions were to be managed, but no longer an integral part of disease management.

The administrative background for the late-eighteenth-century interventions in urban cleanliness and planning can be traced at least to 1696. In that year, Mexico City's corregidor and official (*juez*) in charge of *policía* addressed the need to repair bridges, clean filth from the city's irrigation ditches, repair destroyed paving stones that owners of homes and convents had neglected, and regularly clean streets, all matters of interest to *salud pública*. The Protomedicato blamed corruption of the air on vapors from poorly buried human cadavers and recommended deeper burials, removal of animal corpses from corners and businesses, cleaning of streets, irrigation ditches, and cesspools, and segregation of *indios forasteros* (rural migrants to the city) in hospitals if sick, or returned to their villages if not. (The medical officials left subterranean and celestial causes aside, they remarked, as these were not subject to human will.)[86] But little funding was allocated for these projects and in 1728, shortly before *matlazahuatl* arrived, city ordinances were revised to include similar rules on cleanliness. Municipal officials threatened fines of two pesos for any resident who improperly disposed of trash or human waste in city streets, plazas, and fountains, and a further ten for the improper disposal of animals, "because of the bad odor that results from leaving them in the streets and plazas, and since they are a cause of sickness."[87]

With lax enforcement and municipal funding shortages, an emergency of considerable proportions was often necessary for such regulations to have any effect. Cabrera saw the 1737 epidemic as propitious insofar as it had induced visibility and order among the urban Indian population. God had done what city officials had attempted after the 1692 insurrection in Mexico City, when more than seven hundred Indian scoundrels "who had given neither to God nor to Caesar what was owed them" came out from hiding. The prolonged epidemic lured out many more, "occasioning happiness by their misfortune, making good with God, receiving the sacraments."[88] For officials, nothing threatened order and cleanliness in the urban environment more than water flooding streets full of pedestrians, foodstuff, and animals; infection infiltrating homes and bodies without regard for distinctions of social hierarchy; the poor congregating around the doors of churches to plead for alms; and a stream of rural peasants arriving in the city in search of aid during emergencies.[89] Crisis might paradoxically lead to temporary improvements in public order that administrators so desired but that repeated statutes and threats failed to achieve.

Sporadic institutional efforts to regulate public spaces in the 1770s and 1780s again coincided with disease emergencies. In the smallpox epidemic of 1779, in which more than eighteen thousand people perished in Mexico City, councilmen observed that the quality of air around churches grew worse each day as cadavers piled up, some abandoned at night by the poor, which released fetid vapors into already corrupted air. Noting that cows consumed some of the discarded reed mats used to wrap the cadavers, and that their milk would be harmful to the poor and sick who depended on it, the city council pressed the viceroy to move ahead with plans for two *camposantos* (cemeteries) to accommodate the extraordinary numbers of deaths each day and alleviate the public health crisis.[90] The first cemetery, consecrated by the archbishop on November 8, 1779, received hundreds of corpses in the first week, primarily from among the most impoverished sectors, who lacked the means to pay for church burials anyway. Councilmen stressed that the cemetery was for all who perished and that the policy should be extended accordingly. The archbishop issued orders to this effect but admitted that, while the provision was in conformity with "the ancient discipline of the [Church] Fathers," too many factors conspired against it. Among them was the fact that the king had not yet ordered the provision for Spain, that residents of the *país* were averse to cemetery burials even in their own parish churches, and that almost all would request exemptions as "distinguished persons."[91] In Puebla interest in urban sanitation likewise spiked at this time. A meeting of physicians recommended cleaning and watering streets daily to thwart transmission of contagion, banning cadavers from vestibules and other public spaces, and burning infected clothing. In the San Juan del Rio and San Pablito cemeteries new, deep plots were dug to accommodate overflow from churches and avoid atmospheric contamination.[92]

Though interest in cleanliness was long-standing, something was indeed in the air. Recent studies of Mexico City argue that the late eighteenth century saw a turn toward virtuous restraint—an interiorization of piety—against showy funerals and the processional baroque described above. Among the factors cited for this turn are urban growth, changing conceptions of the city, and the late Bourbon emphasis on secular planning.[93] In the view of self-identified *sensatos*, the physical environment should be more strictly regimented and instrumentalized to discipline human activity and ensure order and good health. During the tenure of Viceroy Revillagigedo, officials and private residents spent vast sums to drain, pave, and illuminate the primary thoroughfares and plazas leading off the Plaza Mayor. This was the old *traza*, the most prosperous part of the city, with rents and property values several times higher than elsewhere. Productive and commercial establishments (just over half of all registered in the capital were concentrated here) brought housemaids, porters, and others from the lower classes to labor.[94] While much of the city, especially the indigenous barrios and the blocks east of the plaza, were neglected, the old market stalls in the plaza were removed, making way for public fountains. Reformist energies were directed at street vendors, bakers, bathhouses, and problems caused by refuse from the old markets, slaughterhouses, and butchers, as well as stagnating waters and perilous streets, with broken cobblestones that impeded commerce, detracted from urban order and beauty, and threatened public health.[95] Renewal programs in other Mexican cities and towns were frequently modeled on those in the viceregal capital.[96]

Along with this rationalization in the organization and use of spaces was an attempt to introduce more effective practices and units of administration to collect statistics and remediate disease emergencies. In 1779, with smallpox rampant, the municipal government split the city into several wards (*cuarteles*) and subsectors for cleaning and administration. Charitable committees of residents of means were established to care for the poor and needy in their homes when hospitals grew full. A printed notice praised the city's charitable efforts during the epidemic, and even invited recommendations from the public for additional measures of relief in the future.[97] Ecclesiastical officials were actively involved in this streamlined system and again in its reestablishment in the following smallpox outbreak. In 1797 the Junta Principal de Caridad, the charitable board rehabilitated by order of the viceroy, communicated instructions more efficiently to *socios* (commissioned heads of each of the 180 subsectors) and worked to distribute medical personnel more equitably. As a result, Mexico City moved from a pluralistic arrangement in which physicians, surgeons, and barbers contracted directly with health committees to a closely supervised system in which eight medical practitioners supervised the medical personnel in their wards. The use of printed forms, on which each *socio* collected information about the number assisted in each subsector, marked the advent of the modern administration that Bourbon-era reformers had long advocated. The data in these forms allowed the Junta Principal to produce tables of statistics for each ward, which were printed and gifted to administrators and affiliates afterward in gestures of gratitude (figure 1.2).

If data allowed officials to make comparisons with previous outbreaks, and plan for future episodes, in other ways the capital had not come far from the older patchwork of impromptu poor relief and medical care. Among criticisms made in an official review of the system was the uneven treatment provided in each subsector, evidenced by disparities in expenditures per patient as a function of the total number of residents in the sector; the unwillingness or inability of some of the *socios* to perform their duties; insufficient medical personnel to supply the subsectors; and

ESTADO DEL QUARTEL MAYOR NUMERO 1.

En que se manifiestan las Sociedades que contuvo para socorro de los pobres contagiados de Viruelas en la epidemia experimentada en el año de 1797, los Muertos, Sanos, y total de socorridos de cada Sociedad, lo erogado en Alimentos, Abrigos ó Vestuarios, Medicinas, Medicos ó Cirujanos, y Barberos, lo que cada Sociedad hizo á sus expensas, y lo que libró contra la Caxa de socorros.

Sociedades.	*Muertos.*	*Sanos.*	*Total de socorridos.*	*Alimentos.*	*Abrigos.*	*Medicinas.*	*Medicos y Barberos.*	*Gasto de Sociedades.*	*Gasto de la Caxa de socorros.*	*Gasto total.*
				Ps. Rs. Gs.	Ps. Rs. Gs.	Ps. Rs. Gs.	Ps. Rs. Gs.	Ps. Rs. Gs.	Ps. Rs. Gs.	Ps. Rs. Gs.
Núm. 1.	29.	277.	306.	385.	377. 4.	218.	140.	606. 4.	514.	1120. 4.
2.	17.	161.	178.	255. 3.	231. 1. 9.	175.	108.	302. 7. 9.	466. 5.	769. 4. 9.
3.	10.	222.	232.	415. 1.	588. 5.	91. 4.	600.	1695. 2.	......	1695. 2.
4.	7.	111.	118.	113. 2. 6.	114. 7. 6.	170.	30. 6.	145.	284.	429.
5.	13.	103.	116.	84. 4.	138. 6. 6.	70. 2.	122. 3. 6.	80.	336.	416.
6.	9.	73.	82.	111. 6.	19. 5.	60.	28.	31.	188. 3.	219. 3.
7.	9.	82.	91.	120. 1.	171.	22. 5.	76.	194. 7.	194. 7.	389. 6.
8.	17.	172.	189.	194. 1.	165. 3.	68. 2.	111.	7. 2.	531. 4.	538. 6.
9.	27.	273.	300.	314. 5. 6.	152. 2. 6.	200.	145.	25.	787.	812.
10.	16.	304.	320.	339. 7. 6.	235. 7. 6.	270. 6. 6.	121. 2.	68.	899. 7. 6.	967. 7. 6.
11.	14.	178.	192.	106. 3.	183. 5.	200.	87. 4.	21.	556. 4.	577. 4.
12.	13.	158.	171.	164. 5.	238. 3.	153. 5. 6.	101.	......	657. 5. 6.	657. 5. 6.
13.	50.	277.	327.	372. 1.	233. 6. 6.	191. 6. 6.	188. 4. 6.	154. 4.	831. 6. 6.	986. 2. 6.
14.	30.	272.	302.	124. 7. 6.	155. 2.	200.	101.	......	581. 1. 6.	581. 1. 6.
15.	29.	493.	522.	272. 4.	293. 7.	180.	228.	3. 6. 6.	970. 4. 6.	974. 3.
16.	83.	695.	778.	315. 6.	503. 7. 6.	212. 6.	154.	......	1185. 6.	1185. 6.
17.	20.	210.	230.	117. 1. 6.	55. 3.	75.	76.	......	323. 4. 6.	323. 4. 6.
18.	40.	311.	351.	206. 7.	230. 5.	318.	130.	......	885. 4.	885. 4.
19.	12.	155.	167.	197. 2. 6.	159. 5. 6.	100.	120.	1. 7.	575. 1.	577.
20.	20.	121.	141.	164. 3.	100. 4.	110.	86. 3.	......	461. 2.	461. 2.
21.	33.	232.	265.	301. 3. 6.	185. 6.	153. 4.	157. 4.	......	798. 1. 6.	798. 1. 6.
22.	197.	1011.	1208.	601. 7.	541. 2.	605.	193.	......	1941. 1.	1941. 1.
23.	10.	72.	82.	100. 1.	58. 6.	42.	60.	......	260. 7.	260. 7.
24.	29.	366.	395.	104. 4. 6.	208. 6.	48. 1.	25.	......	476. 3. 6.	476. 3. 6.
	734.	6329.	7063.	5573. 2. 6.	5344. 7. 3.	3936. 2. 6.	3190. 3.	3337. 3.	14707. 7.	18044. 7. 3.

Figure 1.2 A printed table of statistics from the 1797 smallpox epidemic. Column headings indicate (left to right) subsector; number of deaths, number healed, and total administered; amounts spent for food, shelter, medications, and medical personnel ("physicians and barbers"); and amounts paid by associates from the junta's coffers, and in total. One thousand copies of eight tables and a general summary were printed for distribution to officials, associates, and donors.

SOURCE: AGN Bienes Nacionales, volume 1024.
Courtesy of the Archivo General de la Nación, Mexico City.

the mobility of the population, which in combination with inconsistent reports from *socios* hindered the compilation of reliable data. Above all, the new system still relied on charitable networks and protocols for giving. Officials, corporations, and well-off persons, frequently merchants, were asked for donations and pledged considerable sums (with no lack of pomp and self-regard), while medical practitioners in the subsectors were encouraged to serve gratis, out of a sense of charity. (Each physician received a gratuity at the conclusion of their service, based on how many they treated, and how well).[98]

In this era of urban renewal, perhaps the most surprising continuity is the persistence of the kinds of religious acts featured in Cabrera's plague chronicle. At the beginning of 1787, *protomédico* José Ignacio García Jove reported that the fevers afflicting residents of Mexico City were a less-malignant variety of *matlazahuatl* that had turned contagious and epidemic. In light of this and the previous year's puzzling high mortality, the medical official, a man of faith, recommended on behalf of the public that the city council implore Guadalupe, "who always sends to these inhabitants [*vecindario*] very prompt remedy." Convening days later, the city council agreed to request permission from the Audiencia to spend some 350 pesos on a *novenario* for Guadalupe in her sanctuary, to request through her "that any sickness cease and desist, crops from the land, the happiness of this capital and kingdom, and remedy of all necessities and calamities." The Audiencia in turn reported that it had received a request from a committee of concerned citizens (*junta de ciudadanos*) days before García Jove broached the issue. The committee, represented by three elite signatories, had been considering strategies to mitigate the effects of acute food shortages, which had spurred an emergency planting effort. Believing the capital to be the place where public prayers (*ruegos*) to God should begin, the committee requested that the bishop be entreated to order that in all of the churches of the archbishopric, supplications (*preces*) be made "to implore divine compassion in the calamities that threaten and currently afflict the kingdom, especially from the malignant fevers that have almost decimated many places and are extending in this capital." While the city council deemed supplications beyond its purview, it moved forward with the *novenario*—one of dozens reported that year in the newly revived *Gazeta de México* (1784–1809).[99]

The processional mode in public health emergencies, with its saints, prayers, penitents, and rosaries, appears not to have gone underground or faded from public view in this period of intense reform. In fact, the processions organized by officials in Mexico City represented one peak of a range of activity across New Spain, as documented in the pages of the gazette. A survey of issues in two distinct periods yields a tally of devotional acts reported by local administrators (table 1.1).[100] In the first period, years of devastating drought, crop failures, food shortages, and epidemic outbreaks (of fevers and *dolor de costado*, pleurisy or pneumonia), the number of distinct *novenarios*, *misas rogativas* (petitionary masses), and processions topped thirty in consecutive years. Though most were in the provinces, even in Mexico City, according to the February 25, 1784, issue, "there is no image of miraculous repute in the city to which a *novenario* has not been celebrated."

The crisis-resolution structure remained a common feature: emergencies hastened communities to invoke divine intervention, with sudden, definitive reversals of fortune. The miraculous crucifix of the parish of Xiquipilco, north of the Valley of Toluca, had barely been brought out in procession on the evening of September 18, 1786, when the sky began clouding over and rain fell the next night.[101] In Real de Catorce, newly prosperous after a silver strike, drought threatened to starve the population. The image of Guadalupe "had just been placed on the altar" of the

Table 1.1 Number of devotional acts reported by year in the *Gazeta de México.*

Year	*Total*	*Mexico City*
1784	36	7
1785	39	1
1786	34	3
1787	13	4
1794	6	1
1795	2	1
1796	1	0
1797	5	3
1798	1	1

church for a *novenario* when "an abundant downpour burst forth that lasted an hour, and continued as light rain for another three."[102] In Toluca, the Christ of Farmers (Señor de los Labradores) was processed to the cathedral for a *novenario*. The same evening "an abundant rain lasted for an hour and a half," and with it the epidemic (*peste*) ceased, which moved residents to sponsor a second act, in thanksgiving.[103] In Celaya, a town of textile and agricultural production in the Bajío benefiting from Guanajuato's silver boom, residents staged a *novenario* and procession for its Marian patron, an Immaculate Conception, as the "scourge of *peste*" gathered strength in 1785. "The hopes of the people were not in vain (as they have never been), because the next day the epidemic took flight as if it had never been there."[104]

Many cities and towns synchronized the power of their patrons, as in Pachuca, where half-a-dozen images appeared in two processions in 1786.[105] A drought in the summer of 1794 saw Nuestra Señora de la Soledad (Our Lady of Solitude), patron of the provincial capital of Oaxaca, in procession with three other statues—of Christ, Mary, and Saint Vincent Ferrer—while others emerged from convents in a grand marshaling; following an earthquake, a sure sign of supernatural intervention, the rains finally came.[106] By means of "innumerable" public rogations to end an especially devastating epidemic in Chihuahua, which struck down cattle as well as people, "the Heavens already appear more benign, and the contagion less severe."[107] Occasionally these actions were too effective: years later, petitions for rain reportedly led to ruinous floods in Chihuahua and its surroundings.[108]

This landscape of miraculous activity, hiding in plain sight in an official and public paper, was reported in a time when religious politics dictated a cautious stance on the matter. Ecclesiastical officials were wary of publicizing miracles that might contribute to expanding the popularity of a shrine or image beyond the control of authorities. As evident in table 1.1, the number of reported acts in fact declined in the second period, beginning in 1794, perhaps reflecting this trend. Is it also evidence that the bonds that linked celestial patrons to cities and towns had weakened? That people were turning to these saints less often during emergencies than even a decade earlier? The 1790s were a decade of warfare with England and revolutionary France and growing preoccupation with Atlantic developments. Reports of battles and other news from the international arena, often reprinted from European papers, filled the gazette's pages, along with public ceremonies in cities and town to mark victories. In addition, fewer submissions arrived from New Spain's provinces, and there was an overall decline in the frequency of publication. In 1788, the editor, Manuel Antonio Valdés, complained about the lack of submissions from those entrusted with the task, and again in 1800, observing the paucity of news arriving from beyond Mexico City and Veracruz; in 1798 months elapsed without a single issue. While it is possible that devotions of affliction were no longer viewed as newsworthy—or that the emergencies and disasters of the 1790s, including a widespread smallpox epidemic, were perceived as less acute—changes in reporting and publishing practices warn against concluding that the drop-offs in numbers reflect a decline in enthusiasm.

In detailed municipal records of planning, these public acts of remediation remain central. Repeatedly, viceregal and municipal authorities demonstratively approached celestial advocates to mitigate or end public calamities, of their own volition and at the urging of the people they ruled. As in Mexico City in 1787, they appear as composite efforts, reflecting the plurality of agents that might intervene as benefactors or sponsors in times of disease crisis. During emergencies *ayuntamientos* or *cabildos* (municipal councils), whose members ordinarily worked on behalf of the public good to regulate the price of food, oversee matters of cleanliness, including street cleaning and garbage disposal, and sponsor public works projects, joined with *audiencias* (royal courts, in Mexico City and Guadalajara), ecclesiastical officials and cathedral chapters, viceroys and alcaldes (ward officials), medical authorities, and "charitable" residents and corporations who might contribute to relief efforts (and in the process protect their honor or boost their reputation).

The emotion and urgency informing popular requests for aid was encapsulated in the word *aclamar*, which evokes simultaneously the *clamor* for intervention, the *acclaim*, or public fame and miraculous repute, of the image in a community, and the *crying out* of people in need.[109] For instance, in Puebla in 1736, as crops withered below clear skies and people perished from typhus, residents concluded—from the ineffectuality of the *novenarios* and *rogaciones* (petitions) to images of Jesus Nazareno (Jesus of Nazareth) and Nuestra Señora de la Soledad sponsored by the city council—that more needed to be done and reportedly "affixed signs on all the doors of council members and in various other public places" urging (*aclamando*) the intervention of Saint Joseph. Officials of the city bent to public pressure for another devotional act.[110] In 1786 the gazette reported that the populace of Guanajuato "has not ceased to cry out [*clamar*] with repeated *ruegos*" for the Virgin of Guanajuato to intercede with God on its behalf.[111] Residents and devout groups signaled this acclaim by paying for or otherwise sponsoring ceremonies. Far north of Mexico City in the Villa de Cadereyta (environs of Monterrey), "residents and farmers [*vecinos y labradores*]" sponsored and paid for a *novenario* to petition the local advocation of Mary to bless the population's quest for rains and a favorable harvest of maize and *frijoles*.[112] A penitential procession through Zacatecas, with a *novenario*, for the miraculous Christ of the Parroquia was carried out at the request—and expense—of "el piadoso Público."[113]

Why did these publics continue to clamor for religious images in emergencies? Devotion was not simply a second-best option, necessary because medical science had not yet developed an alternate framework by which to explain, predict, prevent, or actively mitigate epidemics. In addition to the material ends often cited—rainfall, abundant harvests, safety, and good health—there was an affective and aesthetic dimension: spectators were said to receive comfort and pleasure from viewing these acclaimed images in processional garb, including rich capes and jewelry. With Guanajuato battling contagion in 1786, residents swarmed the streets to see their patron, the Virgin of Guanajuato, in procession for the first time in a rich indigo cape, "made in Rome, and blessed by Pius VI."[114] These regal figures had acquired their own reputations over time as powerful intercessors, with established relationships to communities. This fact complicated the matter of which was most appropriate for the occasion. As smallpox gained strength toward the end of October 1797, Mexico City's *cabildo* proposed a "novenario de rogación" for Remedios, its special advocate, to beseech her intercession as on previous occasions.[115] The city council deputized two members to consult with the archbishop in his role as president of the Junta Principal de Caridad, who agreed that some kind of public petition was urgent in light of mortality rates. But the parties disagreed over which intercessor should preside. Would it be Remedios, "trusted in her special patronage" of the city, as the council put it, or the famous Cristo Renovado, the Christ of Ixmiquilpan, venerated in the convent church of Saint Theresa? The crucifix had intervened conclusively in 1737; the archbishop added the "confirmed experience in the previous epidemics of smallpox in 1779 and of *dolores de costado* in [17]83" when he expressed his preference for it. In the end a diplomatic truce allowed that either would be acceptable.[116]

The viceroy put the act on hold, noting that the epidemic was not as devastating as in the past and arguing that acts of thanksgiving for this grace would be more suitable. Far from a sign of dissatisfaction with the processional approach, it acknowledged how closely these acts were watched and associated with critical disease moments: *rogativas* required special care, he thought, not because they were unruly but because the suffering public (*público afligido*) might, upon witnessing them, become upset and imagine that the deadly year of 1779 had returned, which was "indelible in the memory of these residents and of the entire kingdom." Stationed in Orizaba to coordinate war efforts, Branciforte responded in almost identical terms to a request there to appeal to an image of Christ crucified (el Señor Crucificado del Santo Calvario), arguing that the time for public *rogativas* had not arrived, worrying that they would lead residents to perceive a real epidemic disaster (*una epidemia devoradora*) and sadden or upset unnecessarily.[117] Soon after, however, convinced by the worsening state of affairs in Mexico City's parishes, he consented, for the public's consolation. He opted for the Cristo Renovado, with an additional *novenario* for Guadalupe in her sanctuary to follow. The last was "to satisfy many devout who have asked me for it," as well as his own professed devotion to this powerful protector, "whose patronage is felt whenever it is implored."

Remarkably, given her widespread fame, Guadalupe appears in the correspondence only at this point, as her December festival approached. The viceroy claimed to be following the lead of the *vecindario* in this, to whose "general *aclamación*" for an act soliciting her patronage he gladly consented, by combining his *votos* with those of the public (*el público*).[118] While Guadalupe's *novenario* was postponed (her church would be occupied by Indian residents for their special festival at the proposed time), Baltasar Ladrón de Guevara, senior *oidor* of the royal court, recorded enthusiasm for the Cristo Renovado. On the evening of Friday, November 17, "innumerable crowds gathered in the many places of transit," he reported, remarking on "the great tender devotion and gratitude with which they look upon this prodigious image."[119] A footnote in the gazette's reporting referred to a host of convalescents among the spectators, present for the occasion to worship (*alumbrar*) the miraculous Christ "in thanksgiving for having been given their life."[120] The presence of these grateful survivors can only suggest the depth of existential investment in divine intercessors during Mexico's Enlightenment and the gifts the faithful believed they had received.

Not everybody saw these well-lit undertakings as worthwhile expenditures. Much money was spent on wax for candles placed on altars, carried by officials and image porters, lining the processional route, and for priests and ministers. Judge Guevara himself, exemplary of the liberal critique of these expenses, had in fact proposed physical monuments or plaques as one way to redirect the financial contributions of Mexico City's guilds, confraternities, and other corporate bodies away from the refreshments, fireworks, and celebrations on which they typically spent, and toward public works projects that were more "useful to society." Guevara envisioned a commemorative "sign or distinctive inscription" placed in visible sites and thoroughfares announcing sponsorship, "sparing no expressions of distinction such as 'illustrious, honored, generous,' which cost nothing but indulge one's self-love and affirm his achievement."[121] Municipal officials responsible for supplying clean water, food, and medical care were instead planning acts of penance and supplication, which diverted limited time, money, and other resources, left discarded wrappings, food, and other waste, and might well have provided a supportive environment for contagion.[122]

Yet devotional strategies in practice did not contradict or preclude a broader relief effort. For a long time, municipal strategies to combat drought, food shortages, or disease had combined sponsorship of devotion with sanitation campaigns, hospital care, and other forms of aid.[123] In the great famine and pestilence of 1785, relief efforts included not only *rogativos* and *novenarios* but also loans from the bishop of Michoacán to purchase supplies of food, the establishment of granaries in regions without them, coordinated emergency plantings of irrigated fields of maize and wheat in Michoacán's *tierra caliente* region, and instructions, some published in the gazette, on how to make tortillas with *maguey*, rice, or barley substitutes.[124] In Durango measures included public fasting and penitential processions attended by officials and residents, Christian acts that "implore [God for] the remedy of the unprecedented calamity that has afflicted these inhabitants for the past year." At the same time the dean and clergy of the cathedral distributed alms "to feed, three times a day, more than a thousand persons of all ages and sexes, without ignoring the sick and incapacitated, who without this assistance would have perished from want."[125]

During the same outbreak of pneumonia, readers of the gazette learned that an autopsy performed in pursuit of more effective medical treatment by Juan Nepomuceno López, physician and surgeon in one of Durango's hospitals, had revealed the victim's bronchial tube and trachea full of fetid liquid. The very next paragraph reported a *novenario* for Our Lady of Guadalupe in the church of San Francisco, sponsored by Durango's city council, with a penitential procession attended by "many people of all estates and *calidades*."[126] Both modes of relief were newsworthy, and occasionally sponsored by the same corporate bodies, as integral components of a coordinated response (and pleasing to God, according to the gazette, which subsequently reported heaven-sent rains).[127] The same combination of strategies was pursued in Mexico City in 1797, when the Junta Principal coordinated physicians in barrios along with celestial aid, and in Guanajuato in the summer of 1813, with organized "procesiones y rogaciones públicas," plus collections of alms to care for the sick poor, and the division of the city into twelve sectors under the care of a councilman, respectable civilian, priest, and medical doctor (the last assigned to every two sectors, "owing to a shortage of these *facultativos*").[128]

At the pinnacle of Bourbon interest in urban planning and sanitation, some elite Catholics in Atlantic-oriented cities were surely disillusioned by spectacles of religious life. But patronage of public acts was still publicized in formal statements and by conspicuous attendance; despite some signs of creeping disaffection in the archive, officials took their role as custodians seriously.[129] Authorities generally did not find it sensible to decline to sponsor or otherwise support requests for devotional acts, which came from various corporate groups and reflected multiple urban identities.[130] In fact, candles, prayers, vows, charitable donations, and religious images were some of the ways that corporate duty found expression and fulfillment in critical times that demanded broad relief. Late in 1779, when members of the elite confraternity of the Gentlemen of the True Cross, in Mexico City's parish of Veracruz, sought permission to bring out in procession their Christ of the Seven Veils in the epidemic, the *mayordomo* (principal officer) stressed that the devotional image had not been out in many years. Providing the populace with visual access to this embroidered Christ not only showcased the wealth and social position of its fairly prosperous merchant members, it converted the image into an advocate for the city, and in this seemed like a fitting and generous act of charity (one that was also socially aspirational, as members pursued higher status).[131] Urban corporations frequently expressed their conviction that by making available the miraculous images of which they were custodians, they would ameliorate the plight of victims in the community and beyond.[132]

For these reasons, in the fall of 1779, while officials struggled to purify the capital and prevent pestilence from propagating by means of burial reforms, street cleaning, and fumigations (with volleys of gunfire and luminaries of pinewood), religious *deprecaciones* took place on a regular basis.[133] Among these was the elaborate citywide procession for the famous Cristo Renovado, which, as in 1737, was credited with the capital's miraculous recovery. Again, in 1797, residents accompanied this crucifix through Mexico City's newly renovated *traza*; Guevara noted its decorum—"great order was preserved [*se guardó mayor orden*]" all along the route—in a nod toward Enlightenment sensibilities, which preferred that ceremonies be seemly and sedate when they needed to take place.[134] As officials rerouted processional routes for sanitary reasons, delayed novenas, or tried to regulate disorderly crowds, the ceremonial complex remained intact.

There were dramatic changes in these years, but one that has been little discussed was the sudden ability to make the sacrifices of the people, or the "gifts" granted by celestial and terrestrial benefactors, more publicly known. After 1784, reports of processions, charitable acts, and divine aid regularly appeared in the revived gazette, as "monuments of piety for prosperity," to paraphrase one article, that bestowed glory on a city, town, benefactor, religious order, and, less often, confraternity.[135] It may be that the apparent burst of activity in these years was as related to social perceptions of the power of publicity as it was to actual increases in processions during periods of extreme hardship. Coinciding with a blossoming culture of devotional literature, with thousands of novena booklets, sermons, and printed engravings being published to document the miraculous repute and wondrous beauty of images, these experiences—of choreographed response to crisis—were easily translated across space and time because people in so many urban and rural settlements still turned to celestial mediators in moments of personal and communal stress.[136] If not all people saw such gestures as worthy of time and energy, those reading or hearing reports might recognize powerful miracle-working images and their own participation as part of an imagined Catholic community: a mental image articulated through print but formed in the nonliterate, embodied habits of public space.[137] Crisis propagated a shared ceremonial language in an ethnically and linguistically diverse place.

Retrospectively, we pick out differences between medicine and the sensorium and habits of a baroque Christianity as though they were hostile combatants. A more inclusive reading of Mexico's late colonial history shows how medical and technological advances might sustain, rather than delegitimize, this living corpus of devotion, with the state apparatus not only tolerating but drawing on its grammar of mediation, charity, supplication, obligation, and thanksgiving—both emotionally satisfying and rationally sound—as new projects of health care took shape.

CONCLUSION

Far from Mexico, a great plague outbreak in Moscow in 1771 compelled Catherine the Great to write her friend Voltaire a letter, in which the enlightened monarch described an unfortunate incident involving a miraculous icon of Mary, the Bogoliubskaia Mother of God. With tensions high following weeks of harsh anticontagion measures and restrictions on public processions, crowds of people, as Tsarina Catherine condescendingly described them, "had for several days been gathering before an image which was supposed to heal the sick" but "were in fact dying at the holy Virgin's feet." When the archbishop tried to redirect for charitable purposes the substantial donations given by the faithful for a silver image cover, a riotous crowd tracked down and killed the prelate. With its mocking depiction of the fanatical devout, Catherine's report to the French *philosophe* established a familiar opposition between reason and religion, between the enlightened elite and the benighted people they ruled—one not unfamiliar in their time, or since.[138]

In colonial Mexico there were vocal skeptics who made private and public pronouncements of their feelings about processions and other displays of celestial-oriented action. Some have taken their insistence to indicate that the modernizing sensibilities of monarchs, natural philosophers, and professionals did not accommodate the faith claims or dispositions of common people; others assess change by measuring the extent to which either a religious or a scientific mode of action dominated.[139] But scientific periodicals and bouts with disease in Mexico frequently perpetuated religious voices, idioms, and genres. It points up the risk in following the most combative, intolerant, and polarizing views: as one historian concludes, despite a growing commitment to reason and secular solutions by Europe's social elite, "plague exemplified the persistence of monumental irrationality in nature and society."[140] In the face of such uncertainty, many suspected that tradition and innovation should be reconciled and tried to do just that.

Evidence from epidemics and other disasters shows that the growing disenchantment of the world that scholars have found for Europe did not in any case prevail in Mexico.[141] Not only were Guadalupe and Remedios unifying protonational symbols for the upper classes; many other intercessors continued to enjoy broad appeal during Bourbon reformism and through Mexican Independence.[142] In 1833, some thirty years after the introduction of vaccination in Mexico, the first outbreak of cholera morbus brought national wars to a standstill. In Mexico City the liberal statesman Guillermo Prieto recalled passing "churches with their doors wide open and a thousand lights on altars, the people kneeling with arms crossed and shedding tears," while carriages with cadavers rumbled outside and the sick thronged pharmacies. Inside dwellings, residents deflected infection with astringents and images of saints: "everything was fumigations, spraying of vinegar and chloride, vinegar-filled gourds behind doors, the solitary pan with rice and the grill over the coals, and candles burning before the saints."[143]

Why did these practices endure? The culture of image veneration was at once patriarchal, sponsored and coordinated above the barrio, monastery, or district level, and popular, in the sense that public acts reflected local and communal patterns and purposes. Devotional acts might reaffirm the identities and status of urban corporations—municipal, religious, and Indian—and draw alms from residents of means who were invited to gaze on images beyond the usual moments in the liturgical or festival calendar. The act of seeing was part of coming to terms with disaster: devotional images were affectively pleasing and contained memories of past patronage and intercession. Their vitae were written on the topography of cities, and people, in the midst of uncertainty, sought stability in shrines and churches, which became pure and pestilential nodes of activity that people moved into, out of, and around.

Finally, the domestic patrons observed by Prieto were celestial rulers, kings and queens. Principles of obligation, reciprocity, and justice were periodically negotiated and enacted on a vernacular scale, and many manual workers, peasants, and artisans who had no interaction with a viceroy or bishop experienced regal power repeatedly through images.[144] Properly understood as political, image devotion cemented bonds of obligation, in ways that surpassed the imposition of the will of the ruler on the ruled (even if the result was sometimes to reinforce public order). For these reasons administrators who disagreed about the aesthetics and propriety of performances would have paused before ruling in ways that would disappoint expectations. To paraphrase Erasmus, it was better to tolerate excesses than engage in unnecessary acts of destruction.

These rituals were as integral to the enactment of royal authority in colonial Mexico as those involving priests, bishops, viceroys, and councilmen, and administrators who pursued reforms knew that they would be undertaken as much in this arena of public opinion as in the mastery of medical learning. Upon departing New Spain, Viceroy Revillagigedo conceded that not all were yet convinced of the wisdom of the cemetery reforms in Mexico City, Puebla, and Veracruz. Confident in the effectiveness of administration, however, he thought that even the worries of the less enlightened (*gentes menos sensatas*) might be assuaged. When it came to public health, emergencies provided the crucible in which the preferences, perceptions, and embodied habits of laypeople were reconciled with what was new. By 1794 this reconciliation was under way. Much remained to be done.

CHAPTER 2

Periodically Healthy

The Nature of Medicine and the Fashion of Science

I confess that in matters of medicine I am entirely a pilgrim and foreigner. The desire to remedy the misfortunes of others has moved me to place the sickle in someone else's harvest.

—Juan Caballero, friar and amateur botanist, Oaxaca, 1786

Under the patronage of powerful figures like José de Gálvez and Viceroy Revillagigedo, the Swiss doctor Pedro Puglia traveled the region around Real de Catorce, where he lived, to inspect and collect plants, despite the objections of the director of the Royal Botanical Garden. In the fall of 1790, with no demanding medical cases to treat, Puglia interviewed "the poor Indians of the Sierra" of Guanajuato about the plants commonly used as simple remedies in the area. Puglia's informants, probably members of a band of Guamares, told him about one whose root produced a resinous sap, used to treat stomachaches and prolapses. With their help, Puglia located the plant's seeds and root and, in a report to the viceroy, asked to remit his sample to the capital, with the plant's common name.[1]

Puglia's search for medicinal plants was in a long line of those investigations conducted by Dutch, English, French, and Spanish colonists beginning with the dawn of colonization in the New World. With the critical involvement of Amerindian and African collaborators, friars in missions, city physicians, slaveowners, and administrators sought to collect, explain, adapt, and exploit the materia medica of the Indies. In the eighteenth century, with renewed Bourbon interest in the empire's exploitable resources, a commerce sprang up in plants for lucrative applications and industries, including medications, dyes, fibers, and foods. Samples were sent to gardens in London, Madrid, Mexico City, Paris, and other metropoles by an assortment of amateur collectors, clergymen, naturalists, and medical professionals who roamed the interiors of the Americas and the Caribbean in pursuit of reserves of botanical wealth. As scholars note, they tended to credit themselves for the discoveries, becoming the experts who verified, amended, and perfected information, while their informants formed a vaguely discerned backdrop for the discovery.[2]

The manner in which disease emergencies generated demand for remedies and brought communities together to supply it has received relatively less attention in the history of medicine in the Spanish colonies. By the time Puglia wrote, the pages of Mexico's nascent periodical press conveyed foreign works in translation as well as original writing on scientific discovery, instrumentation, and practice and provided a virtual forum in which to debate and amalgamate diverse information related to disease, medicine, and health. Print was inscribed in the larger process of collecting and classifying carried out by communities of healers, experimenters, and readers who submitted for scrutiny specimens from the natural world with potential medicinal virtues. In the process, print culture also made visible problems of disease and medical practice in the viceroyalty and the means for achieving a cure.

These activities were in many respects tangential to the institutions officially created to address perceived inadequacies in matters of medical practice, disease control, and human health. The Royal Botanical Garden in Mexico City (where Puglia's plant sample was likely sent), along with the Royal Botanical Expedition (headquartered in New Spain from 1787 to 1803), exemplified Spain's imperial ambitions to compete with other European states and inventory its American possessions. After 1788 the garden became a lively center of instruction, collection, classification, and study that organized a community of professionals and amateurs to improve medical training and health care. It also exacerbated rivalries between creole patriots and peninsular scientists, which compromised the institution's propagation of the new chemical and botanical sciences, including the Linnaean system of classification and Lavoisier's studies of chemical reaction and nomenclature.[3] It was in any case exceptional in New Spain as a center to support Enlightenment learning. Most hospitals remained underdeveloped and dependent on the patronage of the Crown.[4] New Spain had no medical society like the Société Royal de Médicine (Royal Society of Medicine), established by the French state in 1778 to lead the battle against epidemic disease by assembling people, publications, and information on medical theory and practice.[5] The already limited authority of the Protomedicato, New Spain's licensing medical body, was further circumscribed in disease emergencies that demanded broad response by viceroys, town councils, local administrators, and practitioners.[6]

As a result, besides occasional *tertulias* (salons) to debate matters of industry, commerce, and agriculture, the printed page emerged as the primary means by which a literate public could convene over matters of health, population, and medicine. With merchants, miners, artisans, and bureaucrats seeking out practical applications of enlightened knowledge, public utility was a defining feature of most specialized publications on scientific and technical matters, before these topics gave way, during the insurgencies of the early nineteenth century, to politics in the narrower sense.[7] By employing vernacular Spanish, or Portuguese, instead of Latin, the language of classical learning, "enlightened Latin Americans made clear that secrecy is not one of science's qualities, that communication is essential to scientific learning."[8] If industrial matters invited lay participation, health care was even more inclusive. The nascent medical sciences formed a porous "science of man" in which the object of study was anthropological in the broadest sense: individuals and their social organization, in their interaction with their environment, and in their constitution as physical, emotional, moral, and theological beings.[9] New Spain's periodical press assembled information about anatomy, affect, intellect, lifestyle, and passions, and invited contributions from groups with relevant experience on the radical assumption that an enlightened society benefited from the participation of a majority of its members.

In this conviction the creoles responsible for the rise of a scientific press conscientiously emulated European models, which no less aimed to "civilize" and educate.[10] New Spain's journals resembled French and British encyclopedic projects, including the seventeen volumes of Diderot and d'Alembert's *Encyclopédie*, the most ambitious attempt to compile and classify everything known about medicine, natural history, and the plant world. Less systematic in their organization, more ad hoc and cumulative, literary journals in New Spain juxtaposed accounts of domestic experiments and investigations with medical treatises by the Spaniard Benito de Feijóo (1676–1764) and the Dutch physician Herman Boerhaave (1668–1738), as well as the latest news from European academies and scientific institutions. In this way, these journals facilitated exchanges and conversations inspired by patriotic feeling, a sense that the New World had been unfairly excluded from the Republic of Letters.[11]

In following these developments, this chapter proposes that features of this periodical press, unprecedented in eighteenth-century Mexico, were not in fact novel, but rather integral with forms of emergency relief in the colonial past. The forerunner of this initiative can be traced in the medical self-care manual, which first appeared late in the sixteenth century for regions of New Spain that lacked medical practitioners but abounded in acute and chronic infections. European versions of this genre have been characterized as examples of "medical popularization," or "the process by which regular medicine is diffused to the wider lay public." This view assumes that medical knowledge and expertise flow outward, or downward, from the social elite or institutional centers of medical authority to the masses.[12] For early colonial Mexico, which lacked a sizable literate class, developed markets, and medical professionals, the hierarchical model was never the norm; instead, humoral medicine coexisted, at times antagonistically, with local knowledge from indigenous and African communities on the assumption that remedies for the diseases of the land had been providentially given and that local populations knew them best. The situation was such that learning was not a matter of linear transmission, but instead reflected what was implicit, incipient, and customary in numerous places, or what was "vernacular," taking shape as a mosaic of skills, frameworks, and resources.

The claim to break with the past in the Mexican case conceals this and other continuities. Mexico City's journals, even as they tended to distinguish the enlightened opinions of the primarily educated, literate men who consumed news or debated in print, worked at the interstices of regions, classes, and cultures in collaborative pursuit of relief from the saga of periodic sickness.[13] On one hand, Mexico's deep social stratification and low literacy rates meant that the most idealistic view of a discerning, informed, healthy public to validate scientific knowledge propagated through the population could not realistically be fulfilled. On the other hand, contemporaries believed that they were forging a new age in medical and scientific practice. For them, the culture of print promised to organize information such that it would be easily accessible to laypeople who lacked resources and information, and thus facilitate contact with more rural populations than ever before. Owing to the general threat of infection, which rendered knowledge of therapies, technologies, and cures immediately relevant, it was from this perspective not so odd that publishers, experimenters, and clerics anticipated reaching audiences beyond the narrow stratum of educated, cultured readers, or seek conscientiously to bridge learned and unlearned, urban and rural, and geographic and racial divides. In the end, older genres of vernacular literature morphed into a more supple format that made available prodigious amounts of healing knowledge of local provenance, even as it reiterated social difference and redacted indigenous sources. In this, Dr. Puglia was in good company.

HOW TO HEAL IN NEW SPAIN

In the wake of the devastating *cocolixtli* epidemic of 1576, King Philip II circulated a questionnaire to the Indies to gather information about the political, social, and geographic features of the territories in his domain.

In addition to items on trade, industry, social organization, and natural features, officials were to provide information about "the sicknesses that commonly occur and the remedies employed for them" as well as "the herbs or aromatic plants that the Indians use to heal," with their "medicinal or poisonous properties." A reader of the sixteenth-century *relaciones geográficas* (geographic reports) written in response is struck by the murk of information about illness and medicine. In the southern province of Oaxaca the caciques, *principales*, and elderly residents who were gathered to respond referred to roots, plants, or trees, but vaguely. They knew that they drank medicinal herbs for their illnesses, but not the names; that to cure *calenturas* (fevers) or *viruelas* (smallpox) they had Indian healers who collected wild herbs ("yerbas del monte"); they were able to recognize the herbs by sight, but not by name.[14] Some had recently divulged their plants and roots to the king's physician, *protomédico* Francisco Hernández, who traveled through the region on a related collecting expedition.[15] When they were described, the herbs were "hot" or "cold" and most often purgative in their effects, like *chichicpatl*, the "bitter medicine" decocted from the bark of a local tree and consumed hot.[16] In an exceptional instance of recall, the elders of Tecuicuilco generated the names of herbs for headaches, purging, and fractures, the last applied topically.[17] For the most part, informants demurred when pressed for the special names of their plants. Although disease was ever-present, what was being requested was specialized knowledge, practiced but not expressed, within a setting of rituals, sacred spaces, and deities from which the plants were not easily distinguished. As one Spanish official remarked, the Indians healed "by good sense," without needing to say why.[18]

Those who coveted these remedies and plants had other ways of getting them. Plant specimens were conveyed to the Old World in the writings of *protomédico* Hernández, in the *relaciones* written for the king, and physically in crates destined for European consumers. One was the *raíz de Michoacán* (root of white jalap), the only indigenous herb reported with a Spanish name in Oaxaca (in Tetiquipa), presumably because it was already known in Europe through the increasingly lucrative Atlantic trade in American goods.[19] Those in New Spain interested in these natural remedies, on the other hand, had additional options. They might consult a guide to health and healing, which directed readers to incorporate them in healing regimens and for a range of common ailments. In the early modern world these self-healing guides were cheaply printed, simply reworked, and affordably repackaged versions of more expensive editions. Their format allowed authors to reach mixed audiences and served, as one scholar writes, "to transgress presumed boundaries between high and low culture."[20]

Vernacular medical literature treated such topics as conception, delivery, childrearing, women's beauty, marital relations, and other health matters, and in the process shaped a relationship between those with special expertise and a broader lay readership presumed to need it. In the novohispanic versions, New World plants and foods formed an integral part of healing advice. *Problemas, y secretos maravillosos de las Indias* (1591) (Problems and marvelous secrets of the Indies), by the Spanish physician Juan de Cárdenas (1563–1609), was intended for interested readers who knew only Spanish ("curiosos romancistas") rather than men of science and *letrados* (learned people) who knew Latin, and accordingly drew out explanations and repeated lessons for the benefit of this unlearned audience. The first part explained the laws of nature in the torrid zones of the Indies, whose extreme humidity and heat posed dangers to the bodies of persons unaccustomed to its climate and rendered the trees, animals, plants, and people radically different from those in Europe. A survey of the properties of the fruits of the land included chocolate and vanilla (*tlixochil*), chiles, *tuna* (prickly pear fruit), *maguey* cactus (Mexican agave), the prodigious tobacco leaf, American honey, bezoar stones, corn-based foods like *atole*, coca leaf, and *mecasuchil*, a purgative and additive in prepared chocolate. Occasionally Cárdenas featured indigenous modes of preparation, as with the yucca plant (consumed by the Chichimecas with the shell). The final chapter reduced the hallucinatory effects of peyote and tobacco to their physiological dimensions, explaining that while some plants were used for diabolical or superstitious purposes, they possessed divinely ordained *natural* properties. Paraphrasing Ecclesiasticus, Cárdenas wrote: "God gave [medicinal] virtues to the herbs and things of the land so that mankind could be preserved and freed from its ailments."[21]

In these guides a coterie of doctors and clerics tried to discern this providentially ordered system, clarify its laws, and make its bounty available to lay audiences in the years following the disastrous *cocolixtli* epidemic. Printed in quarto or octavo for transport, written in Castilian by men who had practical healing experience, though not necessarily trained physicians, the guides appeared in some six titles in eleven editions over two centuries.[22] Combining theory and manual practice, they strove to vulgarize—in the sense of making general—specialized knowledge about health. Readers might have wanted to know about the marvels and curiosities of the New World, but in practical terms they would have been anxious about their health and eager to learn from a trusted source how to go about preventing illness. As one scholar has noted, Cárdenas and others writing in this genre were especially oriented toward the ailments and dietary excesses of the leisure classes, who presumably shared the same healing framework and assumptions about the importance of lifestyle, and whose education enabled them to follow instructions, take charge of their own care and treatment, and extend their lives.[23] In early New Spain this often meant returning to ancient authorities, including Galen and Hippocrates, who thought that prevention and treatment of diseases entailed care of diet, exercise, sleep, emotion, and environment (the "non-naturals"), and occasional therapies such as bleeding, purges, and poultices, to achieve a balance of humoral substances and prevent their corruption in the body.

At the same time the diseased environment of the Indies affected many more sick and suffering non-Europeans. Although this context was least pronounced in Cárdenas's work, he alluded darkly, in a chapter on syphilis, to the effects of *cocolixtli*, "which infects Indians without touching Spaniards" and presented "with terrible pain in the liver, and great bloody discharges from the nose."[24] Others were more attentive to the health and diseases of these other classes. Alonso López de Hinojosos, the surgeon of San José Hospital in Mexico City, brought out his *Summa, y recopilación de Chirugia, con un Arte para sangrar muy útil y provechosa* (1578, 1595) (Summary and compilation of surgery, with a very useful and beneficial art of bleeding) after living through the *cocolixtli* epidemic (detailed in Chapter 1). He remarked in the prologue on the need he had witnessed, lamenting that the surgical books that he knew in Spanish (*en romance*) were still too difficult, prolix, or otherwise inaccessible to common people (*gente vulgar*), unless the person happened to be learned in the matter already. "And being saddened by this and by those outside of this city, in mines and ranches and remote regions that lack the necessary remedies," he explained, "I made this book so that whoever knows how to read can find the remedy for the passions and sicknesses mentioned herein, and know its cause and of what it consists and how it should be treated." He offered the reader of his "small volume" instructions for purges, cures for sores and wounds (*llagas*), scabies, ringworm, and "salty phlegm" (*flemasalada*, a respiratory infection), and simple and compound medications based on experience and on the remedies given by God specifically for the diseases of the land.[25] The native herbarium he described included, among other plants, *maguey*, *árbol del Peru* (*Schinus molle* L., pepper plant), and pills from the Michoacán root ("tabletas de Michoacán").

Not to be outdone, Agustín Farfán (1532–1604) expanded the final chapter on common stomach ailments from his earlier (1579) manual on anatomy and surgery into a more comprehensive healing manual, the *Tractado breve de medicina, y de todas las enfermedades* (1579, 1592, 1604, and 1610) (Brief treatise on medicine and on every infirmity). In the opening lines Farfán informed readers that he strove to write clearly and to feature homemade remedies (*caseros*) that might be used by those for whom the book was designed: people who lived far from cities, in villages without physicians or pharmacies. For this audience Farfán featured in abundance medical plants that might be found and applied locally, including not only the common *raíz de Michoacán* but also *cacalosuchil*, whose flowers were classified, in the *relación* from Tetiquipa, Oaxaca, as a powerful purgative. Farfán described its fragrant flowers and prescribed a concoction of its stalk for abdominal pains, stomachaches, interrupted menses, and syphilis, referring to his own personal experience with this remedy "in the city of Antequera in the Valley of Oaxaca."[26]

A doctor and a graduate of the University of Mexico, Farfán was also a member of the Augustinian order and had a good idea of the religious communities and estates where a simple guide like his might find use. The tonsure and dress of the figure on the title page of the 1592 edition—perhaps Father Farfán himself—speaks to the monastic locus of medical expertise in colonial Mexico and the way the value of the remedies gathered within drew on the reputed sanctity of the healer (figure 2.1). Theoretically, if no other healer was available in an emergency, authorities or intermediaries might with a copy of the work function as surrogates, looking after the health of patients in the missions and parishes of the countryside just as their authors, men of singular faith, charity, or devotion, were alleged to have done. *Florilegio medicinal, de todas las enfermedades* (1712) (Medical anthology of all infirmities), by Juan de Esteyneffer (1664–1716), adopted wholesale Galenic principles prescribing the importance of the non-naturals (especially diet) in the promotion of physical health. Its Jesuit author worked in the missions of the northern frontier, among indigenous populations, and wrote for other Jesuits who labored in similar diseased settings.[27]

The epitome of this model was Gregorio López (1542–1596), reputed author of the *Tesoro de medicinas, para diversas enfermedades* (Treasury of medicines for diverse infirmities, 1672, updated 1674). After migrating to New Spain at the age of twenty, López spent six years as a hermit along the Chichimec frontier at Atemayac, in Zacatecas, before moving on to the Huasteca region, the northeastern terminus of the Mesoamerican empire and Mexico's archbishopric. A severe bout of dysentery forced him to return to Mexico City, where he received permission to remain at the hospital in Huastepec (also Oaxtepec or Huaxtepec), run by the Order of San Hipólito, at the site of Moctezuma's botanical garden. A devotee of the Virgin of Guadalupe, it was at the hospital, following his "various pilgrimages" (as related in the prologue to the *Tesoro*), that López found his calling, charitably assisting its sick poor and composing in "silent retreat" a manuscript to compensate for the shortage of physicians and medications.[28] The priest Francisco Losa, his friend and biographer, proclaimed that the manuscript was the distillation of "many experiences and the great knowledge López had of the properties and natural virtue

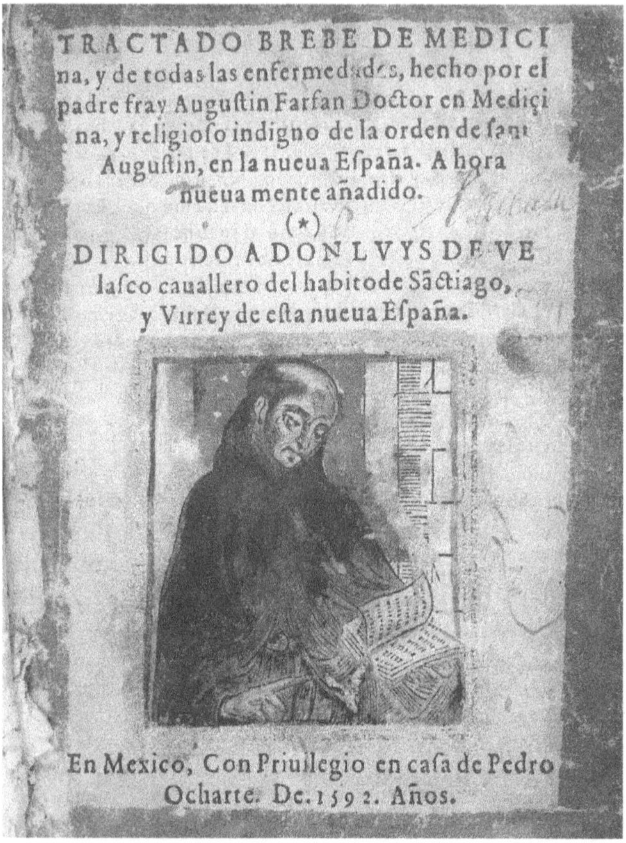

TRACTADO BREBE DE MEDICI
na, y de todas las enfermedades, hecho por el
padre fray Auguſtin Farfan Doctor en Mediçi
na, y religioſo indigno de la orden de ſant
Auguſtin, en la nueua Eſpaña. A hora
nueua mente añadido.
(*)
DIRIGIDO A DON LVYS DE VE
laſco cauallero del habito de Sãctiago,
y Virrey de eſta nueua Eſpaña.
En Mexico, Con Priuilegio en caſa de Pedro
Ocharte. De. 1592. Años.

Figure 2.1 A tonsured friar on the title page of a colonial healing manual. Agustín Farfán's *Tractado breve de medicina* (1592) features its learned author, or perhaps a reader applying its lessons, with tonsure and robe signaling membership in the Augustinian order.
SOURCE: Courtesy of the Huntington Library, San Marino, California.

of plants." Losa noted that the manuscript was intended for the care of the hospital's patients and for men of the countryside (*campo*) and the poor; that the brothers of San Hipólito used it to heal in the hospital; and that copies were sent to other hospitals for use. The remedies and medicaments worked wondrously, Losa averred, "as if the author had studied medicine for many years."[29]

Whether López himself was allowed to practice medicine at the hospital is unclear. He seems to have cobbled the manuscript together from books consulted during his stay. According to one scholarly study, the version of the *Tesoro* published in Mexico City in 1672 corresponds closely to the second section of the manuscript, "Remedies Ordered by ABC." Largely a collection of basic remedies, in alphabetical order, for headaches, stomachaches, cuts, scorpion stings, indigestion, and other common afflictions, the published version apparently derived from a notebook in the possession of Captain Alonso Raboso de la Plaza, the bailiff (*alguacil*) of the city of Puebla. The first section of the manuscript was a close summary of Andrés Laguna's translation and annotation of the *Materia Medica* of Dioscorides, with the addition of New World botanicals; the final section, "Medicinas de Indias o Nueba España" (Medicines of the Indies or New Spain), a compendium of herbs with entire sections lifted from the illustrated dual-language (Nahuatl and Latin) collection of Mexican medicines undertaken by Martín de la Cruz and Juan Badiano (the Codex Cruz-Badiano, 1552) of the Franciscan College of Tlatelolco. The designation of López as sole author can be explained by the fact that the publication of Father Losa's 1613 biography had extended López's fame across the Atlantic, lending powerful cachet to any learning plausibly attributed to him.[30]

The trajectory of the work prior to publication reveals much about medical authority in the early modern Spanish world. That a work of botanical remedies had circulated for decades in manuscript form, in Mexico and Spain, indicates how much medical knowledge moved outside the commerce of printed matter, guarded by institutions like convents and hospitals, often at the geographic peripheries of Spanish authority. These institutions were repositories where learning might be applied and distributed before some of it was made available in print, in institutional and cultural centers like Mexico City. The published versions were the product of significant editorial efforts by contemporary physicians in the viceroyalty, working from a manuscript compiled from ethnobotanists, linguists, and medical practitioners in Mexico City and beyond. The attribution of authorship to López yoked the name and repute of a saintly man, and in the process rendered singular what was a thoroughly collaborative endeavor.

By the end of the eighteenth century, new healing manuals entering markets in New Spain shed this monastic connection. Not only that, influential works by two Europeans with no firsthand knowledge of the Indies largely omit the American materia medica that had featured so prominently before. Samuel-Auguste (S.A.D.) Tissot (1728–1797), author of *Avis au peuple sur sa santé* (Advice to the people on their health), was a country physician trained in Montpellier who achieved fame for his treatise on the dangers of masturbation to physical health. Drawing on his anatomical, surgical, and clinical experience to address the depopulation of Europe, a pressing concern at the time, he observed that this decline was the result of faulty healing methods, which further robbed the countryside, already depleted by urban migration, of hardy farmworkers.[31]

The manual was intended "for those who, finding themselves far from physicians, cannot make use of their assistance." Minimalist and concise, the work was compared to the catechism a parish priest might use for children. Nevertheless, Tissot had no illusions "that this book will be an essential furnishing in the home of every farmer [*labrador*; in other versions, *lector*, reader]." The vast majority were unable to read or comprehend its contents so that it was rather destined for "intelligent and charitable persons who live in small villages and who by some kind of providential vocation are called to assist, with their advice, any and all who seek it." This included priests, whose vocations moved them to provide the sick among their flocks with physical relief, even as they prepared them spiritually for death, and well-to-do residents, landowners, and schoolteachers, who might enlighten their employees and pupils. Tissot allowed that there were talented, charitable farmers, some of whom he knew, who would also enjoy, understand, and apply its lessons.[32] The Spanish translation, with the subtitle "Treatise on the most common sicknesses of people of the countryside [*campo*]," appeared in Pamplona (1773), Madrid (1774, 1775), and in a new, annotated, expanded edition in Madrid (1776, 1778, 1781, etc.) that situated Tissot's references to the Swiss countryside for a Spanish audience, added common Spanish names for ingredients, and included in an appendix the Spanish equivalents of the mineral waters and sulfuric baths that he recommended.[33] Priced between 22 and 26 *reales*, copies arrived with a stream of technical and specialized pamphlets, books, and journals from England, France, and Spain, propelled by more liberal trade policies and the esteem in which some creoles in New Spain held this foreign learning.

That these moderately expensive manuals were known among New Spain's literate classes is suggested by a notice in Mexico City's gazette, written by three certified medical practitioners with experience healing in the 1786 epidemic. The authors cited Tissot's guide and a passage from William Buchan's *Medicina doméstica* that advised not bleeding at the first signs of fever. Following its 1769 publication, Buchan's *Domestic Medicine* became one of the most important books on health regimen and simple treatments in the English-speaking world. In contrast to Tissot, Buchan addressed literate classes assumed to employ servants and the upwardly mobile middle sectors in cities. He assailed the mistakes of midwives and nurses, the use of charms and other superstitious practices, and the dangers of sedentary urban living.[34] The Spanish translation, with some adjustments for the climate and habits of the Spanish audience, underwent numerous re-editions in Madrid beginning in 1785.[35] The practitioners who cited it claimed to have based their diagnosis of *fiebres pútridas* (putrid fevers) on symptoms described by Tissot, who had himself recommended Buchan's work, which was "so well received that within a few years there are seven English editions, three of the French translation, and two in Spanish."[36] By this means readers in New Spain had access to some of the insights of Tissot and Buchan, but in piecemeal fashion, as their opinions were selectively applied in an emergency.

The creole physician Juan Manuel Venegas, author of *Compendio de la medicina* (1788) (Compendium of medicine), was decidedly less impressed with the foreigners' ignorance of New World practices and botanicals. The *Compendio*—with the subtitle "Practical medicine, in which is briefly treated the most useful things, which the author has observed in these regions of New Spain, for nearly all the infirmities that assault the human body, arranged in alphabetical order"—was the only vernacular healing manual published in New Spain in this period. At a cost of 4 pesos, an early advertisement in the gazette to solicit subscriptions clarified that the forthcoming book was not exclusively for professors of medicine but rather those in "places with a shortage of practitioners." It had the advantage of being "conceived in this Kingdom, tested in it, and [full of] simples that are familiar and produced here" and, as such, was more useful than Tissot or even Esteyneffer's *Florilegio medicinal*.[37] The volume, printed "in quarto" and "succinct," was delayed, as readers of the gazette learned, because the author had taken ill healing in the interior (*tierra adentro*) during the 1786 epidemic.[38] When it appeared, Venegas summarized his complaints and critiques of previous works in a prefatory "Warning to the Reader." European editions were excessively and confusingly long and often impractical; Buchan's work, only recently available in Spanish, was clear in explaining the importance of hygiene for good health but neglected medicine, omitting indigenous medicaments and basic rules adapted for common usage ("que necesita el Pueblo"). Tissot's book was beyond the comprehension of the masses on some topics, and on others said nothing; and the charitable manuals for the poor by Esteyneffer and López, which remained "in everyone's hands," revealed a lack of knowledge of basic medical principles on the part of the authors.

Venegas claimed to have observed in his travels through New Spain medicine's shortcomings and accumulated useful knowledge about what worked for the sick, which encouraged him in his dismissal of these and other authorities. The study of botany was useful but too disconnected from practice, he thought, while the medical profession's textbook training and exclusivity concealed from the people useful remedies (he cited the ongoing debate over the medicinal value of lizards [*lagartijas*], which would, he thought, be in common use if their therapeutic properties were the deciding factor). Often physicians guided by esteemed treatises were exceeded in their practice by empirics, who were guided only by "the great authority [*magisterio*] of their experience." This experience, Venegas explained, surpassed the physician's "crude speculation." The risk of error and malpractice in moments of exceptional need, when remedies were prescribed for everything, "from the mouth even of the most ignorant plebe," necessitated his informed, experience-ripened manual. In sum, despite the libraries full of books on chemistry, botany, and philosophy, and committee meetings overflowing with the pompous voices of professors, "a naive old woman, a poor peasant, or a fool Indian often mock them with the happy use of a spurned [local] drug."[39] By implication, Venegas would provide access to this homespun knowledge.

The structure of Venegas's *Compendio* reflected the enlightened sensibilities of his time. The book's entries were arranged alphabetically by disease name, in Latin, but the index dispensed with Latin in favor of Spanish so that the pueblo could find the relevant entry quickly and easily. Venegas provided complete and easy-to-comprehend conversion rates because precise measurement allowed readers to apply the book's remedies uniformly.[40] He shared with his European competitors the view that healers should allow nature to do its work: like Tissot, Venegas targeted Madame Marie Fouquet, director of hospitals for women and girls in Paris, whose popular books of remedies offered excessive treatments that "hinder the healthy action of Nature," if they did not outright kill the patient. Medicine was merely to guide nature, to overcome "disorder" in the patient's eating habits by "a very stable life regimen."[41] For smallpox, Venegas prescribed light bleeding, emetics, and diaphoretics until the eruption stage, in which healing "should be given over entirely to nature," whose healing power was manifest in the pustules forming on the surface of the skin.[42] Unlike Tissot, however, who clarified that his instructions were only to be used when a trained physician was unavailable (otherwise readers were to defer to expert judgment), Venegas exercised no such restraint.[43]

In this and other ways he walked the same path as Dutch physician and chemist Herman Boerhaave, the radical practitioner of medicine based in anatomy and body mechanics. Venegas was similarly suspicious of secrecy, textbook learning, and complicated language, thinking that medical knowledge should derive from discerning experience in local settings, that it should be held in common, and that clear communication was as important as what was being communicated in preserving health. He also resembled his predecessors in New Spain (although he disavowed them) by privileging local botanicals and insisting on his attunement to suffering, to humankind's ameliorative capacity, and to the constraints and opportunities of the land, whose diseases (and natural cures) were not those of the Old World. Here, Venegas describes the dearth of care he had recently witnessed in Mexico's countryside:

> What heart could endure seeing men seized by fever, consumed by pain, convulsing, anxious, suffocating, and in the anguish of serious illness, surrounded by other miseries, tossing and turning in bed, shouting, or begging (often wordlessly) for relief that others could so easily provide? Consideration of these evils is horrifying, but they happen in the world, and principally in our America, where the dispersion of its populations, the vast expanse of its landscape, the inaccessibility of its mountains, and the diversity of its climates militate against an abundance of qualified physicians and deny access to skilled practitioners.[44]

These circumstances compelled Venegas to reach beyond his own professional class to address the problems of those without training. The impulse was not unprecedented; Venegas simply thought that he had done it better.

The early guides to health, often produced by Europeans living and working for extended periods of time in New Spain, were all-purpose works that defy easy categorization; they embody the blurry disciplinary division of the Renaissance, between medicine and other fields. As such, they have helped scholars explain the dietary habits of Spanish colonizers; suggested how racial discourse took root in assessments of differences in the bodies of Amerindians and creole Europeans; and shown how, by policing the uses, abuses, and diabolical associations of chocolate and tobacco, they facilitated the transcultural incorporation of Mesoamerican goods.[45] For their peripatetic authors, with the possible exception of Cárdenas, the most salient reality was that of critical disease infection. The guides were intended to transmit canonical but especially context-specific practice, to city dwellers as well as to literate residents who found themselves as primary caregivers in regions without practitioners. It was this tradition that the Enlightenment versions sustained. Nevertheless, by 1788, Venegas, Tissot, and Buchan had competition. For several years contemporaries in Mexico had been sharing and recycling healing knowledge by means of the periodical press, a more responsive medium by which to address health and discern the secrets of New Spain's people, climates, and land.

SCIENCE IN TRANSLATION

In 1772, with a typhus outbreak in the capital threatening to spread beyond the city, the cleric and creole polymath José Antonio de Alzate y Ramírez (1737–1799) undertook his own investigations into its nature and origins and reported the results in his newly launched periodical, *Asuntos varios sobre siences, y artes* (Various matters on the sciences and arts), in a "special notice to the public." A principal figure of Mexico's Enlightenment, Alzate told of how he had observed the decimation of

San Miguel Nonoalco barrio, in Santiago Tlatelolco, its houses shuttered and hearths cold. He had sought out an Indian resident, described as *muy* ladino, or acculturated, who confirmed *matlazahuatl* in San Miguel and in the barrio of San Juan. When Alzate wondered why other neighborhoods nearby had not succumbed, the informant noted that the deceased in Santa Ana parish were no longer interred in the church but rather in the cemetery, a measure that had presumably slowed transmission. But the buried corpses lay along the causeway that connected the city to Guadalupe's shrine to the north—"the most heavily traveled thoroughfare of this city" during the epidemic. Alzate wondered: "Could this not infect many who walk there?"[46]

By the time Napoleon's invasion of the Spanish Peninsula sparked an imperial crisis, Mexico had not experienced the revolution in reading practices and literacy rates found in Europe. While Mexico City enjoyed the first printing press in the Americas, preceding by centuries those in Boston, New York, and Philadelphia, residents generally did not use print culture to engage with political intrigues or debate matters of state.[47] The endogenous printed matter that circulated in New Spain consisted mainly of the vernacular medical manuals written by friars and physicians (their numbers were paltry in comparison to Britain or France), official histories, royal edicts and decrees, and a range of literary and religious works, including catechisms, vocabularies of indigenous languages, hagiographies of saints and holy people, chronicles, and devotional chapbooks, some with fine engravings of saints.

Innovations in technology and format brought new content to Mexico City and began to invigorate a literary market with topical material.[48] The first two iterations of New Spain's gazette, the government's official periodical, ran intermittently in 1722 and again from 1728 to 1742. It was a compendium of information in the usual manner of the times, with articles on royal births, arrivals of officials and religious orders, military movements, commercial activities, and ceremonial life. Although the paper was not an arena for political debate of royal policy, mercantile and intellectual sectors traveled throughout the world, associated in *tertulias* to discuss matters of science, industry, and policy, and corresponded with academies in Europe. Eventually some in New Spain appropriated print to pursue a "religion of science," taking as axiomatic "that scientific knowledge leads to happiness and virtue."[49]

By 1772, when Alzate arrived in the barrios north of downtown Mexico City, the ambition to explore useful discoveries, instruments, and materia medica was becoming reality, in part through his literary journals. The premise, at once patriotic and philanthropic, was that New Spain, principal "kingdom" of the New World, should be endowed with a repository for the storage and retrieval of useful knowledge along the lines of those being constructed in Europe. While Alzate frequently intervened in urban sanitation projects and consulted with viceroys, he intended these journals to be a collaborative, social endeavor, as evidenced in the way he combined firsthand observations with the remarks of an Indian resident, and in doing so subjected official measures to broader public scrutiny.

Alzate resists study in these terms because he was such a sharp polemicist.[50] His modest claim to be a novice in the sciences was belied by his habit of signing himself as a correspondent of the Royal Academy of Sciences in Paris, or the Royal Botanical Garden in Madrid. His formal education, at the Jesuits' Colegio de San Ildefonso in Mexico City, culminated in bachelor's degrees in arts (1753) and theology (1756). Soon after, his father endowed a chaplaincy with 3,000 pesos for his ordination, which allowed Alzate to commit himself to literary and experimental pursuits that were otherwise prohibitively expensive.[51] Over twenty-five years, Alzate edited four literary journals, in which he introduced subscribers to translations and extracts of published work; he contributed more than seventy translations and original articles to the *Gazeta de Mexico* from 1784 to 1797 (particularly when his own publications were out of circulation); and he produced original research on topics ranging from Mexican antiquities to astronomy, botany, electricity, chemistry, engineering, geography, geology, geometry, hydrology, medicine, natural history, physics, and surgery. He was central to the new sciences in colonial Mexico, but he also sought to place himself at the center of spokes of correspondents and interlocutors of different backgrounds and scientific capacities.

In the prospectus to the *Diario literario de México* (eight issues, 1768) (Literary journal of Mexico)—Spanish America's first journal expressly dedicated to the sciences—Alzate invoked the general good (*bien general*) of the Spanish nation and deemed periodicals like his useful to the Republic of Letters. He promised excerpts from European works, especially those concerning agriculture, mining, geography, natural history, and medicine, but also welcomed contributions from "less cultivated persons," "having dedicated myself to serving not only the literate public [*público de los literatos*], but also the most unlucky country people."[52] Subsequent undertakings were in the same populist spirit. The *Asuntos varios sobre ciencias, y artes* (thirteen issues, 1772–1773) offered extracts of European works in translation, which reflected Alzate's wish to be useful to his patria: "we were born not only for ourselves, but also for our fellow man."[53] *Observaciones sobre la física, historia natural y artes útiles* (fourteen issues, 1787–1788) (Observations on physic, natural history, and useful arts) gave way to the long-running *Gazeta de literatura de México* (1788–1795) (Literary gazette of Mexico), a more ambitious project (139 issues over six subscription periods) brought out by the prestigious publishing house of the Zúñiga y Ontiveros family.

The *Gazeta de literatura* took on a range of social issues and relied on the assistance of at least two coeditors, the botanist José Mariano Moziño (1757–1820) and Mariano de Castillejo, Moziño's "disciple," who, along with his father and brother-in-law, contributed botanical and meteorological reports.[54] While Moziño departed after the first volume (of three) to join the second leg of the botanical expedition under its director, Martín de Sessé, numerous other editorial "assistants," and many personal acquaintances, including physicians, surgeons, friars, secular priests, and lawyers, contributed findings and advice. In the prologue, Alzate paid tribute to principles of objectivity, transparency, and public utility, conceiving the printed page as a conduit of knowledge, to be evaluated blindly, without reference to personal vanity, pride, or other selfish motives. Alzate would not accept submissions that satisfied "self love, irreligion, vengeance, etc.," but he would publish the good ideas of those too humble to broadcast their successes or those put off by high printing costs.[55]

The emphasis on self-education, self-realization, and self-care was a product of the belief that other institutions, including those of public education, did not adequately fulfill these pursuits.[56] *Mercurio volante, con noticias importantes y curiosas sobre varios asuntos de física y medicina* (1772–1773) (Flying Mercury, with important and curious news about various matters of physic and medicine), edited by the physician José Ignacio Bartolache (1739–1790), had the distinction of being Spanish America's first journal dedicated exclusively to medicine. Like Alzate, Bartolache was a staunch critic of the unreformed scholastic system in New Spain's universities (having been expelled from the Royal Pontifical University for reading the "modern" works of such authors as Melchor Cano, the controversial Dominican theologian).[57] He was among the circle of collaborators around Alzate and the natural scientist Antonio de León y Gama, whom he helped observe Venus passing in front of the Sun in 1769 (a phenomenon that produced a global sensation from Mexico City to Paris). The sixteen issues of the *Mercurio volante* represented Bartolache's attempt to introduce the new mathematics and science and transmit his own medical studies in lay terms. The lead issue, which appeared during the typhus epidemic, announced that the journal would "bring news to all parts, like a swiftly moving messenger," using "our ordinary Spanish." In the past, the lack of affordable printing had hindered popular access to useful reports, as did "the mysterious ceremony that everything to do with the sciences comes out in Latin." Latin, Bartolache insisted, "is only needed to understand Latin books, but not to think well, or to acquire the sciences, which are accessible [*tratables*] in all languages." He promised to dispense with this pretense and publish excerpts from worthy authors, translated from Latin and Greek (revered "superstitiously"), including those of Spanish origin.[58]

These were literal projects of translation, and translations in the sense of switching from learned syntax to everyday terms. Both Alzate and Bartolache believed that the latest scientific approaches to anatomy, atmospheric conditions, and therapeutics should be adapted for the common good and communicated so as to be understood by lay and professional readers at once. Though a trained expert, Bartolache urged his readers to challenge him, insisting that no received wisdom or medical truth was absolutely certain and that together they would serve the greater community (*común*).[59] Individuals not typically included within the Republic of Letters, "those we call commoners, people who the world over are considered ignorant and coarse," might nevertheless contribute and be redeemed from their neglect. "Because a common countryman, even of the lowest plebe," Bartolache insisted, "finding in his hands some document by which he can easily be instructed in matters of interest or concern, will without fail apply himself and achieve it; certainly the desire to know is equally breathed into all men." This desire was breathed into women, too, who had been all but dismissed as useless for the sciences by learned men. "Women and simpletons can console themselves with having in their bodies a soul endowed with the same potentialities, perhaps greater than the souls of those university graduates so respected for their public repute."[60] With rational souls, poor and rich, noble and commoner, old and young alike might attain good health, and all would soon play a part in the improvement of society by informing themselves about medicine, most useful of the natural sciences.[61]

This redemptive mission, tied to a patriotic defense of Mexico and its inhabitants, shared some thematic terrain with the manuals and recipe books of old. But the advent of medical journalism, "that special engine of data-recording and sounding-board of opinion," accelerated the rhythm of knowledge production.[62] Whereas it was possible to update the manuals over the course of several editions to reflect criticisms and transformations in practice (though they rarely were), serials revised knowledge and addressed concerns in monthly and even weekly iterations and worked to fashion the image of a public for these pursuits. Alzate was especially interested in the recovery and vindication of knowledge indigenous to the New World, among populations that he construed as authentically *indio*. In a 1791 essay on the "moral and physical character of an Indian," he condemned those who, without any knowledge of indigenous language, had taken the plebe found in cities to stand for all Indians: the real Indian, he maintained, was in the countryside, far from the corrupting influences of whites and *mulatos*. Alzate had learned this in his formative years in Ozumba, when he was exposed to the vernacular of his playmates. "Part of my childhood I spent on an hacienda belonging to my parents; in that retreat, free of other castes, I was joined in my childish games by the small Indians, my contemporaries; at that age, when first impressions are so often made, I imbibed what I saw and heard, and with this it can be said that I underwent a kind of apprenticeship [*noviciado*] to be able to speak with some authority."[63] While Alzate eventually left for the city, the implication was that he had retained a genuine appreciation for and understanding of indigenous populations.

Even as Alzate imported the latest science from Berlin, London, Madrid, and Paris, his patriotic agenda inclined him to collect, publicize, and preserve knowledge from this autochthonous culture. His chauvinism is well known, but in the realm of medicine it was justified by the theory that illness was inextricable from climate. Following this logic, those with experience healing elsewhere might not anticipate the effects of their medicines and therapies in the Indies because they did not understand how climate affected human bodies there. The corollary was that foreigners had something to learn from locals and that simple (rather than compounded) medicines, whose effects were less variable, should be used whenever possible. Alzate lamented that knowledge of natural remedies that the Mexica had accumulated through centuries had been lost. The botanical expeditions under way would help to recover some, but because contemporary Indians had largely forgotten their customs and practices, canonical sources on American pharmaceuticals, particularly those by Spanish authors (who were best acquainted with the New World) would supplement current knowledge.[64]

Among these indigenous drugs was the commonly used *pipiltzintlis* (cannabis plant), which Alzate defended by weighing its medicinal value. Although he conceded that its associations with diabolical visions made for potentially harmful consequences in the spiritual realm, its narcotic effects were of nature.[65] "Happy is he," Alzate lectured, in an article on the medicinal value of the *axolotl* or *ajolote* (an amphibious creature still found at the time in the lakes of central Mexico), "who for the benefit of humanity inquires of the Indians their practical knowledge of simples used to combat sicknesses!" The *indios* of Ixtacalco, neighboring Mexico City, were offered as an illustration: although tertiary fevers continued to confound medical professionals, Ixtacalco's inhabitants were known to recover from the ailment fully invigorated after three or four days, without the side effects of the best-known remedy, quinine.[66]

Toward the end of the *Gazeta de literatura*'s run, two medical practitioners debated in its pages the medical virtues of roots and other botanicals in the context of a discussion of *cebadilla*, a plant commonly used to provoke nosebleeds. The army surgeon Juan Pablo Cancino described using it as a vermifuge to treat Marcos Antonio, of Tacuba, whose abscessed nasal cavity was infested with worms. Cancino cited, among other authorities, Esteyneffer's *Florilegio medicinal*, where it was prescribed for the same purpose. Esteyneffer had repeatedly referred to the fact that the plant was known as *raíz* or *cebadilla de la sierra* by the Tarahumara (or Rarámuri), the borderlands people among whom he ministered as a priest. As tempers flared, the physician Juan José Bermúdez de Castro invoked this association, remarking snidely in his final communication that he had learned from Martín de Sessé, director of the botanical garden, that Sessé had seen the plant in bloom in Orizaba and Córdoba, which supplied the pharmacies of Mexico City. Perhaps this would be of interest to Cancino, who would not have to accompany Father Esteyneffer "to look for it among the Tarahumara."[67] By the end of the century the old healing guides appeared to some quaint or in need of update.

Alzate presented himself as an impartial facilitator of these debates in his paper, even as he actively promoted experience-tested remedies. In the *Gazeta de México* he reviewed the evidence related to a concoction of boiled cockroaches, used by Indian villagers beyond the capital. The previous year don Joseph de Cañadas, resident of Tlayacapan, was struck by an acute case of *dolor de costado* in an unnamed village in Cuernavaca. With no other assistance available, he placed himself in the care of its residents, "who healed him in three days by administering *agua de cucarachas* [cockroach water], and applying to his side various aquatic herbs." Though "a single cure does not a rule in medicine make," Alzate conceded, news had arrived from San Antonio Hacienda, in Coyoacán, where servants and managers suffering from a similar ailment were saved by the cockroach water and a salve from the sediment fried in oil. Meanwhile, on an estate of similar size in Apa, employees were dying in droves. "Given this account," Alzate pressed, "should not *facultativos* examine this remedy from the medical practice of the Indians?" He issued a call not for blind acceptance but for further study: "What is certain is that the Indians are the ones who have taught us the use of the only two medical specifics of the vegetal world that medicine recognizes as such: I refer to quinine and ipecac."[68]

There was an obvious debt to European philosophes and savants, who championed the notion that journals were collaborative and egalitarian and should serve as repositories for useful, tested knowledge. It was a model held up in the French *Encyclopédie*, whose volumes of essays continued to appear in the years leading up to the launch of New Spain's literary journals. Taking Francis Bacon as their inspiration, Diderot and d'Alembert had imagined their work as a useful repository forged by many in a free commerce of ideas.[69] Alzate was clearly inspired by these models.[70] At the same time, the American editors handled matters of race, gender, and health in ways specific to their context. Bartolache's modest efforts to include women in the sciences paled in comparison with England, where by the mid-eighteenth century no fewer than three scientific periodicals were targeted at women.[71] Still, with his insistence that gender difference was not ineradicable and should not blind contemporaries to the intellectual capacities of women and laypeople, his vision was a countervailing force within New Spain's institutional culture, and even worked to oppose a European "science of difference" in which gender categories were being naturalized through the study of human anatomy.[72] Moreover, while both Alzate and Bartolache insisted that they would not treat "matters of State," they pursued and endorsed projects relevant to their political and social setting, in which "private persons" contributed to matters of governance.[73] The appeal to universal reason, with its implicit critique of official institutions and the social order, would, taken to its logical conclusion, inform independence movements and the overthrow of monarchism in Spanish America. At the time, the implications for health care were more innocent, if no less potentially subversive for the medical establishment: with reason innate in everyone, anyone might grasp and use the tools of science for experimentation, prophylaxis, and treatment.

These publishing efforts were thus more than patriotic defenses of the reputation of creole inhabitants, although Alzate has been well studied in these terms. The result was a new patois of medical science: an eclectic collection of theories and experiences of observation, discovery, and treatment from across the viceroyalty and abroad that was vernacular—common and everyday—in part by virtue of being held together in the pages of the periodical press. When it came to medical doctrines and frameworks for infectious disease, contemporaries subscribed to several, and most were assembled in print: corpuscles emanating from desiccated lakebeds, which vitiated the atmosphere in surrounding areas; the inflamed substance identified by the iatrochemical theories of Gerard Van Swieten (1700–1772) and Anton de Haen (1704–1776); and "bad smells," a catchall cause and consequence, whose combat indoors and outdoors was thought to alleviate the propagation of disease.[74] Each theory was presented with the caveat that notions not submitted to critical judgment (*juicio crítico*) would be discarded. A science of healing had to be constructed on the solid grounds of anatomy and physic, assisted by other branches of science, such as chemistry and botany, and rooted in a methodology of close observation, quantification, and experimentation. Typical of his time, Alzate privileged authors who had "read" the natural world for clues by means of tools of measurement.[75]

In the same experimental vein, Bartolache endorsed the study of anatomy and physiology in medicine through experiments on cadavers. In the final two issues of the *Mercurio volante* he published an anonymous medical *memoria* (report) that called cadavers "the truest book that nature affords." Anatomical investigations of the vascular structure of the eye, the location of salivary glands, the structure of the ear and nervous system, and the circulation of blood might reveal the very cause of death, the *memoria* advertised, by showing how a hardening of fibrous tissue in old age restricted blood flow (and produced lethal retentions of impurities in the body). In an editorial note Bartolache disclosed his attendance at postmortem autopsies in the anatomical theater of the newly opened College of Surgery, in the Royal Indian Hospital, which allowed him to comprehend and supplement the great written works on anatomy.[76] Against the devastation recently inflicted by typhus, Bartolache sought to normalize hands-on training and empirical study in the reformed medical curriculum.

Good health meant reading the "books" of nature in an everyday way as well. Weather vanes, barometers, thermometers, and hydrometers facilitated precise quantification of air speed, weight, temperature, and water content; measurements could be fixed and subjected to comparison and critical examination of atmospheric conditions in different locations, which might have consequence in matters of agriculture, sanitation, and various industries. In health care, the eudiometer promised to gauge "good" or "virtuous" air by measuring the diminution in a volume of normal air when mixed with nitrous air, which was thought to release phlogiston (the hypothesized combustible element ever on the minds of eighteenth-century chemists).[77] As in Paris, where cemetery reform in the 1760s followed the thinking that airing out buildings and neighborhoods addressed the transmission of harmful exhalations and restored the air's virtues, campaigns in Mexico City to reform burial practices used the nose as a point of departure for what was healthy and unhealthy, to track down and avoid or correct "foul" airs.[78] But the nose was fickle. Alzate embraced eudiometry, along with other sciences of measurement, in the belief that mechanical observation and quantification of the temperature and quality of atmospheric air might confirm, or override, the data provided by the senses. Possible applications included not only health care and disease management (with air quality gauged, inhabitants might be shielded from insalubrious regions), but also agriculture and mining, where noxious airs enfeebled miners. As Alzate put it, air was the principal support of the human body but also occasionally the cause of serious harm. Its regular observation promised significant benefits.[79]

In repackaging medical science to address society's problems, these publishers were among many who stressed pragmatism and applicability. Like their counterparts in England, France, Germany, and Prussia, who were writing on the unhealthful conditions in jails, lazarettos, and hospitals, amateurs and public intellectuals, natural philosophers, and savants in New Spain carried out a great deal of collecting, counting, and measuring.[80] Good health required that adherents of the new sciences identify and interact in some manner with other members of society, including sectors habitually excluded from scientific practice. To this end, instruments of measurement were endorsed and placed into the hands of readers who were unfamiliar. In two installments Bartolache discussed the principles and applications of the basic thermometer and barometer—both indispensable for anyone wishing to measure daily atmospheric states with precision and thereby protect the health of the human body. He then provided detailed instructions for their fabrication, as neither was as readily available in New Spain as in Europe. He offered metaphors comparing the thermometer's components to pen stems and violin strings and enjoined readers to make use of them for the sake of the public good and "the furtherance of studies beneficial to the nation."[81]

In practical terms Bartolache imagined that residents might monitor the temperatures of public bathhouses (*temascales*). These therapeutic spaces, popular fixtures in cities and the countryside, were largely unregulated and drew the occasional scrutiny of secular, ecclesiastical, and medical officials. Following a *cédula* prohibiting public baths in 1688, New Spain's viceroy initiated an investigation into their medicinal value and whether they might be demolished without harm to Indian tributaries. In their report physicians Ambrosio de la Lima and Joseph de Oliver, citing Greek and Roman thermal baths and classical authors, confirmed that heated waters, by opening pores, allowed nature to do the work of expelling waste. This was especially important for indigenous inhabitants, with their closed pores and pernicious humors, and castes with similar constitutions. In effect the report vindicated the healing knowledge of Amerindians, whose bathing practices were congruent with nature; as Ambrosio de la Lima marveled, "without medical writings, with only fuel and natural reason, they do the same that Galen, after considerable study, prescribed for his patients."[82] The medical experts argued against prohibition in this moment, while the problem of oversight remained unresolved.

In the next century, anxieties about social comportment and the possible scandal arising from the mixing of sexes mingled with public health concerns.[83] In his 1788 essay on urban reform, Baltasar Ladrón de Guevara addressed the pathway leading from Mexico City, through San Lázaro, to the famous thermal baths at Aguas del Peñón. It was barely passable owing to muddy patches and potholes, yet numerous unfortunates (*pobres miserables*) traveled on foot to seek out relief and medication there. He recommended that the Protomedicato take charge of maintenance of the thoroughfare, because physicians prescribed the baths and occasionally even traveled to them to consult with patients.[84] Within the city some twenty-four segregated baths suffered other hygienic

Table 2.1 Content breakdown by number of pages for the *Gazeta de literatura*, 1788–1795.

Subject	*Pages*
Natural history (botany, chemistry, zoology)	352
Health	203
Education / belles lettres (philosophy, language)	192
History and nation (censuses, eulogies, Mexican traditions)	167
Technology (mining, hydraulics, architecture)	142
Physics (astronomy, meteorology)	108
Commerce / agriculture	91
Topography (geography, geology)	86
Total	1,341

SOURCE: Clark, "*Gazeta de Literatura de México* (1788–1795)," and personal correspondence with the author, November 6, 2012.

problems, with some flooding with fecal matter when drainage pipes backed up. Into the 1790s they lacked adherence to any formal measures of sanitation, as Viceroy Revillagigedo observed in a 1793 decree. It was a shocking admission given that, as the municipal council observed, "the *temascal* bath is viewed as medicinal in this capital."[85] Public sweat baths, where residents of all classes attended to their physical health, thus offered frequent reminders of deficiencies in oversight and administration, no less than disease outbreaks, filthy hospitals, overcrowded cemeteries, and lax licensing practices. As spaces in need of reform, they were an opportunity to educate and enlighten the public on the proper way to care for themselves—here, by avoiding excesses of heat and use.

One measure of the interest in practical matters of health in these journals is statistical. Of the nearly four hundred articles published by Alzate in his own journals and the *Gazeta de México*, some eighty-two (22 percent) explored problems and proposed solutions relating to the health of the human body.[86] A tabulation of topics in the long-running *Gazeta de literatura* reveals some 15 percent by page dedicated to health, surpassed only by natural historical topics (table 2.1). While topics covered were often technical, Alzate was confident that his contemporaries might bring the best scientific opinions and practices to the level of the common person's understanding. Benjamin Franklin was the model. Alzate lamented that an inexpensive method of engraving with copper plates, based on techniques developed by Franklin, had not been adopted in New Spain, where printing images remained prohibitively expensive. Perhaps recalling the many devotional paintings and prints then in circulation, Alzate ruminated that even plant specimens, including flowers and leaves, might be faithfully reproduced by means of this inexpensive mechanism, with incalculable benefits for the public: "A simple method to print the image of a machine, plant, etc., at low cost, would be the happiest of discoveries, because it is well known that one learns more with a glance at a printed representation of a machine than reading and reflecting on even the most prolix and perfect description of it." Though a technical aside, it went to the heart of Alzate's didactic agenda, which included attracting an audience for science and making useful information available to those of lesser means. Magnificent editions were fine, "but because literate people [*el pueblo literato*] are made up (as in all societies of the world) of poor and rich," it was necessary to print economically so that publications might be had at a moderate price. The wealthy had their Peter Paul Rubens or Esteban Murillo, he noted; others should have more humble "painters," because a print of a plant or drawing of a device, rendered inexpensively, would ensure the propagation of advantageous knowledge (*conocimientos*) to everyday readers.[87]

In retrospect, journalists in the Age of Reason may appear overly optimistic in their belief that all reasoning persons might grasp and apply instruments of measurement. But the intricacies of health, in contrast to more abstract questions of physics, were of direct interest to New Spain's inhabitants, who were already looking after their bodies, environments, and health (as the advice proffered in healing manuals had long supposed). It required only modest corrections and adjustments, in this view, before they were doing it in a more informed manner. At the same time, a value-free scientific method was hardly canonical, with the moral, homiletic, and allegorical mixed in with the experimental. Bartolache published in his journal a Spanish translation of the renowned European manual on regimen, the *Discorsi della vita sobria*, or *Discourses on a Temperate and Sober Life*, as it was known in the English-speaking world. First published in Padua in 1558, at the height of anti-Lutheran sentiment, the manual was concerned with how to live a long life, narrated as a Catholic redemption story. In the tale, as the Venetian Luigi (Luis) Cornaro (1475–1566) approached middle age, he fell so ill that he was convinced he would die. The best physicians of Italy examined him and concluded that the only remedy was to leave behind the laziness (*holgazanería*) to which he was accustomed in favor of a temperate and orderly (*sobria y arreglada*) life. "It seemed to me quite natural," Cornaro muses, "that a different manner of living would similarly produce different effects, knowing that the art of healing can very well supplement, correct, and perfect nature, and also debilitate and destroy it, according to the good or bad use made of it."[88] It was a conversion story worthy of Saint Augustine's taming of the worldly senses: assisted by physicians,

Cornaro renounces wayward impulses in a transformation he calls "my resurrection." The lesson was that how one lived and what one ate (and how much) had moral implications that affected physical health. One had to live temperately, which meant exercising restraint against disorderly appetites (*apetito desordenado*). As editor, Bartolache approved Cornaro's religious cum medical moral; for him, moderation was the golden rule (*regla de oro*) and healthiest precept (*precepto más saludable*).[89]

This was familiar terrain in New Spain's creole medical culture. The first installment of Cornaro's story appeared just two days before members of the Protomedicato issued an official report on the epidemic raging in the capital. According to their investigation, the illness, characterized by high fevers, remained confined to the indigenous barrios of Santiago Tlatelolco (where Alzate had undertaken his inquiry). But it would undoubtedly spread, they warned, if precautions were not taken. They observed differences in susceptibility that correlated with lifestyle, in language resembling Cornaro's: those "not badly complexioned" (*no mal acomplexionados*) and living an orderly life (*de vida arreglada*) suffered only a mild cold (*una general constitución catharral*), and recovered with warm clothes and beverages; but the fevers of those with "some morbid disposition" or of a disorderly lifestyle (*de una vida desarreglada*) effloresced into the malignant variant *tabardillo* (typhus) that threatened the population.

"Señor Eminentísimo," they lectured, "are there any people more *desarreglada* than the plebe of this City? Their foods are crude, including the pepper they call chile, which is exceedingly harsh and abundant; their living quarters tight, with many dwelling around the *tecuile* or 'coal hearth,' in the center; their nakedness pronounced; their illnesses treated with a thousand absurdities; and others are without medicine or food. Then there is their daily drunkenness." It seemed that "only the infinite Mercy of God" could liberate the population from continuous outbreaks of epidemics, a consequence of "the depraved life of this unhappy people." In conclusion, the experts recommended fumigations with resinous wood, aromatic herbs, bonfires, and liberal use of gunpowder, proposing that the militia relocate artillery drills to affected neighborhoods to counter noxious miasmas in the air.[90]

If it suggested certain terms and phrases, the medical officials hardly needed the most recent issue of the *Mercurio volante* to prime their diagnostic inclinations. They were, with Bartolache, part of the same social network; shared similar training, acquaintances, and correspondents; worked in the same context of urban inequality; read the same medical treatises; and drew on similar paradigms to understand the etiology of disease. In their recommendations to the viceroy or the reading and self-healing public, their advice defaulted to the most hardened ideas about disease as a matter of diet and regimen, sobriety and excess, conditioned by factors of class, race, and gender.[91] When Bartolache reported on a mass outbreak of *mal histérico* (hysteria) among women of the upper and middle classes in Puebla and Mexico City, he identified as principal causes the abuse of alcohol and sweets, tight clothing (it encouraged inactivity), and the custom of going to bed late and rising late.[92] Though the tremors, weeping, fainting, *saltos* (jumping), convulsions, contortions, and other gestures resembling "a spell's effect" that characterized the illness were also thought to be inheritable from mothers, it was lifestyle that Bartolache isolated, proposing that women eat fewer sweets, take exercise, and ventilate their rooms (particularly in convents where many lived together).[93] Depicted as constitutionally weaker and more prone to ailments, women were also expected to manage their own recovery through vigilance. The same law of temperance, applied to the barrios of the poor, became a harsh lesson in neglectful excess. The social elite of Mexico City glanced into the dwellings of lower-class inhabitants in search of explanations and saw disorderly consumption of harmful foods and beverages, the corollary of which was that the sick and impoverished were responsible for their illness, and accordingly blamed for their condition.

The form and content of New Spain's scientific periodicals thus reaffirmed some of the tenets of Enlightenment medicine. Bartolache's discussion of hysteria, with its origins in the uterus, reproduced ideas about gender and class, and naturalized them in anatomical terms, which implicitly negated the enlightened universalism he pursued elsewhere. Alzate's on-the-ground reporting in 1772 was constrained by social expectations: the anonymous informant who appears in his reporting was emphatically ladino, his appearance and behavior telegraphing acculturation and reliability and in this manner bolstering the value of the testimony he provided. Attempts to shift the epistemological weight of perception toward tools that might better discern and evaluate the secrets of the environment were no less fraught, yielding data by means of culturally specific judgments and interpretations of what was worth seeing, representing, and studying—far from a "neutral" or "value-free" practice.[94] It was evident in 1762, when the viceroy, hoping to identify the cause of spreading typhus, ordered the surgeon and physicians of the Protomedicato to dissect the cadaver of a deceased *mulato*. They sliced open the abdomen, inspected the liver and gastrointestinal lining, and carried out experiments with nitric acid, sodium carbonate, lime juice, and pulque on the exceptionally yellowed bile (*cólera*) of the gall bladder. The doctors briefly considered the effects of the season and the stars before reasoning that there were sufficient sublunar causes to explain the illness. Joining Galenic ideas about corrupted humors to new interest in chemical and anatomical experimentation, they cited a lack of natural vigor in the subject, apparently on the basis of his race, and concluded (from their experimental observations) that an acidic beverage with volatile sulfuric particles like pulque would likely exacerbate illness.[95]

It was the beginning of an era in which the viceregal government increasingly turned to the rising surgical profession to study causes and treatments of disease.[96] In reiterating the harms of pulque, however, medical practitioners transmuted social biases into a register of anatomical study and clinical observation that taught contemporaries little they did not already know about the causes of disease, the "lack of vigor" of the lower classes, and the popular use of fermented beverages to fight illness.[97] Aided by the new anatomical sciences and instruments, medical culture in New Spain might seek and find the cause of disease in the machines of bodies and the books of nature, but did not manage to restrict diagnosis to anatomy's supposed facts. The irony, remarked before but no less true, is that the intellectual atmosphere and publishing practices of the Enlightenment engendered a science that helped justify and perpetuate social inequalities down the road.

Nevertheless, what was being attempted in the nascent literary forum was complex. Alzate and other *letrados* supported a temporary bracketing of social hierarchies of class, caste, gender, and education as the condition under which useful information must be communicated. This principle, with its counterpart, the accumulation of facts from empirical study, came into conflict with understandings of pathology and disease transmission, above all in epidemic outbreaks, when social distinctions were accentuated and professionals diagnosed people whose physiology, susceptibility, and living habits seemed to mark them as irredeemably different.

A REPOSITORY OF NATURE'S CURES

What effects did this journalistic experiment have in the management of infectious disease? Like the healing manuals, which left few traces of their use, much of our understanding is speculation from statements about intended application and audience. In the case of the periodicals, however, some people actually responded to calls for greater participation, if not on the scale that their creole editors might have hoped. Especially in emergencies, periodicals became public repositories, as dispatches from across the viceroyalty sought to inform other residents about food shortages, devotional acts, and successful remedies. Those who wrote in helped shape and stimulate a community of amateur naturalists, for which there was no precedent in New Spain.[98]

In his 1772 notice to the public, Alzate moved on from his Indian informant in Tlatelolco's barrio to the matter of medical personnel. The shortage of physicians in New Spain would endanger populations should the epidemic spread to distant pueblos ("sumergidos en los montes") presumed remote from adequate care. Alzate appealed to any healer who worked in the 1762 epidemic to publish the method he had found most useful, or to send it to him for publication in his periodical. In this way interested subjects would have these experiences at hand, "free of any kind of erudition that does not serve to alleviate the sick." In response, a learned resident of Mexico City submitted a text that clarified the mechanical effects on the human body of bathing in hot and cold water.[99] While waiting for an experience-based method, Alzate ran a "Recipe against the plague," from the December 1754 issue of the *Jornal económico*. It was a tincture of Castilian vinegar with rue, sage, mint, rosemary, sage worm, and lavender that was rubbed on the lower back, temples, and forehead, rinsed in the mouth, and inhaled through the nose in times of pestilence. The concoction was called "vinegar of the four thieves," after the men who reportedly confessed, at their sentencing for pillaging homes and murdering their pestiferous inhabitants, that they had been saved from contagion by using it.[100]

The determination to improve the healing arts in remote regions of New Spain was communicated in the prologue to the second volume of the *Gazeta de México*, which had been re-launched during the famine of 1784. Manuel Antonio Valdés, the editor, stipulated the kinds of news he would publish, to be written in a simple and efficient style, before elaborating a vision in which the paper would not only memorialize newsworthy occurrences for future generations but address problems in the present: "How grateful Place A would be knowing that in Pueblo B there is an abundance of such and such fruit that it needs, that has no calculated value there. The one would sell what is leftover; the other would have what it needs, and both would benefit."[101] Herbal remedies might similarly be publicized and exchanged within this interregional economy, in which those possessing special or excess medical resources were bound together with others in need. "How much good would mankind receive by saying that Herb H, which grows in such and such place, has this or that previously unknown virtue to cure such illness, which has already been verified as useful to many sick poor? By means of the *Gazeta* this work of charity can be practiced."

To the extent that they could, by transmitting valuable knowledge across dispersed terrain, periodicals fulfilled this Enlightenment vision of relative resource scarcity. A tradition of secret remedies, recycled healing methods, and domestic tonics was revived in the process. To the March 24, 1784, issue of the gazette, Alzate contributed an antidote first published in Europe, distilled from the manuscripts of a physician from Besançon, France, who over years curing pestilential patients had managed to avoid infection. Alzate claimed that it worked equally well for smallpox and measles: boil equal parts water and sulfur in a clay pot, soak articles of clothing in the solution, and wear them as prophylactics after they have dried.[102] Valdés confessed that he could not confirm whether an especially foul antidote intended for infected regions beyond Mexico City—a poultice of bran, horse manure, chamomile, and salt boiled in a white wine, vinegar, or horse urine base applied to aching regions of the body—had come from a certified physician. With this caveat, he published it anyway.[103]

A submission by don Joseph Mariano Acosta Enriquez, resident of Querétaro and "a well-known subject," was prefaced with this assurance: "Given that one of the most significant goods is health, whatever news is communicated to this office to conserve it or restore it will be received happily, and never be seen as excessive." Two cases known to the reporter were cited. First, a man with pleurisy's swollen lungs covered himself in an emollient of the roasted stalks of *maguey* cactus; he began sweating and felt relief immediately, and the following day urinated "great quantities of clotted blood and lumps." The other was a *teniente de justicia* (deputy official) in the pueblo of San Pedro Texopilco, in Sultepec mining district. When the usual medications proved ineffective during an outbreak of colds (*fríos*), he tried a concoction of whiskey, orange juice, lukewarm water, and sulfur, which apparently relieved him and an additional three hundred people "in hot and temperate climates."[104] Santiago Maureta, surgeon of the provincial regiment of dragoons of Valladolid, submitted a healing method that drew on his thirty years in the profession and recent experience in the outbreak of *dolor de costado* there. The treatment was "useful, beneficial, and relevant to any and all sick poor afflicted by the nearly general epidemic contagion," and especially for those "helpless persons" on estates and in settlements without access to medical practitioners. Four printed pages advised that healers dispense with bloodletting, of little use in the epidemic, in favor of an emetic with almond oil, a general massage with the same oil and alcohol, and a salve, along with a daily regimen of an infusion made of white *tequesquite* (mineral salt), poppy, borage, and other herbs, boiled and strained for use and consumed hot. Maureta invited criticism but accented his bona fides and reasons for submitting, which included the experience he had acquired curing more than a hundred patients, and the obligation of every person "to serve his neighbor with whatever aid he is able to give."[105]

There is a sense of desperation in these missives as contemporaries faced ruinous suffering. The district governor of Igualapan (Guerrero) wrote in 1786 describing a *peste* so fatal that people were suddenly falling dead "without any sign other than a hand on the stomach." Lacking surgeons, the ill were subjected to barbaric treatments, with bleedings carried out "with a nail or piece of glass," thus inflicting further harm. He hoped to arouse the spirits of *facultativos* so that one might relocate to Ometepec province after learning of the numerous inhabitants of its pueblos and their great need, implying the fees to be collected.[106] At the same time, emergencies inspired a far-flung network of correspondents to pursue, test, or publicize local remedies: medically trained men and clerics, if not exclusively so, who directed their scientific proclivities to the study of the natural world. In 1785 the gazette offered a detailed description of a plant found growing among barley and wheat fields in the humid regions of Oaxaca. Don Mariano Carranza, a practicing physician, first conveyed this information in a letter to a colleague in Mexico City, who imagined that "rephrased in a simple style," it might be usefully made known to the public (*el público*), and he forwarded it to Valdés. Called *expule*, the plant was a powerful, benign purgative "frequently used and celebrated there for its excellent virtues" and "so well received among [non-]practitioners in Oaxaca that they consider it a panacea" for fevers.[107]

The same year Fray Juan Caballero wrote from Oaxaca to report the results of experiments with another wild plant that turned out to have a range of medicinal applications. A man of letters, amateur scientist, and avid reader of European periodicals and medical writings, Caballero made several noteworthy contributions to New Spain's gazette in these years, including a detailed description of the cochineal insect that yielded red dye in Oaxaca, and observations on atmospheric pressure and the properties of gas, following the experimental launch of sixteen aerostatic balloons in Antequera, in June and July 1785 (most ignited in flames, which provided onlookers with a surprise spectacle). At Trapiche San Antonio, in Miahuatlán, Caballero had taken note of the use of a plant by the mill's employees. He wrote: "Having heard from the mouths of some field workers of the many and nearly miraculous effects attributed to a wild herb (known among them as the fever herb [*hierba de fiebre*]), who claimed that it freed nearly all who used it, even those in a wretched state, from all kinds of burning, dangerous, and malignant fevers, I resolved to verify the truth for myself and ordered a portion of it brought to me to distribute among people in need, according to their illnesses."

Not only did the virtues of *hierba de fiebre* correspond with the report of the workers, they included other serious maladies, which Caballero cataloged. In the course of the epidemic, the plant had cured more than two hundred cases of *tabardillo* and fevers, a small child close to death from an intestinal blockage (*empacho*), another with a lung abscess, others with severe abdominal colic, and women with interrupted menses. With properties that rendered it effective as a thinner (*diluente*), aperitif, diaphoretic, purgative, and diuretic, the plant worked by helping nature to expunge the sickness (*expeler el mal*) through blood, sweat, urine, and other means. Whereas, in the simple method employed by workers, a quantity "without a fixed dose" was crushed and dissolved in cold water, strained and administered to the sick, the friar preferred more precise measurements: half an ounce in two *tazas* (cups) of water, covered and boiled until reduced by half, and administered still warm. Caballero included a detailed description of the plant, including root, stem, leaves, and small orange flower, comparing it to better-known medicinal plants (e.g., *hierba mora*, *hierba del pastor*, and myrtle) in the belief that it might be located and administered elsewhere. The friar hoped that these experiments might be continued by "medical practitioners and those able to observe with the greatest precision the medicinal virtue of this prodigious herb."[108]

These dispatches were on another level from the philological, philosophical, historical, and theoretical debates being carried out by creole scientists like Antonio de León y Gama and Alzate about the reasons to preserve indigenous names in botany. They were offered in the belief that knowledge of materia medica, generated through practical applications, outside the circuit of standard pharmacopeia, might save lives and provide relief. By the same token, as journalists, administrators, and amateur naturalists sought to bring disjointed methods and information to a common healing sphere, much epistemic insight, experience, and information was left behind. In Caballero's exuberant reporting, the laborers who had informed him about the fever herb appear only obliquely, as background figures. Though they had already verified its medicinal value, what mattered was its rediscovery by a literate person conversant in the arts and sciences. The friar becomes intermediary, amender, and corrector of everyday knowledge, even standardizing the dosage, as he seeks out others who might similarly mediate on behalf of their communities. The economy that Valdés described so neatly in theory, in other words, was laden with power inequalities in practice, in which parties pursued self-interested ends or declined to divulge information and otherwise transformed knowledge into forms, languages, and frameworks more likely to "travel" across a textually integrated space.[109]

Print provided a more realistic alternative to sending plant samples, given shipping costs and other complications; on the rare occasions when they were sent, such physical translations were first carried out on paper. An announcement from Real del Rosario, Sonora, about *cardón* (elephant cactus, *Pachycereus pringlei*), reported on its application as a balsam and antidote against wounds from poison-tipped arrows. The reporter offered to send a sample of the plant, the balsam, and an instruction for its use to any curious reader wishing to experiment.[110] In the fall of 1784, Juan Palacios de la Campa, chaplain of the general hospital in Guadalajara, reported on his experiences with an infusion of the leaves of a shrub reputed to cure hydrophobia among rabid patients. After reading in Spain's *Mercurio volante* about a treatment developed by the surgeon of the king's army in Naples, who in Calabria had used the bite of a viper to cure the hydrophobia of a rabid dog (following the Hippocratic aphorism, "like cures like"), the priest, having assisted some dozen rabid patients in his twenty-two years at the hospital, sought out a less dreadful remedy. Apparently unaware of or unsatisfied with other common treatments—applying the hair of the biting dog, cauterizing the wound, ingesting European specifics—he found one in his own backyard, in the form of a shrub growing on the hacienda next to Mochitiltic ravine.[111] Described as roughly three *varas* (yards) in height, with leaves and seeds resembling those of a laurel tree, it was known colloquially as *el arbol de la margarita* (daisy tree) or *la flecha* (the arrow) in the adjacent town of Ostotipaquillo. An infusion of its leaves cured his rabid patients, and a priest residing on the hacienda confirmed its virtues.

Valdés agreed that others would be interested in the possibility of relief. He suggested that contemporaries had at last found the long-sought cure for rabies and encouraged further experimentation, on animals, to discern the plant's prophylactic properties. The following winter, readers learned that Palacios de la Campa had collected samples of the plant and sent, at his expense, an entire crate of it to Mexico City, which was stored at the publisher's office "and will be provided to anyone who needs it." A subsequent article added that the plant's identity had been confirmed by an anonymous subject, someone trustworthy ("digno de toda fé"), who had sent leaves from Guatemala that matched the sample. The informant maintained that it could be found in the mountainous regions from Querétaro all the way to the province of Sinaloa, and that it was effective in cases of typhus and smallpox as well, owing to copious sweating provoked by ingestion.[112]

It intrigues to imagine residents, healers, and naturalists arriving at the printing house of Felipe de Zúñiga y Ontiveros downtown for a sample of the plant. Whether anyone did, information about the natural world was most often collated in print, to locate and apply allegedly efficacious species independently. With remedies described, effects observed, and the height, size, weight, and appearance of specimens quantified, reports became primers in collection, measurement, and observation. In response to Fray Caballero's detailed botanical report, a *teniente de cura* (lieutenant priest) in Pachuca, Julian Antonio González, wrote that he recognized the plant as one he had used himself as parish priest of Ixtapalapa during the epidemic of 1737, on parishioners and to self-medicate when he had fallen ill; in the 1763–1764 epidemic, in San Andrés Epazoyucan parish; and most recently in the smallpox epidemic, when he healed some thirty patients on Santa Rita de Cadena Hacienda. Although his method varied, on the basis of Caballero's descriptions, González identified the plant as the one known in the region by the names *mirto cimarrón* (wild myrtle, *Loeselia mexicana*), *espinosilla*, or *hierba de la Virgin*. Additional applications reportedly included hair loss (for which some still use the plant today).[113] In response, Caballero clarified that *mirto cimarrón* was known by locals in Oaxaca as *espinosilla* or *hierba del tabardillo* (typhus herb) but was not the one he had identified. Because this plant was also effective against fevers, the friar proceeded to describe its size, shape, and color so that subjects could locate it and distinguish it from his own contribution to this repository.[114]

There were advantages to this endeavor of not yet uniformly adopting Linnaeus's method of classifying species. In February 1788, on the eve of the opening of the Royal Botanical Garden, Alzate fired the first shot in a public debate (broadcast in the pages of the *Gazeta de México* and the *Gazeta de literatura*) with peninsular botanist Vicente Cervantes, who arrived in Mexico City as part of the Royal Botanical Expedition. A proponent of the Linnaean system, Cervantes applied it to the botanical collection and in instruction at the university. Aligning with the celebrated French naturalist Georges-Louis Leclerc, Comte de Buffon (1707–1788), Alzate argued that the system was deficient insofar as it highlighted sexual features as essential at the expense of everything that was known about the plants' medicinal virtues and applications; he preferred an anthropocentric classificatory system that accounted for these, in place of laconic naming of the plant world.[115] This approach to nature was the one already taken by chaplains, friars, parish priests, physicians, and surgeons when describing local plants. A novice naturalist, Caballero was aware of botanical terminology but opted to avoid it in favor of local usages. That contributors made little use of Linnaeus's binomial system did not render their descriptions deficient. To the contrary, because this depository was meant for public withdrawals, some verbosity was useful and even necessary (as Alzate and other creoles subsequently advocated in their patriotic defense of ancient Mexica learning and practice). It might even lead to serendipitous "discoveries," as in confusion over the identity of *mirto cimarrón*.

Recognizing that findings might be confirmed, modified, or overturned in this medium, the friar intervened once more in a letter to Valdés, published on May 16, 1786. As the mysterious epidemic of the past year began to subside, Caballero now argued that the epidemic was not *dolor de costado* or pleurisy (theories he was able to discard after studying a published description of similar symptoms among patients in the writings of a Mr. de Rochard). Following Tissot, the friar hypothesized that the epidemic was a variety of rheumatism, the result of the obstruction of pores and suppression of transpiration that expelled superfluous humors. Observing patients in the town of Zaachila, Oaxaca, had confirmed his hypothesis: treated with the fever herb (*hierba de calentura*), the sick had recovered their health after copious sweating. Caballero hoped that Valdés would communicate this to the public, so that medical practitioners might discuss the best approach to end the outbreak, "because of its great interest for the health of all." He concluded by excusing himself for presuming to address these rather different audiences; he had been moved by the urgency of the situation to "place the sickle in someone else's harvest."[116]

To transgress the imperative to tend one's own garden acquired new significance in these years as periodicals realized, to a degree, Bartolache's vision of a shared healing community, in which those in possession of medical knowledge offered it to "remedy the misfortunes of others," as Caballero wrote. The novel mode of communication of information about disease, gleaned from settings of prophylaxis and treatment, depended as much on the medium (still constrained by cost and readership) as on any fundamental break in the medical paradigm.[117] Now correspondence from Colima's priest to the bishop of Michoacán, informing the prelate that in the province many had been healed of malignant fevers by drinking boiled tamarind water, or infusions of the fruit they called *chocoguisles*, or *tumbirichis* (bromelia plant) in Michoacán, acquired public dimensions as the epidemic unfolded.[118] Print likewise publicized a report from the parish priest of Teipan, twenty leagues from Acapulco, that despite the great sickness there, residents survived thanks to simple uncooked animal fat (*sebo crudo*) mixed with salt and *rosa de Castilla* and massaged into the joints of arms and legs and the pads of feet, which induced sweating and lowered fevers. An editorial hand connected and revised these contributions. Here, a note determined that experience with this simple remedy confirmed the May 16 issue featuring Caballero's report.[119] An anonymous informant from Matehuala (San Luis Potosí) reported that in the outbreak of *tabardillos* in the valley, consumption of a yellow-flowered plant, known there as *guachichile*, had saved lives by provoking copious sweating, along with purging and other "natural evacuations." It was distinguished by its characteristic flower from the plant known as *hierba de calentura*, but its use was the same. Readers were again referred to the issue in which Caballero described his experiments with the fever herb.[120]

Writings on nature's bounty by creoles in and beyond New Spain served to defend Spanish America's culture, inhabitants, civilization, and flora and fauna from deprecating European ideas about American degeneration. From the perspective of disease emergencies, dispatches about the natural world served rather different, if not incompatible, purposes. Publishing constraints meant that nature was made visible not in engravings but in descriptions by local informants, governors, priests, and practitioners, who joined a community of patrons (who subscribed to and underwrote these papers), readers (and auditors), occasional healers, natural philosophers, and laypeople in need of relief or in possession of local plants.[121] If not on the scale of the multivolume *Encyclopédie*, clerics, physicians, and other healers and midlevel administrators living far from each other contributed to the interregional production of information about medicine, yielding a "vernacular science" based on their experiences in the field.[122] Their reports, phrased in a simple style ("en estilo sencillo") and compiled by means of the printed page, were vernacular in multiple senses: produced in accessible translations; ideally reproducible in different healing communities; and adapted from everyday, ordinary practices.

They were also domestic, as distinct from official or institutional. Nevertheless, the viceregal government played a part in this activity by supporting the naturalists and other residents who assembled and remitted information, simply by issuing orders to subalterns to this effect. As editor of the gazette, Valdés was constantly aware of the government's interests and the propriety of the news that he printed.[123] If discussion of public health seemed politically neutral, even recommendations about a cure for rabies might make a political point about the way in which the government did or did not control canine populations. This raised the matter of censorship. Announcements with bearing on the health of Spanish subjects were technically the purview of the Bourbon state. When the Protomedicato intervened to indicate the potential dangers of the method expounded by surgeon Maureta in the gazette, the viceroy ordered that henceforth Valdés would first submit for review any item pertaining to the health of Spain's vassals before publication. (Members of the Protomedicato were to proceed with caution in undertaking reviews, especially when reports came from credible practitioners, as Maureta was.) Print was not a free marketplace of ideas: there were medical experts and novices, and although the former did not always agree, they would help the government police the court of public opinion.[124]

In practice, even censorship might further the cumulative emendation of healing knowledge. At the end of 1797, as the smallpox epidemic spread, Valdés returned to the colonial manuals in hopes that one, tailored to the ailments of the viceroyalty, might again provide relief. He thought that the *protomédico* Hernández and the Augustinian Farfán (who was mainly celebrated by reputation, "because his medical works are only known in certain very scarce reports") were deserving of future study, but that Gregorio López's *Tesoro de medicina*—written specifically to heal the sick in Huastepec Hospital, "where there was neither physician, surgeon, nor apothecary"—was more beneficial. The fiction surrounding its creation was now evoked to warrant republication: López had written about what he had seen and experienced, which made his writings credible and worthy of faith. Valdés reproduced its advice on smallpox, which consisted of sweating the patient with a tincture of *chicaquilitl*, a plant with pink leaves and purple flowers found among *maguey* cactuses. In a note the *protomédico* Juan de la Brizuela cautioned readers against these and other therapeutics aimed to provoke sweating in smallpox patients and recommended instead medicaments that "temper boiling blood."[125] Even in this censure, the collaborative principle of the medium prevailed: multiple opinions, revised, recycled, annotated, and debated, in a composite, provisional medical project.

Inevitably this print sphere served the public health interests of the viceregal state more directly.[126] Insofar as print compensated for the shortcomings of New Spain's medical infrastructure, however, it also usurped the function usually ascribed to absolutist governments. Already in 1785, it recorded private initiative geared toward public instruction and benefit: a cast of pilgrims, as Caballero put it, laboring in new lands on behalf of the people's health.[127]

CONCLUSION

In 1772 a parish priest forwarded to Bartolache a letter he claimed to have received from a cacique named Pascual Ángeles de los Reyes. The priest introduced don Pascual as a university-educated, middle-aged ladino Indian who had occupied all of the positions of authority in his parish. He explained that this gentleman, considered a Seneca in his community, regularly read Bartolache's *Mercurio volante* and Alzate's *Asuntos varios*, and that he had composed a page of objections he brought to the pastor for consideration. The cleric had urged him to publish it after making minor corrections.

The letter provides a rare glimpse, perhaps fictionalized, of a reading community around these journals. Don Pascual thanked Bartolache and Alzate for making news available in a style that was accessible to the common person and explained that he had acquired the first issues when he accompanied his son to seminary in Mexico City. Among the concerns he expressed was the fact that Bartolache's publications seemed to lack faith in the capabilities of Americans, undervalued the healing arts as practiced on this side of the Atlantic, and unnecessarily disparaged

Aristotle, Hippocrates, and Galen. Of the third and fourth issues, on the thermometer and barometer, don Pascual wrote, in prose sprinkled with Nahuatl terms: "I have already told my wife and daughter-in-law that they should not bathe in the *temazcalli* [*temascal*] until I can measure, with my *thermometer*, how many degrees of heat the water contains so that the *temazcalixtli* [air vent] can be well regulated, to prevent their blood from overheating." The cacique requested further information on these baths and begged that they not be discredited as beneficial: he rented out two to the village's pregnant women, "and I have seen them work miracles, although it is true that on some occasions the sick are left worse off." As for *pipiltzintlis*, not even a fraction of the abuses that were alleged took place among Indians. With so many *curanderos* in villages using the herb as a cure for a range of ailments, don Pascual wondered why doctors discounted it rather than adopt it.[128]

Bartolache suspected that the talented, discriminating, well-read "don Pascual" was a fabrication and insinuated his friend, the priest, "sensing a hint of fraud." Considering the literary ubiquity of satire, aspects of the letter do appear absurd. Among the friends and acquaintances gathering to discuss the issues in a local store was the storeowner—don Pascual's *compadre*—who becomes so incensed that doubt is cast on the scholarship of the venerable Spanish friar Feijóo that he burns the offending issue and orders dozens more from Mexico City for the same purpose. If Bartolache's suspicion was right, the letter and its portrayal of a critical reading public was a cleric's tongue-in-cheek take on a science of the masses: ironic commentary on an imagined universe in which residents made homemade thermometers to measure the temperature of village baths, shared copies of periodical literature, and discussed what they read in public spaces, in social, critical, emotional terms.[129] Even Bartolache apparently saw the humor in the conceit of an all-inclusive public for modern science, whose time had not yet arrived.

For good reason, studies of public health reform and scientific discourse in Spanish America have tended to focus on socially homogenous groups of upwardly mobile and literate creoles, who staked out debates on sanitation and disease in urban centers like Mexico City as their own, exclusive prerogative.[130] In this view, reading and publishing activities became a means by which this class further distinguished its virtues from the rabble, even to the point of forming a proto-national imaginary. Enlightenment manuals for lay audiences sought "to inform the educated public about medicine and simultaneously to demonstrate for this public the hegemony of healthcare professionals in managing these matters, establishing clear boundaries with respect to other healers, and with respect to what this educated public could do by itself."[131] The periodical press likewise telegraphed an exclusive arena in which science could be debated and performed publicly, in a flamboyant and aggressive manner.[132] Women and the lower classes did not participate in these spectacles, even if they were occasionally invited. This reinforcement of hierarchies is readily apparent even in the less specialized *Gazeta de México*, where erudite medical topics, including botany and technology, were protected as the domain of a few. So concluded Joseph Dionisio Larreategui, a botanist and graduate of the University of Mexico, when assessing the debate over Linnaean nomenclature. "Precisely in disputes about language," he huffed, "is where those who know it, speak it, and use it have a say; and those who can manage none of these do not."[133]

Some Mexican savants nevertheless condemned the exclusion of those not initiated into the world of Latin and technical learning, proclaiming their commitment to a more open and inclusive forum. Why? The historian of science Steven Shapin, observing an aversion among natural philosophers to specialized mathematical language and forms of secrecy in early modern England, has noted that "the circulation of knowledge in public space was deemed vital for securing its veracity and legitimacy. Languages of exclusion were, therefore, out of place in the public forums of truthmaking."[134] Inclusiveness provided the necessary conditions for the verification of claims about medical knowledge, scientific techniques and methods, and the natural world.

Aspirations to neutrality and transparency were at play in eighteenth-century Mexico, but beyond this philosophical and ideological justification, some practical aspects were key. First, knowledge related to health and healing, often centered on the environment and the human body, was best applied through some popular, common, or in the terminology of the day, *public* extension. Don Pascual came to stand for a group on the margins of a textual Republic of Letters, who did not possess specialized training and were not in the professional class, but nonetheless formed the locus of medical practice. In so much of New Spain, knowledge about health derived from nonspecialists working in major cities, towns, villages, mills, and haciendas. These people occasionally formed part of corresponding networks that produced empirically tested diagnostic reports, botanical descriptions and dosages, and household remedies, but they labored under conditions that did not always lend themselves to precise measurement or classification, and they responded to the exigencies of disease rather than the latest scientific debates and fashions.

Journals offered a better option for the delivery of time-sensitive news and the adaptation of knowledge produced in villages, parishes, or haciendas. There were many reasons to contribute. The printed page was a means to personal honor; it might bestow fame and glory, in the eyes of one's peers, or God, and likewise take it away.[135] Some looked to the new print medium to convert demand into financial gain or to reach, teach, enlighten, save, or civilize communities residing hundreds of miles away.[136] For reasons having to do with philanthropy, professional development, patriotism, suspicion of traditional scholasticism, profit, and ideas of race and redemption, the effect was to redraw the bounds delimiting rational participation in medical and scientific practice. The involvement and conversion of broader sectors of society to new practices and notions of public utility would ultimately happen beyond the printed page, but optimism led some to believe that this substitution of a new order for the old was imminent and that they were preparing the ground.

From this perspective, nationalism, elitism, and the professional and class aggrandizement to which these contributed were only part of the story, and not irreconcilable with a less institutionally restricted literary and scientific practice that was pursued for reasons that were at once ideological, personal, and pragmatic. Looking back, this experiment seems destined to fail, but there were tangible results from efforts to involve a more geographically and socially diverse community. As vernacular texts multiplied, more people might draw on some homegrown herb, remedy, or method to assist in intractable illness, correct or supplement outdated or ineffective medical traditions, or simply stand witness to the spirit of discovery that infused these works. This was England's virtue, according to Judge Guevara, where there was no project or idea pursued to benefit the nation that had not first been birthed in a free press, from whose books and periodicals the government adopted better practices.[137] In this view the synchronization of private interest and enlightened governance was the wave of the future. As its precursor, Mexico City's print culture served as a brief experiment in a science by, of, and for the people who were known to possess cures that the professors of medicine did not. If not in these literary forums, they too would have a say.

CHAPTER 3

"Massacre of the Innocents"

Preventing Smallpox, 1796–1798

No one can know the real boundaries in a *monte*.
—Bernardo Ruiz de Conejares, Villa Alta (Oaxaca), 1797

In the summer of 1796, outbreaks of smallpox in the Audiencia of Guatemala, the province of Oaxaca, and the ports of Acapulco and Veracruz moved the viceroy, the Marqués de Branciforte, to declare a state of emergency. Administrators in Guadalajara, Guanajuato, Oaxaca, Puebla, San Luis Potosí, Valladolid, and Zacatecas received orders to isolate infected individuals and populations immediately, "without excuse or exception of any person."[1] Adapted from Spanish surgeon Francisco Gil's treatise on smallpox, the emergency measures resembled those implemented in Europe beginning in the fifteenth century to combat leprosy, plague, and other infectious diseases. When plague struck the walled Tuscan village of Monte Lupo in 1630, for instance, public health authorities in Florence ordered the construction of a pesthouse for the sick, a cemetery for plague victims beyond village walls, and quarantines on households.[2] In 1788, hundreds of copies of a printed extract of Gil's work were circulated to bishops, district governors, medical practitioners, hospital personnel, and parish priests with orders to follow its instructions and begin constructing provisional infirmaries.[3] The measures were not without precedent in New Spain, as officials of the Protomedicato defensively informed the viceroy. In the 1773 *matlazahuatl* outbreak, they noted, afflicted persons arriving from the countryside for medical care had been quarantined and attended to in a convalescent ward (*hospedería*) established at the outskirts of the capital.[4]

Atlantic ideas about enlightened governance, fixated on human population as a measure of industrial growth and geopolitical strength, dictated a more rational and uniform approach than the sporadic infirmaries of the past. With an epidemic on the horizon, the government extended countermeasures to most of New Spain, prescribing quarantines, cordons around infected communities, and infirmaries to segregate the sick. Infected homes were to be clearly marked, patients isolated and scrubbed, clothing and bedding washed and fumigated, and cadavers interred in remote chapels or fields.[5] Complications came to light as local administrators struggled to implement measures in hundreds of towns and villages along the epidemic's path.[6] From Pachuca, where an outbreak was imminent, the district governor requested clarification. Were nursing infants to be among those removed from their homes and, if so, should their mothers be allowed to care for them? Should force be used to separate others? And how would the necessary items—medications, physicians, beds, clothing, foods, and the full-body linen gowns used by caretakers—be paid for?[7]

Challenges arising from this experiment in disease control became salient for many affected communities in the south of colonial Mexico. The region is often written out of studies of public health reform, whose prevailing urban focus has unintentionally obscured the scope of the experience and implied that rural people were either not much affected or that they did not contribute to the resolution of disease emergencies. Research on the smallpox episode, in particular, leaves the impression that the eventual reversal in official policy was the result primarily of the political pressure applied by merchants and deliberations carried out at the highest levels of government.[8] But many more of the pesthouses and cemeteries prescribed for burial outside (*extramuros*) of settlements were constructed for towns and pueblos, where pathogens and people spilled over quarantine lines and discontent fueled protest between Guatemala and Mexico City. Officials faced cynical maneuvering for profit, tormented indecision, covert subterfuge, foot-dragging, principled stands against meddling by outsiders, alarm over the separation of children from parents, and obedient deference, along with less dramatic instances of resignation.

This chapter highlights these responses as it follows the transition from the contagionist approach to disease, still officially endorsed, to one that placed immunization at the center. The partial overturning of the anticontagion regime, and the grassroots adoption of a new medical paradigm, was catalyzed by weeks of protest in the rural south, where Indian tributaries expressed broad-based sentiments of moral outrage and communal concern. Technological change provides the overarching storyline, but divergent interests, reactions, and perspectives on healing and governance—gleaned from depositions in criminal cases, petitions from villagers, reports from priests in charge of more than a hundred *pueblo de indios* in the district of Villa Alta (see map 2), satirical texts, and bureaucratic correspondence—are not easily reduced to their political or medical effects. Neither does a multi-sited approach lend itself to the kind of contained narrative that a focus on elite policymaking and literate debate is likely to produce.

Nevertheless, complaints revolved around three broad areas of frustration and anxiety. First, communities registered repeated objections to the impact of quarantines on village boundaries and subsistence, in a region where trade spanned districts and where sown fields were often located well beyond inhabited settlements. Like their Tuscan counterparts, indigenous producers, consumers, and traders in Mexico were highly mobile. They sold goods at market, tended herds and fields, and went on pilgrimage to local shrines, and they chafed under regulations that complicated these activities. We are left imagining what local vendors and the faithful in the valleys and sierras thought when they learned that the annual October festival in honor of the miraculous Christ of Tlacolula would be suspended in 1796. People ordinarily came from all around to sell fruits and goods and enjoy this "singular pleasure in the year," and the social and economic import of the event weighed on Oaxaca's secular and religious officials. Ultimately they agreed that it would be impossible to keep infected communities away from the sanctuary should the event proceed.[9]

The prescribed infirmaries struck many as especially harsh. The epidemic coincided with attempts to transform urban hospitals into cleaner, more therapeutically effective and socially desirable places. But reform was up against the common perception of the hospital as a pestilential, overcrowded environment of last resort, where the destitute went to die.[10] In the previous smallpox epidemic, when some industrious and charitable estate owners ("hacenderos caritativos") established infirmaries for workers and residents in barrios surrounding Oaxaca's capital, the royal governor alleged that Indians "preferred a pitiful straw mat [*un mal petate*] in their homes to the beds that were prepared for them."[11] At the end of the century the prescribed infirmaries, often little more than hastily built or converted huts, inspired little confidence in parents who learned that their children would be removed from their homes and transported to them, sometimes over long distances.

As for *camposantos* for more sanitary burials, medical theories of contagion dictated severing the deceased from the community of the living, which shocked the system of social relations and challenged communal possession of church grounds. These sites were respectable places that kept the deceased close to living members. The habit of burying bodies in sanctified grounds, not infrequently near the altar, might demonstrate social status, corporate privilege, and wealth. Death was the moment when

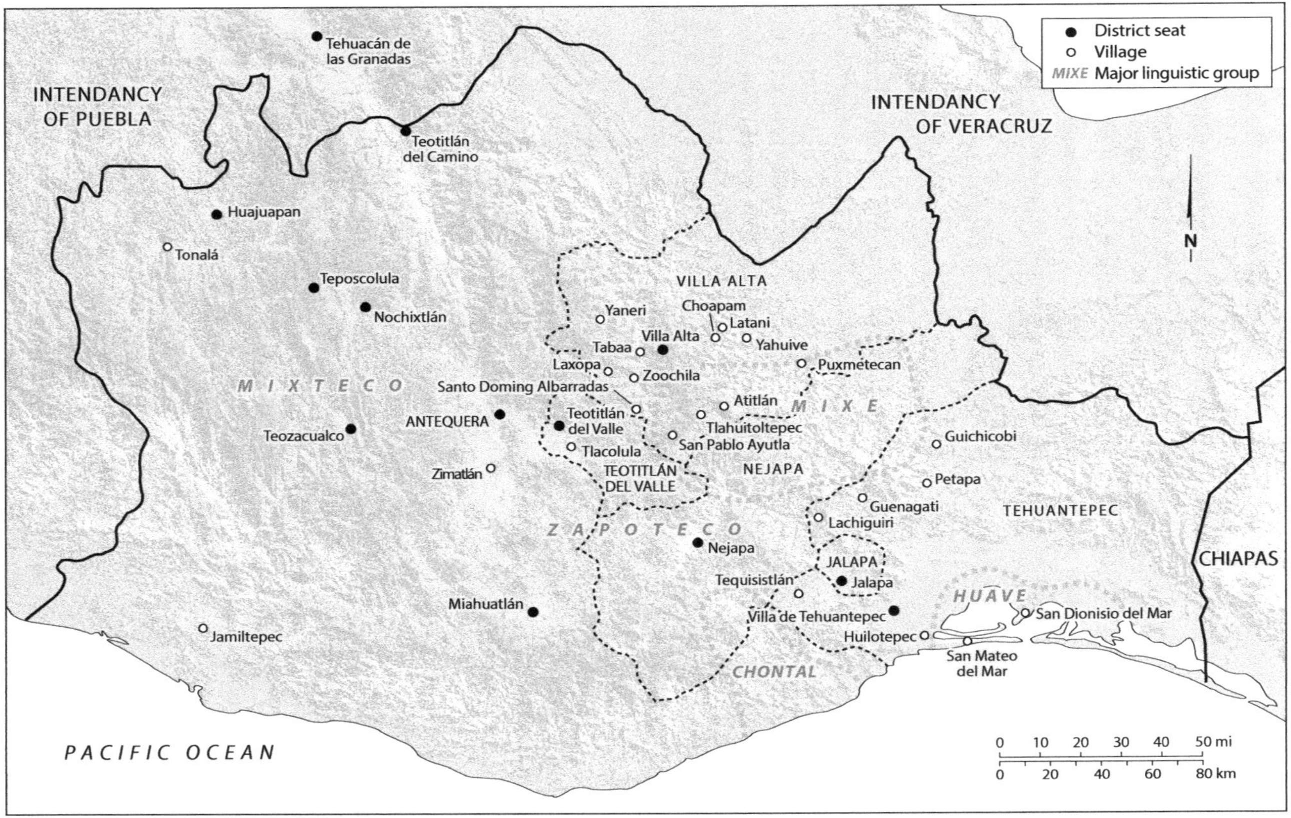

Map 2. Intendancy of Oaxaca.

a mobile people came to rest, and some balked at burial in remote places that were seen as little more than a wilderness.

The crescendo of dissent reverberated across the Atlantic when news of troop movements in Oaxaca reached Spain. Yet the resolution of the crisis came not by force but through sporadic experiments with new medical practices. Inoculation trials in Tehuantepec and elsewhere turned villages into laboratories that provided the data needed to confirm the viability of the practice. The government's unsteady navigation of an alternate path forward in the face of local conventions, politics, and knowledge prefigured the ambiguous revolution in preventive medicine to come.

"EVERYTHING IS A ROAD"

The two mountain ranges of the Sierra Madre, running parallel from the United States through Mexico, form a tapering high plateau that carves Oaxaca into dozens of ecological zones, ethnicities, and linguistic groups. Fragmented by this mountainous terrain, the human geography of the south of Mexico was characterized by communities that lived in isolation, farmed in scattered plots, and identified by village. Fewer large estates here than elsewhere in New Spain meant that people were less likely to be pulled away for work, particularly in the remote sierra Zapoteca and Mixe regions.

By the end of the eighteenth century, efforts to mitigate ethnic distinctions, consolidate Spanish administration, and incorporate communities into the monetized economic sphere had achieved partial results. Reformers placed *doctrinas* (protoparishes for Indians) under the care of diocesan clergy and transferred instruction of children from priests and Indian *fiscales* (their lay assistants) to designated primary schools under Spanish maestros.[12] French-style intendants and subdelegates were introduced to streamline taxation and tribute collection, maximize indigenous productivity, and prohibit commercial activities formerly carried out by district governors with indigenous communities. Beginning in 1787, Oaxaca's intendant, Antonio de Mora y Peysal, assailed the *repartimiento* system, the monopolistic trade in cotton and finished textiles that underpinned the economy, which channeled profits to local officials, priests, and merchants.[13] But administration still required a certain amount of bargaining when it came to reform. Lacking recourse to physical force, the viceregal government relied on district governors, village leaders, and parish priests to enact policies, whose revisions and recommendations were evaluated by *fiscales* (royal attorneys in charge of civil, criminal, fiscal, or Indian affairs), who made recommendations to the viceroy. This chain of communication and review might take months, which compelled local functionaries to exercise their discretion whenever necessary, and insofar as villagers expected it.

In the summer of 1795 smallpox broke out on the Isthmus of Tehuantepec, a crossroads of trade between New Spain and Guatemala. Fishermen from the Huave village of San Dionisio del Mar had fallen ill and infected numerous nonimmune children after a trip by canoe to neighboring Tonalá. Spurring a prolonged, ultimately futile attempt to save the nerve centers of New Spain, Oaxaca's intendant instructed Pedro Fessar, Tehuantepec's subdelegate, that anyone who wanted to pass beyond Nejapa, in the direction of Oaxaca's capital along the Camino Real, was to pass quarantine first. Even mail carriers were required to submit their loads for disinfection with vinegar, with susceptible persons denied passage and returned to their place of origin.[14]

Almost immediately fishermen, farmers, muleteers, and merchants expressed hardship. On August 7, the governor of San Mateo del Mar appeared before Fessar with two alcaldes and a scribe to convey the suffering of their community: reportedly entreating on their knees, they related that fifty or sixty individuals from their pueblo had been detained by the *salvaguardia* (patrol guard) in Huilotepec, presumably on their way to market in the Villa of Tehuantepec, where in exchange for a chicken or a measure of chiles they might expect a *cuartillo* (half a liter) of maize. Located on the saline coast, San Mateo possessed no *milpas*, which required residents to exchange hens, fish, and turtle eggs, in addition to chickens and chiles, for maize. Representatives added that the neighboring villages to which they were permitted travel (Niltepec in the north, and Zanatepec and Tapanatepec in the direction of infestation) were small and lacking foodstuffs, while no one in Santa María Petapa or San Juan Guichicobi bought what they had to sell. They could not maintain themselves, the officials insisted, and would have no means to pay the next installment of tribute, due shortly.[15]

Complications in production and trade pointed to the close-knit relationship between the smaller villages of the coast and interior and the major market center of Villa de Tehuantepec. Fessar advocated for regular communication between the villa and its surrounding pueblos by stressing that the town depended for its subsistence on producers elsewhere and supplied markets well beyond. The unsold fish brought by residents of San Mateo, for instance, they left with *forasteros* (itinerants) in the villa, who transported the surplus all the way to Antequera, the Spanish capital of Oaxaca. The effects of disease control had already begun to reverberate through a landscape of informal and formal trade in fish, fruit, *achiote* (annatto), cotton, the indigo dye *añil*, and salt, which dominated commercial activity. Production of salt alone facilitated networks of exchange in goods controlled by Indians and *mulatos*, such as shoes, straw hats, *huipiles*, maize, and beans, between Oaxaca and Chiapas, Guatemala, and Soconusco.[16] A crucial input in silver refining, officials and the merchants and miners who controlled salt's trade clamored for an exemption from restrictions. Salt was soon declared less susceptible to contagious elements than other prohibited goods and allowed passage after brief quarantine. Following this exemption, Tehuantepec's merchants sought dispensations for a host of other goods, especially *achiote* and dyestuff, noting the importance of timely arrival of merchandise destined for Oaxaca, Veracruz, and Spain. Fessar, who owed his post to these influential residents, dutifully made their case.[17]

The threat to regional economies grew when, in August 1796, smallpox arrived in Teotitlán del Valle, a weaving center in one of the central valleys.[18] Teotitlán presented an especially dangerous source of contagion because of its location just miles from the commercial and administrative hub of Antequera, where surrounding populations converged every Saturday to sell food surpluses, pottery, salt, fish, cochineal, and pulque at market. In addition to regional trade between Antequera and a network of markets, towns, and cattle ranches, a handful of goods—most notably, red dyestuff from cochineal beetles, silver, and cotton—flowed into viceregal and international markets. The raw cotton produced along the coast supplied a regional textile industry centered inland, with growing populations in the central valleys driving demand for the cotton mantles worn by the indigenous sector. By 1792 an estimated quarter of the male non-Indian population in the capital was employed in the textile industry.[19] Powerful regional merchants and guilds had counterparts in Mexico City, who became vocal in the discussion of the quarantine policy once trade routes were disrupted.

On the ground, administrators were attuned to the needs and worries of tributary Indians. Finding themselves severed from markets and fields, weavers in Teotitlán faced their own hardships. Esteban Melgar, an experienced Spanish administrator charged with overseeing emergency measures, stationed recruits to monitor traffic on the roads into Villa Alta and requested an immediate delivery of some fifty *fanegas* of maize (approximately seventy-five bushels) to be sold at cost to residents who were unable to leave for markets or tend to their *milpas*.[20] A group of poorer villagers proposed an arrangement whereby they pawned their woven articles in exchange for cash. After these weavers were paid a portion of their market value, the articles were delivered to an intermediary, fumigated, quarantined, and sold in Antequera.[21] In the matter of villagers' crops, Oaxaca's intendant proposed that they be placed temporarily under the care of neighbors, to protect them against theft and grazing by cattle while maintaining the cordon until harvest season. According to Melgar, men and women appeared at the municipal building in "great distress" when they learned of the arrangement. They begged permission to tend their fields and care for their oxen, reasoning that otherwise the crops, "many of which still require care because of the late season, would be lost, and many families lived from the maize, zucchini, and green beans they picked daily." They distrusted their neighbors, who they feared would neglect their fields and cattle and even take advantage of the emergency to despoil them of their land and its fruits. A survey on horseback revealed that the village's plots were indeed bordered by Santa Ana del Valle and Macuilxóchitl ("Maculsuchil"), which moved Melgar to station guards there to discourage congregating.[22]

These concerns over sabotage and the defense of land—Melgar called them *canonizado* (timeworn) for Indians—were not so easily dispatched. Although a lively market system integrated communities, strong corporate identities and independence in matters of production and consumption left villages vying for control over parcels of land, elevated parish or market status, and political primacy. The stakes were high, with considerable wealth or prestige accruing to confraternities or producers in the village that came out on top. Land was frequently a flashpoint in intervillage politics. Arable plots were dispersed over large areas and required aggressive legal defense or a steady presence to uphold claims to ownership. Any boundary was provisional and contested, defined by use and vulnerable to transgression.[23] The government turned to teams of villagers to guard the cordon lines that were being raised as the epidemic progressed, with daily wages (2 *reales*, in Tehuantepec) to ensure that only those carrying supplies of food might pass.[24] But drafted villagers remained players in an agricultural landscape that required regular travel to plots of land.

An ethnically tinged intervillage rivalry inevitably flared up at one of the checkpoints on the road leading into the highlands of Villa Alta. Mixe-speaking villagers from Tlahuitoltepec, Tamazulapan, and San Pablo Ayutla *cabecera* convened on October 12 at Lachicocana, a well-watered site in the highlands, to begin construction of a *jacal* to shelter the men who would patrol the road from the valley. The next day, sixteen Zapotec residents of Santo Domingo Albarradas arrived to inquire into the work. An official investigation in the aftermath of the ensuing skirmish uncovered a volatile situation. Villagers had been litigating over a patch of land in the vicinity, until recently farmed by a member of Ayutla, that had been ceded to residents of Albarradas after papers surfaced proving ownership. The latter had sown ("by order of their alcalde mayor") ten *almudes* of maize, roughly a bushel, to help reinforce their new claims of ownership.[25]

According to testimony in Spanish from the imprisoned alcalde and scribes, when members of Albarradas arrived at the site they had found their adversaries, the Tlahuitoltepecos, roasting ears of corn, which they presumed had been stolen from nearby fields. They claimed that the workers had explained that they were building a rancho—suggesting a more permanent edifice—to patrol the road against infestation. After leaving peacefully, they had been pursued and arrested, whipped, and placed in stocks in San Pablo Ayutla. They stressed that they were simple rural people (*campestres*), who needed the confiscated arms to protect their fields against human and animal intruders, including deer.[26] The account offered by Tlahuitoltepec's leaders in Mixe (through an interpreter) cast themselves as victims. They had been resting and lunching when delegates from Albarradas approached them, asking why they were building in their territory, and "if they did not know that the land was in litigation before their subdelegate." Insisting that they knew of no cordon, the delegation returned with a contingent of villagers armed with shotguns, knives, axes, and machetes. The Zapotecos tried to arrest several of the workers on the pretext that the corn was stolen, but one escaped, roused up the others, and together they rushed the armed men, confiscated their weapons, and administered their "deserved lashes" in the district seat before throwing them in jail.[27]

The new regime of disease management had become entangled with village politics and ethnic animosities that went beyond disputes over corn and fields. A document submitted by leaders of San Pablo Ayutla detailed acts of theft, violence, and attempts by Albarradas villagers to appropriate fields and cattle leading up to the cordon's placement.[28] Tlahuitoltepec's elected officials, with pulses elevated from the recent whippings, testified that "these Zapotecos are very wild" and that out of fear they always went in groups to the work site.[29] Construing their foes as temperamentally aggressive, they justified the manner in which they had fended off and whipped them "for being disobedient and foul-mouthed."[30] Assuming temporary control of a contested passage, they took advantage of the emergency to punish their adversaries, who had recently gained legal advantage but saw it slipping away.

The nature of this altercation, presumed to involve farmers defending their fields, was deemed too trivial to merit further consideration, and arms were returned, with warnings, to their owners.[31] Relief that the disturbance had only been about boundary disputes (*disputas de linderos*) suggested that it could be bracketed and managed apart from efforts to intercept infection. Bernardo Ruiz de Conejares, Villa Alta's district governor, issued a judgment reiterating orders to Tlahuitoltepec's leaders that they not impede the transit of neighboring villagers, who "have need of locating their cattle or the path to their fields." He reminded them that the cordon "has no other purpose than to detain those who come from infested regions, and specifically Teotitlán's valley."[32] In a separate note he added that terrain should be considered to identify less disruptive boundary lines for any future cordons.[33]

Months later, when Conejares revisited the episode at the checkpoint, his optimism had faded. He had since recognized that people moved with greater ease than the guards appointed to patrol the roads. Residents with whom he consulted on overseeing paths had confirmed that patrolling mountains was much more difficult than the valleys below, where a guard on horseback might cover great distances along level roads without visual impairment. By contrast, Conejares wrote, the real boundaries (*linderos*) in what amounted to a backlands (*monte*) were unknowable. At every step trees, precipices, and uneven terrain obscured the view, while paths were accessible only to Indians on foot, who could make long detours. As a result, any cordon would work "only for Spaniards and mule trains."[34] The district governor of Tehuacán de las Granadas, bordering Oaxaca and Puebla, pointed out as a practical matter that Indians assigned as guards made a living from their work; given an unbearable or impractical *tequio* (communal task), they detained muleteers on only the most highly traveled roads, leaving open numerous others along which residents traveled on foot.[35] The administrator of Metztitlán (modern state of Hidalgo) echoed these observations, reporting that people used roads that were just trails through *monte*, neither on maps nor recognized officially, "because for them, everything is a road."[36]

Months after the disturbance in Villa Alta, guilds and miners convened in emergency sessions and drafted petitions to amplify these themes and make viceregal orders respect their interests. They appealed to the high economic costs of policy, and to the simple impracticality of policing so many paths and quarantines. Trade and mining deputies in Antequera urged reopening the roads by pointing out that contagion had already spread across the province and that quarantines were harmful, to *miserables indios,* other traders, and to commerce: cargoes of wheat to the mills were being delayed, along with sugar, mantles, straw mats, fruits, and other comestibles, on which the city survived and trade with surrounding populations depended.[37] The first deputy of Oaxaca's mining corps insisted that the provincial capital was "open on all sides," with numerous exits all along its circumference. Because villages along the Camino Real depended on trade with the capital, residents had ample incentive to violate quarantines along numerous secluded paths, which they did regularly.[38]

In their own petition to the viceroy, eleven men representing the agricultural interests of Tehuacán de las Granadas portrayed their town as the navel of a global economy. They noted that most of their products, especially flour, were consumed over the quarantined border with Oaxaca, and that Tehuacán was an indispensable stopover for goods flowing north from Chiapas and Guatemala (cochineal, indigo, and cacao) and merchandise arriving from Spain and Mexico City, including cloth from China and finished clothing from Querétaro and Puebla. Dramatically rendered, this commerce was the lynchpin of regional, viceregal, and even European economies. Emergency measures were excessive, a direct attack on free trade (*la libertad del comercio*), "morally impossible" to enforce, and irrelevant now that smallpox had spread to Antequera and Tehuacán, thanks to numerous Indians who arrived each day after evading cordons. Freedom of movement had prevailed, and they recommended inoculation as a more suitable measure.[39]

In Mexico City the *fiscal* for civil affairs, Francisco Xavier Borbón, noted parallels between the documents arriving from Tehuacán and from the trade and mining delegates in Oaxaca.[40] While the logic and form suggest that Tehuacán's was composed independently (among notable differences, the document from Oaxaca never mentions inoculation), in voicing their interests these parties indicated common knowledge about the interdependence of the regional economy. They observed that Spaniards relied on the goods produced by Indian villages—raw cotton and dyes, foodstuffs, and processed items—and simultaneously rearticulated the perspective of humble producers and consumers that a precarious economy meant hunger and unemployment, stressing the population without necessarily containing illness. Above all, enforceable isolation under a policy of mass quarantine required a population living within fixed boundaries, with established roads and trails governable by the state. Instead, goods and people moved in commercial, agricultural, and territorial borderlands.

With this insight, the keystone in the viceregal program's arch was revealed as defective. Borbón himself, a key player in the coordination of emergency relief, was compelled to see that "there are many and diverse roads and trails by which to enter those populations, as none of them is walled, or has doors to prevent free entrance at whatever place."[41] Roads and borders were the product of local knowledge and patterns of use and not easily discerned or policed, which proved fatal to a program of surveillance. Faced with a morass of geography and the reality of regional economies, administrators had to compromise.[42] Meanwhile, villagers insisted in other ways on the "moral impossibility" of the anticontagion regime.

AN ANATOMY OF PROTEST

To be deprived of one's child was as powerfully felt as being deprived of one's daily bread. Tehuantepec's district governor was among the first to have to inform parents that their sick offspring were to be removed from homes and villages. The news was greeted with incredulity in the villa, the measure considered unprecedented and harsh. "I have just finished gathering the Indians to make known to them the ruling that children who fall sick are to be sent to outlying settlements," Fessar reported. "I see them in a disobedient mood. They claim that where their children die, there everyone will die. And reason does not convince these people, even if I explain that it is for their own good." He painted his Indian charges as unreasonable, disobedient, and stubborn, even though he shared their perspective and had his own reasons to oppose the provisions. Months later Fessar would insist that the population was simply too large to enforce orders, "even if troops were to assist" in removing children from their homes.[43] In effect, the mandate was a dead letter there.

Where administrators did not go so far as to annul impractical measures, they tried to convert their charges to the official view. In Teotitlán del Valle, the quarantined weaving village, some fifty women gathered at the infirmary's construction site on the morning of September 29 to announce their discontent before a captive audience of officials and villagers. The daughter of the Indian governor, Sebastiana Vásquez, who worked in Antequera's main plaza as a *tortillera* (and was later described in criminal depositions as ladina in appearance), announced the assembly's decision that the village's children would not be checked into the infirmary or buried in the new *camposanto* and threatened to withhold tribute and religious fees if officials did not agree. Melgar, joined by Teotitlán's priest, sought to convince the women of the benefits of the anticontagion measures. Enlisted by the administrators for support, the men working on the infirmary warned that disobedience would bring soldiers from Oaxaca to enforce measures and subdue the women, who allegedly replied that "if troops came, they would be more than satisfied, and would prostitute themselves for their pleasure."[44] None of the women held formal office, but they took charge of political affairs nonetheless: their words brought public shame on the men, in a place where honor was carefully guarded, and in effect "pluralized patriarchy" by appealing to sources of masculine authority beyond the village.[45]

Despite this inauspicious start, Melgar pushed ahead. He managed to have sixteen children transported on straw mats and planks to the infirmary, with assistance from a corporal from the provincial militia, the priest, and a soldier from a cordon checkpoint. (Melgar stationed the corporal outside to deter the women who persisted in seeing their children.) Measuring some twenty-two feet on each side, with an annex including a kitchen and rooms for nurses, the interior was adorned with layers of green palm to "refresh the infirmary and please the patients." Inside the children were dressed in clean clothing and fed rations of *atole* and mutton broth with lettuce.[46] Melgar made careful study of Francisco Gil's treatise on smallpox as well as an instruction for treatment authored by José Flores, the president of Guatemala's Protomedicato. Oaxaca's intendant praised the latter as tested and better suited, quoting the title, to the "nature and way of living of Indians and rustic folks," who, he added, "with little difference are virtually the same in all parts." Approved by Oaxaca's physicians, Flores's work extolled "cleanliness and purity of the air" and maintained that the best thing for Indians and other poor people was to prevent the spread of infection to other pueblos, by patrolling movement, sweeping and washing streets, and fumigating frequently with sulfur.[47] An eager convert to the program, Melgar administered the herb *cañafístula*, commonly used as a strong purgative, and released patients once the scabs over their pustules separated (which the experts recommended). Nevertheless, he conceded his shortcomings as a healer. He had requested a *curandera* from neighboring Santa Cruz Papalutla to help manage the infirmary and "administer enemas," because with so few to care for the sick Melgar spent the entire day there "observing novelties in the patients and prescribing medicines" and ignoring his other responsibilities.[48]

The Wednesday after the infirmary opened, a weaver named Francisco Ruiz was warned and turned away after he approached to see his children inside. The following day, residents stopped cooperating with the indigenous authorities who arrived at homes to collect the sick.[49] On Saturday when a boy in the infirmary died, a procession of women, incited by news that he would be buried in the despised *camposanto*, made for the church carrying rocks in their *huipiles*, saying that they would get a church burial from the priest, or riot.[50] After a brief standoff at the church grounds over the matter of a proper burial, according to eyewitnesses, Ruiz announced that he was going to join his son in the infirmary and issued a call to arms with his wife, Magdalena, and Santiago Vásquez, a son of the Indian governor, "saying that once they were together and the fire had been lit, they should not stop until everything was burned."[51] At the entrance to the infirmary a young mother allegedly shoved the town's Spanish schoolmaster, José Aragón, who was working inside as nurse, and entered, followed by a *regidor* (elected official) of the village.[52] Aragón recalled having to throw himself against the door "to prevent the *indias* from entering to remove the sick; but these women, who came loaded with rocks, shoved and slapped the witness, threatening that if he spoke they would kill him."[53] With Aragón dishonored and disarmed, the children were carried out in various states of undress.[54]

In the aftermath two battalion companies arrived from Antequera to seal off the district seat and contain its residents. Seven men and eight women identified by Melgar as ringleaders were jailed, and the twenty-two sick children returned to the infirmary. Melgar posted a rump force to guard entrances and exits and carry out periodic fumigations, but the soldiers began pilfering and deserting in short order and allegedly charged passengers for permission to move through the cordons they were supposed to patrol.[55] Barely two weeks later, three recovering smallpox patients were found hidden in their homes during inspections. On November 9 roughly one hundred women allegedly mounted a second assault on the infirmary and were restrained by the guards. Melgar complained that eloquent words could not turn Indians away from "ancient customs" and "harmful practices [*usos*]" in favor of a rational method of prevention and cure.[56]

A tangle of contradictions and obfuscations, the witness testimony that forms this account generally confirms the impression that this was a pueblo divided over how to proceed in the face of superior orders. Clandestine political agitating in Teotitlán in the days preceding the riot was coordinated extraofficially by one Jacinta Zarate, a sixty-five-year-old widow, who brought together committees of women and men to mount a legal challenge to the measures. According to Melgar, Zarate had been in the lead as the *capataza* (forewoman) of influential convocations of women in two previous moments of reform. In one an ecclesiastical official had tried to restrain musicians in the church and been mocked; the other was the controversial secularization of the *doctrina*. Wary of a recurrence, Melgar had warned male villagers that they alone would be held responsible for any "excesses" committed by the women in this more serious matter of disease control.[57]

In church on the Rosary Sunday preceding the uprising, Zarate allegedly reprimanded a twenty-five-year-old *mantero* (producer of cotton mantles) who was employed washing laundry at the infirmary for not joining the women to obstruct its construction or contest the consecration of the cemetery, "saying that he was not a man."[58] In the village's chapel, Zarate likewise shamed two widows, according to their testimony, telling one that she was "a bad mother to her children" for allowing one to be removed to the infirmary. The women subsequently helped organize meetings in Zarate's home that fateful week, which reportedly drew some forty women and thirty men on Monday. Attendees were scolded, reminded that "the sick in the infirmary were not given anything other than broths and *atoles*," and the men in attendance called shameless ("eran unos sinvergüenzas") for helping to build the infirmary. If they did it for the pulque that Melgar had distributed at the work site, Zarate taunted, she would have gladly provided it.[59] In these meetings villagers contributed the 40 or 50 pesos necessary to retain the services of a Spanish lawyer in Antequera.

Because these assemblies could not draw sums of money from

communal coffers, which required the authorization of *cabildo* members, they relied instead on a variety of *derrama*, a head tax imposed for extraordinary purposes, including legal action. Contributors were likely emboldened by the reassurances of the lawyer, who allegedly informed them that the measures stemmed from the intendant (who feared that smallpox would infect his children) and would be easily overturned. He requested a *parecer*, a formal statement authorizing a legal complaint, in the name of all the officials and elders of the town, which was apparently drafted surreptitiously by an outsider.[60] As though the feeling expressed by parents for their children was incidental, Melgar placed blame for discontent on the lawyer, whom the Indians looked on as a "celestial oracle," and swore that villagers had been obedient prior to his involvement.[61]

But they had not been. Politicking took place in chapels, streets, and private homes, and in the face of determined silence on the part of the ruling *cabildo*. The Indian governor and his alcalde dutifully reported the storming of the hospital on the day of the *tumulto*. A statement claiming to represent the views of elected officials and elders emphatically denounced Zarate's faction, blaming the unfortunate turn of events on ill-advised political and legal organizing by "mujeres plebes." They insisted that only a handful of men had attended meetings in the preceding days, to witness the *parecer* made for the lawyer; reminded Melgar that they had not caused any commotion in his twelve years as administrator; and reiterated their ongoing support of orders. Whether this meant that some were unsympathetic, opposed to the women's encroachment on their authority, or merely flattering Melgar in a strategy of deniability, in declaiming the central issues that so concerned activists, the statement ends with another plea for "the opening up of the road so we can go see *nuestras milpa* [*sic*]" (their crops).[62]

The split in formal masculine authority and its alignment in different configurations with informal female leadership was nowhere more evident than in the family of the Indian governor himself. On the day of the riot, Lorenzo Vásquez, the governor's son, was working in the infirmary kitchen. As the throng approached, he emerged to upbraid his brother Santiago for arriving as its leader. In return, Santiago menacingly hefted rocks and berated his brother for serving under the Spanish administrator.[63] Male relatives and in-laws, some with children in the infirmary, joined the movement, and at least one official, *regidor* José Lorenzo, was among the first to enter to remove his children, even at the greater risk of his position.[64] The fissures typical of village life were apparently exacerbated by measures that reached deep into Indian households. Political activity during the emergency took place beyond the male-dominated republic but not independently of men. Legitimacy within the legal system implicated male power holders, and villagers assigned to those with more formal status, through the petition's legal fiction of a unified front, the roles they were officially compelled to abjure.[65]

Although Teotitlán's experience was exceptionally documented, villagers there were not alone in voicing concerns about the program or in seeking to convince others of its potential harms. As he attempted to straighten out the logistics of cordon lines, Conejares, the official in charge of the sierras of Villa Alta, expressed alarm when he learned about Gil's treatise. If there were obstacles to "making uniform [*uniformar*] its resolutions among cultured folk," his district—impoverished, remote, with poor roads, and of "the most rustic Indians"—presented infinitely more. Chickens were skinny, even maize, the region's principal staple ("fructo del País"), was costly, and barbers, *curanderos*, and medications were scarce. With respect to the proposed pesthouse, the official anticipated the same problems that Melgar had encountered: "Who will take care of them? Who will recognize the [critical] moments pointed out by the author [Gil]?" Even when translated by interpreters, villagers could not be made to understand the most straightforward orders, and it was impossible, without troops, to convince them to do what they chose not to. He concluded by suggesting that new instructions be issued that were more sensitive to conditions in Villa Alta, as Gil "speaks only of cultured and civilized regions."[66] In May 1797, with his district still mostly free of smallpox, Conejares nevertheless issued a circular to priests asking them to enjoin their parishioners to follow precautions in healing, burial, and contagion avoidance.[67]

The eyes and ears of the colonial system, priests played indispensable roles as intermediaries. They confessed, buried, healed, and explained the official program to their flock, while transmitting local sentiments to secular authorities, and were among the first to insist that their parishioners would respond poorly to outside intervention. Indians were prone to states of lethargy and negligence, some priests responded, but also unlikely to carry out onerous responsibilities because these were burdensome for farmers in the middle of harvest season.[68] Tabaa's priest reported that the *república*, apparently eager for relief, demanded additional medicines from Antequera in addition to those being provided by a Spanish healer.[69] Zoochila's priest provided an exhaustive litany of reasons why the measures were simply impracticable. His parishioners were stubborn and viewed the extraction of children from homes "with an inexpressible horror," despite his attempts to persuade them that it was in their interest. Two sick boys in Santiago Laxopa had been hidden by their parents and might have perished without the sacraments if not for the fact that the priest's assistant (*vicario*) paid them a visit after the elder boy failed to attend church functions. The priest thought the result would be the same wherever orders were implemented. He deemed his Indian parishioners, "even the most ladinos," incapable of taking charge of public health, as their commitment to savage remedies (*remedios bárbaros*) rarely allowed the adoption of others, and the sick were poorly cared for. Bringing in *gente de razón* (non-Indians) would prove difficult: they too were viewed with horror, "as all of us who live among them know." The priest proposed that because the homes in his *doctrina* were already dispersed, the sick might safely be left inside with simple prohibitions on entry: "after all, the parents look upon their children and care for them better than any other, whoever he may be."[70]

Now, as villagers in the region set about building and staffing these pesthouses, they expressed the same sentiment about care and family. In San Juan Guichicobi, Fray Joseph Mariano, anticipating opposition by mothers especially, recruited two widows to serve in the infirmary as nurses. The women wondered how the mothers of infants who needed to feed would be summoned. They illustrated their own incapacity by raising their *huipiles* to bare their breasts, and scoffed when the friar replied that he knew how to make a milk substitute from wine and corn gruel (as detailed in the Introduction).[71] If not as colorfully as the widows, others expressed similar commonsense skepticism about the separation of small children. Leaders of Santa María Puxmetecan, east of Villa Alta, questioned the wisdom of taking nursing infants (*a los pechos*) from their mothers. Santiago Atitlán's elders, when called by their pastor, admitted to him that they were not reporting illnesses because sick infants, in their opinion, were too small to be removed (*como eran chiquitos*).[72]

In Tabaa pueblo, where a home at the edge of the village had been converted into a pesthouse, parishioners gathered before their priest to alert him to the abysmal conditions inside. They were willing to proceed with orders, but chaos reigned by the time fifteen children had entered. One could barely move "because in addition to the fifteen there are at least as many more mothers of these patients." Family members had to provide food, since, as the priest admitted, "it is not even possible to find two men or women who could attend to [the children] with the same charity and love" as their parents. Residents pointed out that the nursing infants could not safely be separated from their mothers and raised the possibility that the older children, feeling abandoned by their parents "and ruled by complete strangers, will be stricken by a panicked terror, which without doubt would be enough to cause death." Village leaders journeyed to the district seat about this time to register their complaint before the subdelegate, telling him that in addition to the fifteen children, there were many ill in the pueblo, where they should remain.[73] Parents in San Pedro Yaneri also cited risk of exposure after it was discovered that eight sick children had been hidden away "in the most interior parts of their homes," for fear that they might be removed to the remote *monte* where the priest was preparing an infirmary. Village justices claimed ignorance of subversive acts, but they too petitioned in the district seat to exempt the children (*muchachos*) from the order. Otherwise, "they will die of *fríos* [colds], because here different temperaments reign," and some lacked clothing to cover themselves adequately. Adding to their petition, the village representatives requested that the official not block the road to Ixtlán because it was the route of their *comercio* and by which they remitted tribute ("el real tributos" [*sic*]).[74]

In these communities complaints were raised in ways that resembled what one would expect in male-led Indian republics, where patriarchs frequently traveled to the district seat to formally petition an official. In this case they found a sympathetic audience in Conejares, who had likewise concluded that the measures were unworkable. Only when joined with administrative reports (or criminal files) are the roles of women glimpsed, however partially, alongside them. Usually out loud, women articulated ideas about health, disease, and risk; the superiority of parental care of children, especially small children; the dangers of exposure to the elements; and the power of certain emotional states, especially fear and panic, in compromising health. Their role in Tlacolula, the weaving *cabecera* neighboring Teotitlán, is left to the imagination when village elders and leaders drafted a petition to the viceroy (perhaps because their administrator was unavailable or uninterested). Tlacolula's leaders requested that their children be allowed to remain in their homes for care and reasoned that this would be better than moving the sick into the open country without shelter and under burning sun, dew, or rain. The majority of the men were unable to sign, stressing that because they were the most unfortunate Indians ("Yndios pobres miserables"), they had not sent a procurator to Mexico City to execute their appeal. But they were not ignorant. They well knew that children were at a higher risk of contracting illness, viewing it as virtually inevitable. And without immunization, they were probably correct.[75]

Villagers did not undermine or sabotage, wholesale and forever, public health measures, as some priests, medical experts, and officials predicted they would. Instead, they responded in ways unpredictable even within a community and subject to political maneuvering of the sort witnessed in Teotitlán. When faced with anticontagion measures, residents of the *cabecera* of Santo Domingo Latani converged on the *sujeto* pueblo of Choapam, perhaps encouraged by a pastor who opposed the measures as harmful to his Indian flock. Congregating in the plaza, they publicly mocked residents of the subject village for allowing an infirmary to be built, called them fools (*tontos*), and encouraged them to not to send their children to it. Antonio de Zúñiga, who was there to implement the cordon, singled out a certain Juan Sanchez, who arrived personally at

Zúñiga's home. "I have a son," Sanchez reportedly declared, "and I warn you that if he contracts smallpox, you will not remove him from my arms until he is dead." Zúñiga responded cautiously, suspecting that Sanchez had been sent to test the waters and wary that the agitators from Latani "would ride roughshod over my person, as they have already done with my commission, and its honor."[76]

Political rituals in the sierras and valleys of Oaxaca resembled the "stylized performances" observed in eighteenth-century food riots in England, in which crowd activities were calculated to embarrass and intimidate social betters.[77] In Zúñiga's account, the challenge not only diminished official authority (and demonstrated that there would be no consequence for unruly behavior), but sought to encourage neighbors to embrace a more active and oppositional attitude as a matter of their honor. It recalls descriptions of women in Teotitlán humiliating villagers for cooperating with provisions that violated the community ethos, referring to what women ought to do with respect to their children, how men ought to behave in defiance of unjust orders, and how the sick ought to be treated. Shame, a function of disunity, implied ideal roles that both men and women ought to play in protecting the integrity of the household and the community, drawing on feelings of guilt, disrespect, and dishonor to compel more unified action. It is a reminder that not all peasants had decided uniformly, as a condition of their nature, against the interventions of the colonial state, that not all felt disrespected, or at least not strongly enough to join in protest, and of a moral universe that was only ever imperfectly shared. Instead, by calculated political action, residents strove toward some minimal consensus and conformity.

By tracing the regional purchase of morally charged ideas about disease, kinship, and justice, a common cultural ground in the region comes into view. Oaxaca was a fragmented terrain, geographically, linguistically, and socially, but through it people traveled to market or to consult an attorney, to spread gossip or follow news of the world beyond the village bells. In Tehuacán mothers condemned Teotitlán's infirmary when reports of casualties arrived along with infection, and made plain, according to the district governor, that their *entrañas* (entrails) would be torn out of their bodies before they allowed their children to be torn from their arms. The administrator concluded that he needed troops to separate the village's children from their mothers.[78] The same bodily imagery surfaced six months after Teotitlán's *tumulto*, when the seven men imprisoned in Antequera sent a small masterpiece of image management to the viceroy—a document that seems to move between raw testimony and the massaged appeals of legal counsel.[79] Like the appeal submitted by the female prisoners, that of the men deftly employed the defense of the innocent Indian to claim that an outsider had incited riot. But it went further to frame unjust measures and excuse the women, who as mothers had ceded to momentary impulse in storming the infirmary. After recording the injustices that had befallen villagers, and denouncing the public lashings of at least two at Teotitlán's pillory, it implored the viceroy to appreciate the pain and health risks that isolation had inflicted on families. Like Herod's massacre of the innocents ("ya se parecía la degollación de Erodes"), administrators, it charged, were modern-day incarnations of the malicious king, seizing innocent children and delivering them to their demise. Yet these children were pieces of their mothers' *entrañas* and of their *corazones* (hearts), the language metonymically linking them as sacrosanct organs to the women, who had done no more than reconnect with their offspring, who were in the care of "sinister hands." The consequence of this disruption of the familial order was sorrow, even death: the imprisonment of Teresa Hernández "caused the loss of her son, who had survived the epidemic and been put in the convalescence hospital, and who then died from weeping because he had been deprived of his grief-stricken mother."[80]

In Oaxaca, life and death conditioned both reproductive practices and the language of reproduction. By disproportionately affecting children, smallpox infection (and measures to contain it) only exacerbated the perception of vulnerability, at a time when high child mortality rates meant that many young were lost to gastrointestinal infections and respiratory ailments.[81] The legal defense retreated to a naturalized idiom of maternal desire: mothers, ignorant of superior orders (it was claimed), approached their children reflexively, to restore an ideal, healthy relationship, its violation the basis for their apparently irrational, emotional, and passionate behaviors. Hearts and *entrañas* (the latter used interchangeably with *vientre* to denote the sacred womb of Mary and by extension her son, Jesus Christ) formed a resonant conjunction of meanings in colonial Mexico, one that served this defensive gambit well.[82] The formulation of justice and intimacy through biological idioms and biblical tropes underscored, in effect, the unnatural rupture of the bond between mother and child and couched it in terms that conjured sites of legitimate emotion and instinct but not, crucially, deliberate or premeditated calculation.

The sentiments so carefully shaped were voiced in prosaic, less polished ways by many more who, though hemmed in by emergency measures, were not cowed by the experience. Voicing discontent, they met their overseers in face-to-face interactions in communal spaces including streets, shrines, plazas, and churchyards, to contest the Bourbon scheme, in which functionaries were asked to apply a reductionist version of disease as contagion and sanitation—a view in which infected children and their parents were held apart in separate and opposed categories of unclean and clean. Yet the crowded living conditions of the lower classes might be interpreted according to a different logic by which intimacy and emotional connection were the foundations of good health.[83] By insisting that health demanded the familiarity of a loved one, and would be compromised without it, Mexico's peasants perceived disease within a broader early modern framework, in which the emotions were foremost in maintaining a state of health. (Modern medical science's findings that fear and anxiety, especially, play an outsized role in the onset and prolongation of illness seem to confirm this view.)[84] Pursuing these connections, we find that villagers shared not only forms of governance, devotional practices, and modes of dress and production, but also a cultural logic of disease, healing, and death.[85]

Laypeople moved to preserve the continuum not only among communities of the living and the diseased, but also the deceased. The church grounds remained a traditional site of congregation, ceremony, and sociability where officers and communal representatives were elected, and a proper final resting place. When Atitlán's pastor attempted to bury a smallpox victim recently returned from Antequera in the newly consecrated cemetery, "many Indians came together telling me that the church was theirs, and asking why they had to bury him outside." The community threatened to take up their grievances with the district official, and "with a rebellion on my hands," the priest relented.[86] Yahuive's pastor instructed the Indian justices of the three pueblos in his *doctrina* to bring their deceased to consecrated grounds outside—"even if it is no more than an enclosure of sticks, with a cross in the middle." Village representatives balked, wondering whether such a policy "was being observed in the city and other populations."[87] The seven imprisoned Teotitlanecos described the *camposanto* as even more isolated than the infirmary, "in the mountains" and hedged with thorny shrubs.[88] On the day of Teotitlán's uprising, when crowds of women assembled outside the priest's personal quarters to harangue him and bargain for church burial, they reportedly rejected the district governor's offer of burial in a chapel at the outskirts, saying that "the Indians had built the church and they were not animals, to be buried in the countryside [*campo*]." Retrieving the boy's body from the makeshift morgue, they buried him at the door of the church, where they performed a ritual of mourning and celebration (and ignored the official's advice to sprinkle a layer of lime "to consume the body").[89]

Amplified and exaggerated by administrative reports, protest made explicit certain norms of decency and commonsense rules that had been overlooked in the rush to craft an enlightened policy of disease management.[90] The resulting verdict, appearing more unanimous than it actually was, condemned a policy that not only failed to protect health but actually exposed populations to illness. The effect reminded the government that sacred norms were not to be dishonored without the agreement or consultation of communities.

FROM PESTHOUSES TO HUMAN POX

Months of accumulated complaints by village elders, parents, artisans, merchants, priests, and bureaucrats—all of whom claimed special exemptions for themselves, their charges, their communities, or their trade—all but assured the demise of the anticontagion regime. Ironically, the intendant's mismanagement of the deteriorating situation in the provincial capital of Oaxaca made matters worse. The arrival of smallpox in the surrounding valleys led Mora y Peysal, in consultation with physicians, to split Antequera into eight *cuarteles* for inspection and isolation and more efficient surveillance. Residents were ordered to report any infected individual on threat of punishment (fines of 50 pesos, or two months in jail), while those who denounced them were promised anonymity and a share of the fine.[91] The climate of suspicion and fear was heightened when the intendant, the day after Christmas, dispatched an infected fourteen-year-old Indian girl from one of the city's barrios to the infirmary at Teotitlán.[92] Two more victims followed soon after, which instigated an outcry and rush by residents to hide their sick children or abscond with them to nearby haciendas, ranches, and pueblos.

A cache of reports from the cathedral clergy and commissioned residents conjures an apocalyptic scenario, in which parents undermined authority, healed in secret, and neglected Christian obligations. In the repeated refrain, it was "voz común" (common knowledge) that parents were concealing their sick children in pits in the ground, foregoing sacraments, and abandoning the deceased in public. The reports require cautious reading; because Mora y Peysal had failed to include ecclesiastical authorities in planning, the crisis gave the church hierarchy ample reason to exaggerate the social discord. Nevertheless, some accounts include the kind of detail that suggests firsthand knowledge of events. Senior councilman Diego de Villasante, one of the city's elite mine owners and most prosperous citizens, reported in his capacity as head of one of the wards that of seventy smallpox patients registered there, roughly half had been found hidden under beds, lifted onto roofs, or placed in corners, some wrapped in straw mats behind doors. Those mothers who fled to the countryside, he imagined, preferred death for their children there than in one of the hospitals. Parents were forgetting their Christian duty, abandoning the deceased in the city's churches to avoid punishment, and allowing their children to die without sacraments or spiritual nourishment.[93] The pastor of Xochimilco, one of the city's most populous barrios, described how during inspections parents placed their children rolled into a *petate* in a corner, on the roof, or in crates. Parishioners reportedly informed him that if children were transported to Teotitlán, they would catch a chill, or "if they went well covered, an untreatable cancer from the burning heat" of the sun.[94] One resident, who was commissioned to oversee a sector in which the impoverished homes were still in shambles from an earthquake, estimated that the twenty-six smallpox cases and two fatalities he had found represented a fifth of the real number. It was not easy, he regretted, to avoid the ploys (*astucias*) of paternal love.[95]

Administrators, priests, and parents engaged in months of negotiation over emergency measures as a newly vigilant state sought to locate and isolate diseased children.[96] There were numerous modifications to this system of surveillance as people talked back, left the places assigned them, or rejected quarantine measures. One response was a shift in sacramental practice, with parents foregoing last rites of confession and extreme unction.[97] One lieutenant priest (*teniente de cura*) was approached by parents upon his return from administering sacraments in a nearby pueblo, who begged him to grant church burial to a boy who had perished on the road. The group had apparently left the city with the boy hidden in a cart to return him to his village and, passing the priest along the way, feared to stop him for last rites before he expired.[98] Another priest described the sacristan opening the doors of the church to find an infant (*angelito*) who had been abandoned after succumbing to smallpox, presumably without any spiritual nourishment at all. (The fact that the intendant's inspectors had pursued the infant inside was offered as an aggressive violation of ecclesiastical privilege.)[99]

While the abandonment of the deceased was not uncommon in times of plague, parents improvised other solutions to keep their families intact. During inspections of an outlying settlement of laborers, the prior of the Dominican order discovered a girl of fourteen or fifteen with her face covered in pustules. "Asked if she wanted to be confessed, with a very tender voice and great fervor she told me that was what she wished." Reprimanded, her parents explained their concern: "Father, they say you priests also have been obligated under penalty to report immediately if called to confess a smallpox victim." The family had concealed the girl's sickness not only from the church but from the apothecary, knowing of the rule ordering the denunciation of any residents found to be ill. The mother recounted how, with her daughter incapacitated, "unable to swallow or keep anything down, I put a handkerchief over my face and went to the pharmacy, saying that I had a sore throat. And the remedy they gave me I administered to my daughter." The friar was prevailed upon to send a priest at evening prayer, cloaked in darkness, to whom the girl confessed.

Afterward, the confessing priest was dissuaded from using his small lamp as he departed by the parents. With assistance from these clergymen the family kept their secret hidden and returned to the sacramental routines of the church.[100]

The reports argued that Antequera's harsh decree actually contributed to instances of concealment, as an extraordinary number of residents went underground.[101] Accentuated and multiplied, intimate gestures of care and subterfuge were transformed into a state of mass subversion. The case was sealed with a pair of crudely handwritten pasquinades that "have presently flooded the city," according to Oaxaca's bishop, who remitted a copy to Mexico City along with the cathedral clergy's reports.[102] Remarkably global in perspective, the alarming texts charged the government with violating the law of God by comparing circumstances in Oaxaca's valleys, including the ejection of the sick from the capital, with events in France. The first page, in rhymed verse, identified the intendant as the main perpetrator: "imitating Herod," he had dispatched the infected young woman to Teotitlán's infirmary—on foot, pregnant, and alone—where she had perished "without sanctuary." In this corrupted world, God no longer mattered, only heretics; nor did the king, who did not reign over "disorderly matters." Residents were incited to imitate New France in rebellion against ungodly rule, with volleys of gunfire "on the cited day." The second page, a general call to arms, summoned the masses ("toda la pelbe" [*sic*]) in the event that another child was removed from its home. All priests who wished to escape alive were warned not to resist the "invasion," while the most famous of Bourbon reformers were invoked as enemies in a concluding cry: "All with one voice, death to the relative of Gálvez, long live the law of God."

Wielded with aplomb in the legal defense of Teotitlán's prisoners, the allusion to Herod's biblical slaughter confirms the region's ties to the Atlantic world, where it was a common political trope.[103] The rhymed verses also reiterated and elaborated regional concerns about the government's policies: the expelled Indian girl represented the special vulnerability of the young and the innocence of the child/victim.[104] Though she was not, according to the record, expecting a child, her pregnant figure doubled the sense of children being violated and sacrificed at the hands of a malicious "king." Finally, in describing as heretics the famous Gálvez clan, popular imagination identified the hand behind the measures, or more poetically rendered recent public health experiences an extension of the same reformist impulse experienced in Oaxaca for nearly a decade.[105]

Bishop Gregorio José de Omaña, a strenuous critic of the secular government's handling of the epidemic, added additional details to the evidence being amassed. He claimed that no one appeared to request burial in his or any other parish and that the use of a distant infirmary had dampened monetary contributions to the relief efforts. The bishop criticized the intendant directly for not considering the distance forced upon the sick in several hours of travel, when it would have been more logical to follow cultured nations ("naciones cultas") by providing for a hospital at a reasonable distance.[106] Reviewing these materials, the *promotor fiscal* (chief legal adviser) of Oaxaca's cathedral noted that, although an "infirmary" had finally been established in Jalatlaco barrio, it consisted of a storage shed from which stores of lime had been removed to make space for the patients. There was only one, and the boy was exposed to the elements through holes in the walls.[107] To mounting evidence of a "sudden" rebellious spirit among inhabitants, the legal adviser contributed an incident in which a riotous crowd outside the church of Our Lady of the Snows had forced councilman don José Antonio de Larrainzar to abandon his task when he arrived to register the sick. The recommendation was that the sick be cared for in their homes, "as has always been observed in similar circumstances."

Another option presented itself as authorities reached a consensus about the unworkability of Gil's instructions. Inoculation had been attempted sporadically in preceding years and outbreaks, as when a "peste de viruelas" struck Campeche in 1793 (blamed on the trade in slaves between that port and Havana) and moved Yucatán's intendant to inoculate an unknown number to protect the population from the threat.[108] Several requests to inoculate arrived from many more low-level officials and civilians beginning in 1795, when the spread of infections into New Spain's interiors made human smallpox fluid more widely available. The administrator of *alcabalas* (sales tax) in Nejapa, who oversaw disease measures in Mixes Bajos, dutifully threw up a cordon around Guavicuzas (or Quiavicuzas) pueblo and began hospitalizing the sick. The administrator requested permission from the district governor to inoculate in the event that smallpox could not be contained, having practiced it sixteen years earlier in the previous epidemic.[109] In Villa de Tehuantepec, Captain Luis Joseph de Ribas began inoculating children at the end of 1795; by February 1796, Fessar reported 500 inoculations and 30 fatalities, a significant improvement over the 536 deceased out of 2,574 cases of smallpox in the same register.[110]

Reviewing these cases in Mexico City on April 17, 1796, Borbón advised giving permission to extend inoculations in Tehuantepec to the Villa of Jalapa, Guavicuzas pueblo, and elsewhere by means of persuasion ("por via de exortación, y persuación"). He reiterated that inoculation should not be mandated but adopted voluntarily, and never against the *voluntad* of parents.[111] Oaxaca's intendant communicated these instructions to commissioned individuals and subordinates in the region: inoculation was useful and beneficial when precautions were taken to prevent infection of others, to be introduced by persuasion, and only after all possible measures had been taken to halt transmission.[112]

By then inoculations were ongoing in several parts of Tehuantepec, with varying outcomes. In Zapotec-speaking La Magdalena, the healer in charge of smallpox documented eighteen inoculated children, with no indication of difficulty.[113] A more extensive campaign in Tequisistlan yielded on average forty-two inoculations a day over two weeks in June, overseen by the district governor and a *curandera* named Faustina Baleria, who excelled "despite being a woman over the age of forty."[114] A campaign in San Juan Guichicobi began with a demonstration by Rafael Melo, schoolteacher and tax official, on his children and the previous Indian governor, followed by "others among the more reasonable [*racionales*]" who had been persuaded by religious officials. According to a report submitted by Indian officials, the more "rustic" commoners threatened Melo, forcing him to take shelter in the priest's house, or closed their doors when they saw him coming and shouted for him to leave. Others left in droves with their children for neighboring Sarabia.[115] When another healer with more experience arrived without medications, villagers rejected him. The priest deemed it hopeless: parishioners were uncouth (*cerril*), "some saying that God sends sickness to the people, and not the Spaniard, by taking it from others and infecting the children."[116]

In Teotitlán del Valle, following multiple assaults on the infirmary, the anticontagion regime gave way to inoculation at the urging of the physician summoned there. The protocol involved separating patients in convalescent wards, but Melgar offered villagers burial in the church cemetery as incentive to cooperate.[117] As described by Oaxaca's intendant, twenty-six small children were brought to the new infirmary, where they were purged overnight. The next day, when the inoculator performed a public demonstration on a teenager who was laboring on the huts nearby, the children "ran terrified upon seeing the practitioner with the lancet in his hand." Their mothers returned them, "having been disabused of the idea that to inoculate their children meant mortally wounding them," but the subdelegate insisted on distributing coins and cookies to persuade the children to allow their hands to be washed again; twenty-two were inoculated "without need of a modicum of violence."[118]

By the time infection reached Spanish administrative centers, inoculation was not only technically possible, due to a supply of human pox, but also conceivable as policy, as a result of trials in the infected countryside. Medical and royal authorities were performing back-of-the-envelope calculations of inoculation's risk as the crisis unfolded. In February, with tensions in Antequera mounting, commissioned justices and the city's physicians convened to discuss official measures. They noted, in addition to concealments and the popular belief that sending children to infirmaries meant death, the fact that inoculation had been tested in Tehuantepec and Teotitlán.[119] The physicians, formerly committed advocates of anticontagion measures, now agreed that the situation was untenable: the more than one hundred sick residents in the capital could not be relocated without great harm to public health. They endorsed inoculation, citing a report of nine fatalities out of four hundred operations in Teotitlán as a massive improvement over a mortality rate of one-fourth of those infected naturally.[120] Also taking note of these statistics, the intendant's legal advisers supported a new decree that allowed the infected to be healed in their homes along with elective use of inoculation.[121] The following day, the intendant, his hand forced, reversed most of the measures in place for the last six months.[122] Two weeks later, an edict overturned the cordon between Oaxaca's capital and surrounding regions, allowing immune adults free passage (visitors to Antequera's *tianguis* [market] were still forbidden to overnight with sick residents). "This capital is the shared center of commerce and finance for the entire province," it announced, and "however much caution is exercised one will never achieve absolute severing of communication [with it]."[123]

When rebuked by his superiors for overturning the prohibitions without permission, Mora y Peysal called Gil's treatise an "impossible task" that caused incomparably greater harm than infection itself. The capital relied on surrounding pueblos for commodities and essential goods such as corn tortillas, "whose use is much more widespread in this city than in any other part of the kingdom."[124] If an admission of defeat, already the official could boast of successes: children of all social statuses (*condiciones*), accompanied by their parents and relatives, were flocking to the four physicians who performed inoculations in the capital. Nevertheless, skeptical residents were awaiting the outcomes of these cases, which compelled him to order a thorough investigation—of inoculators, their assistants, and the method of convalescence—to demonstrate that any deaths were caused by other factors.[125]

It was a precarious moment of technological change, and authorities in Mexico City moved to salvage some health policy from the haphazard arrangement that was coming into being. Viceregal officials following reports from Chiapas, Oaxaca, and Puebla realized that anticontagion measures were poorly implemented and broadly opposed.[126] Summarizing reports from Oaxaca written only days earlier (a remarkable feat given additional sanitary measures for mailbags), Borbón had been disturbed by the bishop's report concerning the distance traversed by the sick from Antequera to Teotitlán's infirmary, and in this he sided with residents who had expressed concern about the removal of their children and the dangers of exposure.[127] Borbón followed the advice of Mexico City's Protomedicato in recommending that the upper classes ("vecinos decentes") maintain their sick at home, with necessary precautions, and that only the pestilential poor and destitute, "who in any other sickness would go to the hospital," be removed.[128] He outlined a new plan for Mexico City and other settlements in the epidemic's path: fumigations of corrupted air by bonfires of wood, shrubs, grass, and other fragrant materials; a circular to bishops urging petitions to God and the saints for relief and priests to press their parishioners to accept burial in *camposantos* outside of populated communities; and settlements split into more manageable *cuarteles*, with *juntas de caridad* (charitable committees of secular and ecclesiastical authorities and honorable citizens) formed to help collect and distribute alms, food, and instructions to the sick poor when hospitalization became impossible.[129]

Less definitive than Oaxaca's suspension, the viceregal plan restored and reemphasized traditional approaches, including charitable care and prayer and petitions to saints, while endorsing the new medical technology—in effect integrating it into the fabric of colonial response. Inoculation trials in the south had paved the way: the official order cited inoculation's "advantages and the happy success constantly witnessed in Oaxaca, Tehuantepeque, and in other pueblos."[130] But administrators and healers still had only José Flores's instructions for guidance. An "Important Notice" appearing in the *Gazeta de México* on May 10, 1796, advised that to save "infinite individuals" the only remaining recourse in the event of an epidemic was rapid inoculation, dispensing with lengthy preparation of patients. The notice pointedly compared the low mortality rate following inoculations of 628 children in Tehuantepec with circumstances in Petapa, where the majority perished without it, but did not outline a method for success.[131] Borbón proposed that the Protomedicato compose a "simple and clear" instruction, to be sent to bishops and intendants, justices and alcaldes, urging voluntary adoption of the practice. The Protomedicato responded positively: there would be reluctance, but it might be overcome through early, well-publicized successes.[132]

THAT ALL MAY REASON

Smallpox cases swelled in Mexico City through the summer of 1797. Residents in the capital's barrios and suburbs took to self-medicating with herbs such as borage and other "domestic medications."[133] They studiously avoided priests and physicians, thereby undermining attempts to detect new cases.[134] Corpses reportedly moved with their faces covered and hands gloved concealed signs of pox and hindered burials of victims in the churches and cemeteries designated for each parish.[135] At the end of August, with a full outbreak imminent, frustrated officials launched the inoculation campaign stipulated in the February 28 order. A house in the city center along Santo Domingo bridge was converted for inoculations, and by mid-September several hundred wealthier residents had voluntarily submitted.[136] Reports of deaths and botched operations spurred an investigation that led authorities to Teresa Bastida, a doña from the upper echelons. Bastida recalled hearing "in one of many conversations about inoculation" that the children of certain residents had died. With children of her own to inoculate, and needing to know "with certainty," she had investigated and discovered that one of the boys had actually died of epileptic fits (*alferecía*), while the other was still alive.[137]

More troubling for the fate of the practice was a printed page of *boleros* on inoculation found for sale in the main plaza. The young bookkeeper of the cathedral's choir had purchased a copy for a *real*, a modest price, from a peddler in the Portal de las Flores. He turned the stanzas over to authorities, along with a description of the vendor, an *hombre de fresada* (a man dressed in a cape or cloth poncho, implying his humble origins).[138] "Inoculations are the invention of the most impoverished, needy physicians," it begins.

But it is known that those who are inoculated go with Death.
Those who are inoculated have no judgment, thinking they are made well, which is a ploy.
What is certain is that they are left scarred, and some dead.
I must give you sound advice: do not get inoculated, you are being led astray.
We see that the inoculated are pestilent.
Aching México groans, the impoverished physicians have infested it.
. . .
With this I take leave: Poor physicians, how badly your treatments go.
Soon you will know how the inoculated die.[139]

The crudely composed stanzas lampooned the technology, accused administrators of exaggerating the risk of smallpox, and denounced the greedy and incompetent physicians practicing with their dirty lancets (some were called out by name). Not for the first or last time, parents and others anxious about the matters of life and death were invited to hear and respond to criticisms of the government's relief efforts by way of oral culture.[140]

As opinion threatened to turn, authorities prepared to censor irreverent speech and pursue those who spread rumors. Cosme de Mier, the president of the Audiencia, was a sponsor of these early inoculation efforts, eager to extend their use and furious about the slander. Weighing in on the investigation, he noted that "it is not the pueblo that produces" calumnies against inoculation, "but rather a few secular and religious ecclesiastics," who held some moral aversion and disseminated opinions against it to dissuade those less *sensato*. With some three thousand inoculations performed already, the practice still had far to go among the masses, who would surely refuse it if these ecclesiastics stoked fear. He advised the viceroy to request that religious prelates caution their subordinates not to imbibe or encourage discourses or orders contrary to inoculation, "whose principles require other ideas, distinct from the ones their studies and experiences can provide them."[141]

Cosme de Mier's position coincided with that of royal attorney Lorenzo Hernández de Alva, who was a proponent and early adopter of the technique in his household. Alva had authored a legal opinion in support of a ban on critical speech, referred to by Cosme de Mier as an *apología*, that treated inoculation's history and merits and his own favorable experience. In Alva's opinion, indisputable proof of inoculation's simplicity and utility justified a decree summarily prohibiting any slanderous speech, to ensure "that no one dare criticize, mock, or dissuade the people from adopting inoculation, by word or writing." In this way "tall stories and lies" that began with the upper classes would not trickle down to the commoner (*vulgo*), who was "very easily prone to let himself be affected by the sounds of voices and incidents without first examining them." To permit the upper classes to debate matters of inoculation was one thing; it was quite another to spread rumors, mutter, declaim, and thereby dissuade the inexpert (*imperito*), the gullible, and those intellectually incapable of distinguishing opinions. Those who abused this liberty to discuss would be responsible to God, king, and public for lives lost.[142]

After months of protest over the quarantine of villages and the sick, the colonial state was at last poised to quarantine critical discussion of the new medical program, with public order and public health the ends that justified containment. Not only were the lower classes assumed to be especially vulnerable to bodily contagion, they were susceptible to false ideas and loose talk, lacking the necessary hygiene in the one case, and in the other, the intellectual fortitude to resist. It was the epitome of a colonial regime that categorized a class of *miserables*—the poor, women, children, and slaves, but especially Indians—as specially protected wards of the state. In law and in practice, Indian villagers were granted distinctive legal and fiduciary considerations and placed directly under the patronage of the viceroy, the king's representative, who was expected to defend the defenseless, open his doors to the poor for an audience, and even arrive unannounced in hospitals to distribute alms to the sick.[143] Portrayals of kings and viceroys as benevolent fathers, with vassals as their obedient, loving children, were prescriptive, ritualized, and idealized, and tributaries frequently beseeched them, in writing and occasionally in person.

Throughout the epidemic this figure was repeatedly summoned in defense of local concerns and interests. In Antequera, seditious papers denounced bad provincial government even while insisting that the king did not rule over "disorderly matters" and paid his royal person tribute with *vivas* and acclamations. When smallpox struck Ixhuacán de los Reyes, in Xalapa district (Veracruz), village leaders invoked the viceroy in requesting permission to use communal funds for an infirmary and sick care, "certain that His Excellency the Viceroy, in accordance with known demonstrations of his pious intentions in favor of the Indians, will declare it well done."[144] It was to this same figure that residents of Teotitlán del Valle looked expectantly when they broke the cordon encircling their village, believing, given the terms in which they were accustomed to being governed, that there would be justice and remediation on the other side once the viceroy knew their predicament.[145]

When things turned violent there instead, Fiscal Alva, who was assigned to review the case, upheld the Crown's end of the bargain by ruling that force must only be used as a last, distasteful measure.[146] Citing several Laws of the Indies, the royal attorney argued that rebellious words by unarmed Indians was not a criminal act, that resisters should be persuaded to obey and made to understand by religious authorities using gentle means, that viceroys, as the king's proxy, were expressly empowered to forgive acts of rebellion, even if such acts were against the royal figure, and that even in riots the dispatch of armed men to pacify Indian pueblos was prohibited. Declining to continue criminal proceedings, Alva arbitrated within a long line of strategic appeasement typical of the Spanish colonial system, "a calculated blend of punishment and mercy" that at once augmented royal sovereignty and recognized that peasant production was a linchpin of royal revenue and subsistence: as one contemporary put it, "the Indian's cloak covers us all."[147] A decree of censorship, now endorsed by the same functionary, was not incompatible with this impulse: it was for the protection of the masses, whose health stood to benefit from silent obedience, whether they knew it, liked it, or not.

The viceregal government was of two minds on the matter of critical speech and freedom of choice. Pedro Jacinto Valenzuela, another *fiscal*, adjudged harshly the official investigation into rumored deaths from inoculation, pointing out that the government never prohibited discussion of the outcomes of inoculated smallpox. To the contrary, its potential benefits had to be discussed and evaluated by parents who clearly had an interest in determining whether to submit their children to it. Such discussion was not only inevitable, he noted, but useful to the government as it sought to calculate mortality against smallpox rates and weigh its value. Valenzuela concluded that in light of parents' guaranteed freedom to choose, "it is natural that each person should reason [*raciocine*] about the grounds for inoculation's efficacy, or inefficacy," as the case might be. Ultimately, the viceroy declined to issue the ban on unflattering speech that Alva and others requested.[148]

Fundamentally different schools of thought informed these positions. One, evolved from medieval conceptions of royal sovereignty and the family, and tempered over centuries of colonial rule in New Spain, adopted a view of society in which the father figure, endowed with greater capacity for reason, benevolently governed the metaphorical children. So that the lower classes, under the tutelage of wise patrons, might be instructed in the ways of an enlightened polity, this view warranted censorship of speech and action. It accorded well, incidentally, with the stance of confirmed Enlightenment figures like Voltaire, who declined to include the mass of people among those who ruled: while opinion governed, the reins of government should be held by the select few, he thought, including *philosophes*.[149] Banned in Mexico by the Inquisition, Voltaire's writings were hardly needed for the ruling elite to arrive at a similar conclusion.

On the other hand was a more realistic approach to a technology that had not yet been fully vetted and verified, whose practice remained uncertain. Because all individuals were being asked to make a choice in a matter that affected their households and families, they would be allowed and invited to draw conclusions on the basis of observation and local application. This approach might even, by providing additional information and testimony, advance the cause of empirical truth and improve the government's function. This expectation of a more discerning, civilized public, articulated in the push for rural schools, reforms in parish life, and in the pages of literary journals, received the endorsement of the government, to the extent that censorship was not vigorously pursued. It left open the matter of how immunization would be propagated, practiced, and judged in the following decades of adoption.

CONCLUSION

Prior to the epidemic, signs of social unrest that challenged the prerogative of the Bourbon state to apply reforms were sometimes met with quick, deliberate, violent repression.[150] By contrast, deliberations at the center of viceregal power during a pivotal turning point in the history of medicine suggest significant fissures in the edifice of enlightened absolutism. The model described here—chaotic, fractured, contingent—might more faithfully approximate the nature of the Bourbon reform period beyond disease emergencies. Energies poured into medical improvements and population management culminated in a draconian anticontagion program that yielded, as it deteriorated, a technological shift with an ambivalent stance toward dissent. Repeated challenges to royal authority during the emergency—in seditious papers, stanzas mocking the medical establishment, and a rural rebellion—saw a relatively mild response that must be understood in the context of a volatile Atlantic. This included regicide and revolution, along with self-identified enlightened figures (natural scientists, military men, royal authorities, and regalist prelates) who sought to correct negative images of Spanish imperialism by means of progressive economic policies and philosophies.[151] A roundup and repression was impractical in this moment in any case, as subversive opinion implicated too many to be resolved through the arrest of a few ringleaders.

Explanations that focus on decision-making and intellectual trends at the upper levels ultimately obscure critical local contexts of provision, within which administrators had to acknowledge the concerns of laypeople as they apprehended the realities of disease. In the end negotiated reform was a reality born of on-the-ground necessity and went beyond the influence of landed classes and merchants in Oaxaca. Of many problems animating correspondents in the Republic of Letters, infectious disease was more immediately apparent to families and communities attuned to the repercussions of contagion theory's application. One need only recall the government's failings in respect to medical reform, the study of epidemics, and health care—which compelled journalists, priests, naturalists, and physicians, in conversation with local healers, to step in to observe the natural world, manage outbreaks, and contribute to the common good—to appreciate that study cannot be confined to governmental, scientific, and medical institutions. Knowledge about disease and health was an affair of villages, churchyards, and provisional infirmaries, no less than lecture halls, scientific societies, and periodicals.

Given this reality, bureaucrats and physicians were compelled to bow to what was possible within the geographic, economic, and social frameworks of everyday life. When priests, parishioners, artisans, and peasants insisted on adjustments to enlightened protocols, and even undermined secular and medical authority in public, they went largely unpunished not only because rulers lacked the will, resources, or stomach for it, but because there was some recognition of the legitimacy of the customs and claims of the populace. This is not to say that public opinion was sovereign: even if rulers recognized the force of opinion and drew on it for support, the *público* and its potential reasoning capacity was carefully distinguished from the rabble, the *plebe*, whose capacity was open to doubt. Still, for some, to silence their voices meant not only repressing an unruly mass but violating a rationally judging community. The outcome, in an age when inoculation remained untested in New Spain and practitioners inexpert, was a concession to the need to know more, to the liberty of the king's subjects to contest injustice, and an implicit affirmation of the value of local customs and experiences, alongside statistical analysis and instrumentation, in forging better public health policies

What ensued as a result of compromise was a more viable policy of disease control and an ex post facto confirmation of the bounds of protest and dissent that fathers and mothers, commercial and agricultural interests, municipal councils, priests, ecclesiastical *cabildos*, indigenous representatives, and other civil authorities and professionals carved out for themselves from the entrenched political cultures of the colonial state. Opinion was contested, and more than just the sum of elite creole and Spanish assessments. Commentary from diverse and disjointed publics was admitted by default and necessity. Heterogeneous voices shaped debate, emphasizing the cultural substratum of health, the nature of borders between people and communities, and the importance of kin networks in providing care.[152] The result was a policy pastiche, at once technologically forward-looking and nostalgic for the caste categories, charitable impulses, and devotional practices that contributed to resolving crises in the past.

These bonds and obligations had been overlooked in the anticontagion campaign, but at every turn officials remarked on the omission. When addressing the shortage of income in Teotitlán del Valle, Fiscal Valenzuela supported further acquisitions of villagers' textiles but stressed that the usual buyers should not take advantage by fleecing the community, which would ignore the obligations established by "religion, humanity, and the sacred ties of civil society."[153] The viceroy and his advisers were especially troubled by the lack of cooperation between Oaxaca's secular and religious authorities and reminded the intendant to proceed in concert, "so the public understand that the two powers are united, as is proper, in such an urgent matter."[154] New charitable programs to collect and distribute alms helped ensure that church and state would work in union once again.[155]

Resurrecting familiar rituals, Oaxaca's intendant reported that the cathedral chapter, in agreement with the bishop, had resolved to petition Nuestra Señora de la Soledad, the city's patron, in her limestone basilica, with members of the city council attending processions, as customary.[156] Later that year in Mexico City, as a thousand new parishioners were infected each week, the miraculously renovated statue of the Christ of Ixmiquilpan accompanied the devout once more through the streets.[157] If the immunization campaigns to follow made better use of the "sacred ties of civil society," it was in part owing to experience in this sobering epidemic.

PART II

Immunization

CHAPTER 4

The Gift of Immunity

Domesticating Techniques

> These public demonstrations have inspired even the most impassive individuals, such that when certain black *jovenes* on Raboso Hacienda noted that its owner, don Pedro Azcué, still did not want to proceed with their vaccination so as not to subvert good order and due process, they transferred the fluid from those who had been vaccinated themselves. They made the incisions using only the spines of the tree they call Huichache as an instrument, and achieved with these operations the same happy outcomes as if they had been carried out in the established order.
>
> —Officials of the Central Vaccination Committee, Izucar district (Puebla), 1806

On June 28, 1798, Joseph Esquivel Navarrete, bishop of Durango, took to the pulpit in the cathedral to deliver a paean to inoculation. Thousands had been immunized in the north of New Spain, thanks in part to the distribution of printed instructions and the efforts of public health committees in Durango, Guanajuato, and Monterrey.[1] The outcome in terms of mortality was even better than predicted, and measures taken that year more effective than the alms collected for relief in previous epidemics. But the bishop wondered why so many among the plebe, in addition to distinguished citizens and corporations, were soliciting inoculation for their children and families when in the past these same people had been reluctant to follow the customs of "honorable people." At the confluence of piety and divine mercy, the spirit of general, spontaneous adoption witnessed during the medical campaign could only be counted a miracle. Navarrete recommended the procedure for all newborns henceforth and enjoined the congregation to give thanks to God, to whom a great debt was owed for the divine gift they had received.[2]

The practice of inoculating against smallpox had been known for some time, but its inception and adoption in Mexico marked a radical and, from the bishop's perspective, miraculous moment that required explanation, instruction, and elaboration. The premise was that by infecting a healthy person with a mild case of human smallpox, he or she acquired immunity against a more deadly infection. An oft-told origin story about the arrival of inoculation in Europe holds that Lady Mary Wortley Montague, wife of England's ambassador to Turkey, inoculated her children after she observed local medical practitioners in Istanbul use a needle to make small incisions in the skin, into which human smallpox material was introduced.[3] From this experiment the practice of inoculation spread to London's prisons and to the American colonies in the second decade of the eighteenth century.

In fact, the procedure originated at multiple sites and varied by time and by place. In Boston, Cotton Mather first learned the practice from an African servant, Onesimus, before he read of it in the *Philosophical Transactions* of London's Royal Society, and applied what he learned in an epidemic of smallpox in 1721. "And we have an Army of *Africans* among ourselves," Mather marveled, "who have themselves been under it [inoculation], and given us all the Assurance, which a Rational Mind can desire, that it has long been used with the like Success in *Africa*."[4] In some places cotton impregnated with dried scabs was placed in the nose. Sometimes the procedure was preceded by a period of bleeding, purging, and restricted diet to bolster the patient's constitution, which took parents away from work and required costly medical expertise. Eventually streamlined techniques and improved outcomes encouraged practice by laypeople, including parents and amateur inoculators.[5] While knowledge about inoculation was made and remade globally—in Turkish and African medical practices, the letters of the well-connected wife of the British ambassador, and the pages of the *Philosophical Transactions*—it was validated and applied locally, through trial and error.[6]

Like any mass methodological and conceptual innovation, in other words, inoculation entailed a process of appropriating, elaborating, and contextualizing. Historians of science suggest that instrumental objects in particular require a period of "domestication," when their practice, applications, and place remain unstable. The barometer, for example, now used primarily to measure atmospheric pressure, was in early modern England an oracular tool and an ornamental display of status, brought indoors and incorporated into bourgeois households with other objects of conspicuous consumption. Instruments "tend to be used for purposes not intended by those who originally developed them" and "are made meaningful in specific contexts, by becoming embedded in the practices of their users."[7] The scholar of design Donald Norman has approached this process of social adaptation as a relationship between the qualities of a device or object and the physical, logical, and cultural capabilities of the human agents who use it. Design's "discovery" in something as simple as a chair is not inherent in the object, but the outcome of this bond between people and things, and influenced, sometimes considerably, by the designer's perception of what a community's conventions will permit it to do.[8] For these reasons the design and presentation of a technology is a subject no less rich in possibilities for study than the way an object is actually approached and used by people; often the two go hand in hand.

Though unlikely that inoculation's instruments were displayed as status-granting ornaments in colonial Mexico, one historian found evidence that children on the island of Puerto Rico engaged in play vaccinations at school following early campaigns, bringing to mind the way a stethoscope migrated to the nursery from the clinic.[9] It invites a more sustained examination of how, from the inception of preventive programs, their technologies were displayed in churches and in procession, fixed in ecclesiastical genres, and seized upon by many nonprofessionals who contributed to their design. Durango's bishop, among many who advocated a more permanent public health policy as the epidemic of 1798 abated, expanded the identity of inoculation as a liturgical act, bringing a terrestrial audience (including those who were not yet converts) in communion with a celestial benefactor. His sermon became performative in this way, bound to the marvelous transubstantiation of organic matter, as wine and bread ritually become the body of Christ.

A few years later a more ambitious public health endeavor, the Royal Philanthropic Vaccination Expedition, traversed the four continents of the Spanish Empire to introduce the less lethal cowpox virus to Spanish subjects. As scholars have noted, the undertaking enjoyed an organizational mettle that signaled a more assured and modern enterprise than any before, unsurpassed until the disease eradication campaigns of the twentieth century.[10] Yet its design was no straightforward matter. It involved lay communities in overwhelming numbers, and matters of persuasion and instruction, in addition to the collection and experimentation typical of previous Spanish American expeditions.[11] Beginning in 1804, cities and villages throughout New Spain erupted in lively celebrations marking the *entradas* of medical teams tasked with propagating vaccine (see map 3). Live music, illuminated buildings, fireworks, and bullfights attracted crowds to public spaces to hear decrees and sermons, witness acts of adoration, and sing *alabanzas* in praise of the virtues of Edward Jenner's vaccine. These campaigns, along with gifts of coins and cookies, became part of a decades-long struggle to graft vaccination into the routines of everyday life.

Historians have generally declined to track medical developments

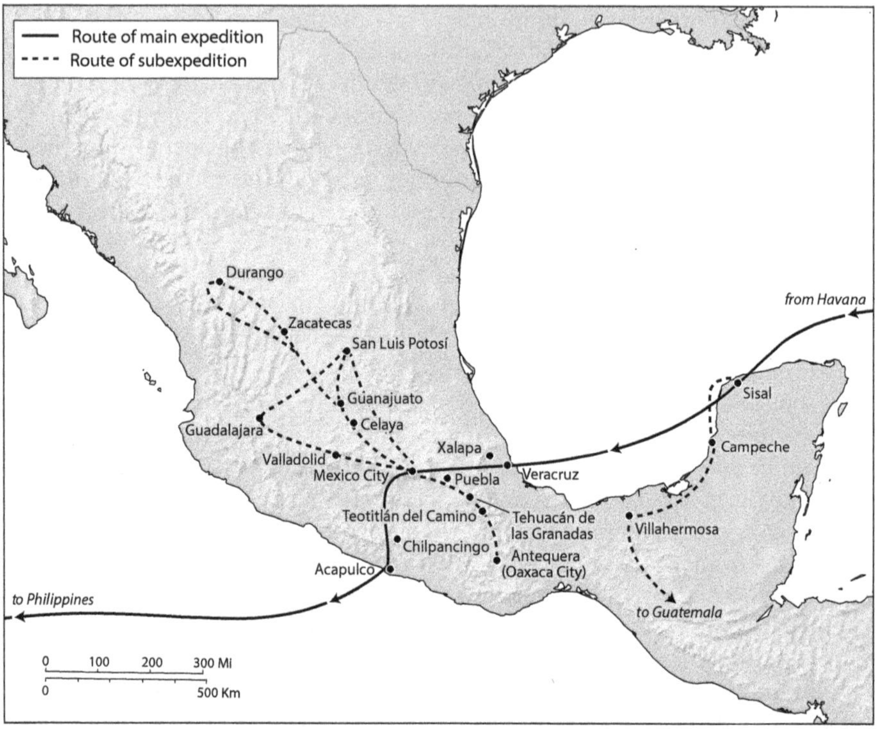

Map 3. Approximate path of Royal Philanthropic Vaccination Expedition through New Spain, 1804–1805.

through such multimedia pronunciations and performances. This approach is necessary if only because, in contrast with England, newspapers in Mexico were in a nascent stage, and the production of knowledge about immunization relied only partially on print. An uptick in periodicals dedicated to scientific matters (traced in Chapter 2)—the initiative of creole savants hoping to augment the public for specialized knowledge—must be put in perspective: they were plagued by high cost and, by implication, low readership, and while the official gazette occasionally conveyed medical developments and royal initiatives, sermons and public demonstrations more often provided the early modern analog to our "media." Knowledge about immunization produced in ceremonies of thanksgiving and supplication composed a vast public relations campaign, carefully stage-managed to shape vaccine's image among literate and illiterate groups.

No less part of this process was the written work of physicians, bureaucrats, physiocrats, bishops, priests, and aficionados in medicine who gave immunization its meanings in the early years of promotion and propagation. Many sought to cast in the most hopeful light a technique still uncertain, dangerous, and unknown, as the most informed experts argued about the bovine source of vaccine, the correct appearance of vaccine pustules, the type of instrument best suited to make injections, how to transport the pus material, where on the body to inject, and whether the vaccine had other therapeutic applications. Observing resemblances between the discharges produced by inoculation and familiar therapeutics like purging, bleeding, and leeching, many contemporaries decided that a shot in the arm similarly worked by evacuating some corrupted humor or poison from the body. While humoral expectations fail to account for the modern biomedical understanding of immunity, the old provided a credible framework for the new.

In New Spain news about vaccination was broadcast to the general populace shortly before the outbreak of insurgency, with all its disruptions—broken communication, military occupation, shortages of public funds—and years of social instability. Before then, promoters sought to demonstrate its relevance in a time when Enlightenment learning found its fulfillment in mines, agriculture, and hospitals, where the population might appreciate scientific innovations in terms of their practical utility in commerce, industry, and medicine.[12] Popular science in a Catholic empire came to look rather different than England's Newtonian revolution—a broad-based cultural movement of a different sort.[13] To see the ways in which domestication invited broader participation requires accounting for the media and rituals that produced the public spectacle surrounding vaccine. Through them, early campaigns had an effect not only in fighting disease but in demonstrating how changes in scientific practice might affect daily life.

THE ATLANTIC DEBATE OVER INOCULATION

Endorsement of inoculation as state policy came late in the Spanish world, with the propagation of a royal *cédula* on November 30, 1798—more than a year after it was granted in Mexico. In the meantime a great deal of informal practice, experimentation, and debate took place, much of it geared toward convincing government agencies to identify the technology as one worthy of adoption. Partisans who wished to calculate lives lost as a result of smallpox versus those saved with inoculation had at their disposal quantitative data from reports, tables, mathematical analyses, and historical treatments.[14]

Yet data could be interpreted in multiple ways. What was known as "political arithmetic" became a powerful political weapon in the hands of Enlightenment critics of government who, like French philosophes Montesquieu and Rousseau, argued that states were in decline by positing a decline in population.[15] Pedro Rodríguez, Count of Campomanes (1723–1802), the influential minister of state and president of the Council of Castile, was an avid practitioner of the new political arithmetic and a prolific writer and reader.[16] In 1774 he reviewed the evidence in favor of inoculation in his *Discurso sobre el fomento de la industria popular* (Essay on the development of popular industry), for which he had nearly half a century of publications and mortality records. For Campomanes these figures (mortality rates falling between one in ten and one in five for natural smallpox, in comparison with something closer to one in one hundred for inoculated smallpox) confirmed the universal threat, and that the Indies suffered its devastation unnecessarily given inoculation's use in Chile, Europe, and even parts of Spain. Campomanes proposed, in addition to industrial development, adopting inoculation as one of the most effective advances in preventive health. As he put it: "What excuse could we have not to give the population such important aid?"[17]

Things were more complicated than Campomanes allowed. As enlightened absolutists across Europe embraced inoculation for its financial and geopolitical benefits, the ongoing debate surrounding the practice pitted doubtful moralists, who might point to the not insignificant risk of death, against utilitarians, who insisted on the margin of success. The most vocal anti-inoculators, including Vicente Ferrer Gorraiz y Beaumont (1718–1792), historian at Madrid's Royal Cabinet of Natural History, have been characterized as reactionary traditionalists, whose writings aligned in the pivotal 1780s with the "general posture of the clergy" in the midst of a "thirst for openness and modernity."[18] Even so, rejecting the technology as against nature (*contra natura*) was not incompatible with objections on practical and empirical grounds. In his *Juicio o dictamen sobre el proceso de la inoculación* (1785) (Opinion or verdict on inoculation's trial), Ferrer, a former member of the Augustinian order, graduate of the University of Salamanca, and professor of theology and philosophy at various Spanish universities, posed these concerns within a framework of conscience and Christian religion. He denounced Samuel-Auguste Tissot and Charles Marie de la Condamine (1701–1774), the French naturalist and author of one of the most famous texts on inoculation, the *Mémoire sur l'inoculation de la petite vérole* (1754) (Essay on smallpox inoculation), for allegedly insisting that inoculation was strictly a medical calculus distinguishable from the moral sphere. For Ferrer, disease and sickness derived from original sin, and those who opted for inoculation contravened the natural order.[19]

Simultaneously, Ferrer and other anti-inoculators expressed fears about the threat of secondary infection, the highly variable circumstances in which inoculation would be practiced, and the responsibility of subjects of enlightened rulers to assess and assume for themselves the risks. On August 4, 1757, some of Spain's most influential physicians gathered in Madrid and voted to deny a license to publish the Spanish translation of Condamine's *Mémoire sur l'inoculation*, citing possible public health risks when necessary precautions, above all segregation, were not taken.[20] In 1774, José Amar, president of the Protomedicato, registered objections in his *Instrucción curativa de las viruelas* (Instruction for curing smallpox) on the grounds that inoculation might harm the patient, particularly in a country where medical professionals were scarce and where contagion from natural smallpox proved difficult to control, to say nothing of the many additional risks of the operation.[21]

In 1785, Jaime Menós de Llena, a Catalonian physician with medical experience in the army, interpreted reports of campaigns in Barcelona, Boston, Madrid, and Paris to mean that inoculation killed as many or more than natural smallpox, that it increased the risk of epidemics by creating new foci of contagion, and that it failed to protect the inoculated from future infection. He also carefully distinguished inoculation from God-given remedies such as bleeding and purging, following Amar and Ferrer.[22] Francisco Gil's contemporaneous *Disertación físico-médica* (the basis of the anticontagion program adopted in New Spain) was no more original. The surgeon cited inoculation's ambivalent reception in France and mixed results in Britain before conceding that while he was not strictly opposed, he preferred another plan, "more certain and less burdensome, by which to undertake not only palliative treatment, as with inoculation, but to establish a radical cure by which to eliminate this *peste*." Gil's plan for eradication would have widespread ramifications when applied in the next smallpox outbreak in New Spain.[23]

If Gil promised to populate Spain with healthy subjects, so too did the inoculationists (with Spain embroiled in conflicts with its rivals over trade and mineral wealth in the Americas) approach the matter in starkly utilitarian terms. One of the most prominent was Timothy (Timoteo) O'Scanlan, an Irish physician with an academic background in Paris and practical experience in the Spanish army who became well known in Spanish America in the 1790s. O'Scanlan dedicated his first practical guide to inoculation (1784, *Practica moderna de la inoculacion*) to Campomanes in appreciation of the minister's advocacy. His subsequent apologetic essay (1792, *Ensayo apologético de la inoculación*) finally came out owing in large part to the support of the Council of Castile, especially Campomanes. The culmination of more than thirty-eight years of study and calculations to determine the number of lives that might be saved by Spain's adoption of inoculation, O'Scanlan's essay appealed to the same geopolitical interests as his patron had years before. It argued that inoculation "is intimately intertwined with the prosperity of the State insofar as it leads to increase in the population, from which derives growth in the arts and industry."[24] Those who had been blinded and debilitated by smallpox, seen roaming the streets of Madrid, incurred considerable costs to state and society. O'Scanlan predicted that Spain would soon follow the example of England, Russia, and others in adopting inoculation. "By it," he wrote, "all without exception will contribute to the good of Society, the growth of the population, and the promotion of the arts and industry. Each individual, as a member of the same body politic, will help bring about this public benefit."[25] Guided by the utilitarian mantra of enlightened political philosophy—development, industry, population, public benefit—O'Scanlan and other promoters sought to harness the salvific powers of science to boost wealth, economic growth, and geopolitical prestige.[26]

In December 1786, Mexico's gazette announced that copies of O'Scanlan's newly published guide to inoculation were available for purchase from the bookstore on Calle San Bernardo, in Mexico City (likely the one owned by the Jáuregui family, prominent publishers and purveyors of international titles). The advertisement offered biographical information about O'Scanlan that included his Irish heritage and his medical service and qualifications in the Iberian world.[27] Beyond these works, which were sold in Mexico City and Veracruz, the transatlantic debate about inoculation's merits was not staged, and is not readily traced, in periodicals, treatises, or healing manuals in New Spain in the years before its official adoption. Despite his active editorial and investigative work in matters of health, the creole polymath José Antonio de Alzate y Ramírez, for instance, printed only two relevant items in his long-running *Gazeta de literatura*.[28] An exceptional expression of anti-inoculation sentiment crops up in a single terse paragraph in Juan Manuel Venegas's *Compendio de la medicina*, which reads: "Not only is *Inoculation* not in use in our America, but it also should be considered harmful, because once a pestilential poison is introduced into our bodies (as we in these regions generally consider the humor of smallpox), it can only wreak havoc." The warning reappeared exactly so in two nineteenth-century reprints of Venegas's guide, despite widespread adoption of vaccination in Mexico by that time.[29]

COLONIAL GENRES OF PROMOTION

Instead, the debate over inoculation began in the streets and homes of residents during tense disease emergencies, whose habits and conventions of speaking and worship informed attempts to promote and propagate the new medical technique. In Mexico City's 1779 smallpox epidemic, city councilmen called on French physician Esteban Morel to perform trials on the population. As related in the Introduction, Morel had years of experience traveling the French Caribbean in the service of the French and Spanish empires as court physician.[30] Initially both the city council and viceroy supported Morel's inoculatory practice, but rumors of disfigurement, dismemberment, and death in the city left the clinic in the convent hospital of San Hipólito empty of patients. The city declined to publish Morel's "Disertación sobre la utilidad de la inoculación," favoring instead a pamphlet by creole physician José Ignacio Bartolache that featured discussions of atmospheric putrefaction and fumigations.[31]

Morel's unpublished treatise contains much of historical interest in this moment of experimentation. It documents the first recorded inoculation trials in Mexico City as well as the promotional strategies adopted by professionals to convert lay audiences to their point of view. Morel's contemporaries considered him an expert, an empiricist, and the epitome of enlightened rationalism, but in his promotional role he leaned heavily on religion and showed a deep attentiveness to the customs of his adopted home. The treatise was prefaced by a letter to members of the city council thanking them for their support and flattering them with observations on the Christian piety and acts of charity and spiritual aid he had witnessed in the streets of the capital. Hoping to secure additional support, he portrayed smallpox's destruction: facial deformities exceeding those of a leper; the sick child physically transformed beyond his own mother's recognition; the learned man who loses his faculties of judgment and reason. Not even the young men of the *cabildo* were exempt, Morel warned: their attraction to a lovely maiden might be cut short by an "intolerable stench, a stench that brings fainting" and "the fury of smallpox engraved on her once beautiful face, now destroyed." By choosing inoculation, such a grim future might be staved off, in favor of one in which children flocked to Minerva, "laughing and playing in their rooms and courtyards."[32]

The text of the treatise begins with a straightforward definition of inoculation, a depiction of the procedure, and a history of its international practice. Among distinguished people (*gente distinguida*) of European states, inoculation "has already become, if I may put it this way, fashionable [*de moda*]." The well-traveled Frenchman stressed that the social costs of smallpox went beyond mortality to the physical disfigurement of survivors, which limited marital prospects (a striking consideration in a society in which marriage and the religious life were the main paths for young people).[33] Following this was the core of the work, a list of frequently asked questions and answers. Morel adapted the arguments and the conversational format provided by his famous compatriot, Charles Marie de la Condamine, whose essay on inoculation (denied publication in Spanish translation for two decades) had addressed the most common doubts and objections of the time. Might someone contract smallpox twice? Might the inoculated contract other diseases through the blood? Did inoculation contradict divine will or providential design? Was it morally forbidden to infect someone who might otherwise never contract smallpox? Even if risk of death was small, how might a parent be expected to assume it? To the ethical and religious objections, the French philosopher famously responded that if inoculation was against God's will, then all therapies used to prevent or treat disease were under the same ban.[34]

Morel placed these objections in the mouth of a loving father, a *padre tierno*, who fears submitting his child to inoculation. This father notes that from 1737 to the present, there had been only three epidemics in Mexico and that many individuals died without contracting smallpox. Why, then, risk inoculation in the absence of epidemic threat? Because the viceroyalty was less isolated than ever before: the recent opening of trade (*comercio libre*) had linked Europe and the Americas in unprecedented ways and, with more direct commerce, there would be more paths for epidemics from all parts of the world.[35] The objection that physicians are unaccustomed to treating smallpox in the lapse between epidemics, which would put the inoculated in grave danger, evokes a comparison with Paris, Montpelier, London, Vienna, and Amsterdam, where "it is observed that fourteen virulent individuals die per 100, even though they are assisted by the most celebrated physicians in the world." In other words, the mortality rates would be even higher in Mexico if smallpox was not prevented.[36] When the father objects that even an inoculated child could subsequently contract smallpox, Morel impugns the character and habits of his source, whose claims are not sound proofs (*pruebas auténticas*).[37] Many practitioners in New Spain, according to Morel, confused smallpox with other sicknesses, perhaps chicken pox, for which he blamed female nurses and *curanderos* who, perhaps wanting the patient to believe their assistance was necessary, encouraged this misunderstanding, which persisted until the patient was struck with the real thing.[38]

If tactless for Morel to disparage the medical expertise of his new home, it was hardly surprising that he weighed in, given his background and training. He moved no less confidently within the theological realm to validate and explain inoculation's virtues. When the father raises the possibility of contracting an illness from inoculation and losing a child anyway, Morel admits the limits of human science, asking the father to have faith in God's will. In the absence of a sure antidote, "inoculation is the indispensable remedy against smallpox, the only one until now sent by the Omnipotent to guard, with time, against the risk of a sickness that mocks other remedies and alone kills a seventh of those killed by all sicknesses combined."[39] In Morel's telling, it was religious zeal ("el celo de la Religión") that inspired parents to take responsibility for the health of children, and "our sacred Religion" that opened the eyes to "other less sensible, and truer goods."[40] In response to the twelfth objection—that if death from smallpox was divinely ordained, immunization would contradict God's designs and tempt His wrath—the physician responds that, equally, Divine Providence has given medicine to humankind. If medicine *does* contradict God's will, then bleedings, purges, mercury treatments, and "other innumerable remedies" popularly used do so as well. Properly acknowledged as a uniquely effective divine gift for human preservation, on the other hand, it was an offense to God to fight smallpox without it.[41] In fact, like bleeding, purgatives, emetics, and *vejigatorios* (irritants used to raise blisters and free the body of dangerous materials), the purpose of inoculation was the same: "to evacuate the cause of some sickness, or at least part of it, through the veins."[42] In conclusion Morel offered a prayer for acceptance: "May God desire that this public recognize the frivolous objections they may hear against inoculation, and that parents, in favor of their children, take advantage of this class of medicine."[43]

Thus Morel sought to normalize an unfamiliar remedy and to show that, far from a novelty, it was already widely known and practiced overseas and even in some form in New Spain. Overlapping beliefs about illness and the body, rooted in a humoral tradition, meant that Morel, in spite of his expertise, might stand on the same plane as his lay audience when touting inoculation's virtues. He claimed that the bare facts supported his science, but he also knew that these alone would not suffice. Only in an appendix did he document what he called the *hechos*, the outcomes of the trials in the capital. Of the six inoculated *indios*, the sickest patient was "Julio," who had fewer than three hundred pustules over his body; none of the others had more than eighty. Of the eight European children, Bárbara had fewer than twenty pustules, "not one of them on her pretty face or any other visible part, with barely a short, slight fever."[44] Because the disease was visible, and its scarring consequential, Morel carefully described the appearance and gravity of lesions on the children's bodies to support the argument that inoculation was far better than the alternative.

In short, political arithmetic was here subdued to arguments at once aesthetic, domestic, medical, and spiritual. From an imagined frontispiece featuring happy children under the watchful eye of Minerva to humanizing descriptions of patients, the treatise was an artfully executed work of persuasion that simultaneously insisted on the value of empirical evidence, couched arguments in a fully rendered providential framework, and presented inoculation's benefits and "facts" within an imaginative depiction of the epidemic apocalypse. Morel's formidable science was enrolled to appeal particularly to New Spain's elite (to the point that he presented inoculation as *de moda*, especially in Europe).

The theological arguments and prayers would seem to indicate that he drew on his deep piety, if not for the fact that Morel was not an especially devout man. He was among some two hundred French residents arrested and jailed at the end of 1794 by the Inquisition, in an atmosphere of paranoia about a French plot among sympathizers of the revolution.[45] By then Morel had amassed a hefty file of denunciations, including charges that he failed to attend mass or take communion, consumed meat on Fridays, cohabited with a woman, and read Montesquieu, Rousseau, Voltaire, and other forbidden authors. Apparently not especially moved by New Spain's devotional practices, Morel was overheard saying, during a procession for Remedios on May 14, 1789, that residents brought out sacred images for rain in seasons when it was likely to rain anyway. He also reportedly said, on more than one occasion, that although one followed another philosophy, one might live safely under the watch of the Inquisition by conforming outwardly to the country's religion.[46] This precept governed Morel's unpublished treatise, in which he made every effort to integrate inoculation into the Christian order: if God had given the remedy to humankind, then it was in human hands, by human agents, that it must be deployed.

Works that introduced medical science to lay communities frequently moved between registers, laced with references to international authorities, unbiased observation, and experimental trials while steeped in personal and exhortatory language and rooted in everyday spaces, practices, and norms. During the smallpox outbreak of 1797, Lorenzo Hernández de Alva, New Spain's royal treasury attorney (*fiscal de hacienda*), was among several functionaries who sought to manage social unrest and popular opinion when rumors and mocking *boleros* about inoculation surfaced in the streets. He composed a legal brief in favor of a viceregal decree prohibiting speech (see Chapter 3), which he justified by arguing for inoculation's proven benefits and absolute safety. Regretting that he lacked time to compose his own proper apologia (*discurso apologético*) for the purpose, Alva instead recommended several European works, primarily from the Spanish and Italian worlds, and cited Campomanes (the former president of the Council of Castile), that without people "'the various operations that civil society requires lack arms.'"[47] He then went beyond these classical works to an experience closer to home.

Having rehearsed the conventional arguments, including inoculation's usefulness for Spanish industry, Alva shifted to personal testimony of its value and safety. Recent successes with the method had moved Alva to inoculate his children, María Guadalupe (sixteen) and Lorenzo (twelve), under the supervision of Dr. Manuel Moreno, professor of anatomy in the Royal Indian Hospital. In the new, simpler method endorsed by the Protomedicato, the patient was not enclosed inside a dark bedroom, Alva noted, "infested with the pestilential exhalations of smallpox," but rather allowed "all the help and comforts that a healthy person enjoys, with certain precautions."[48] Two days before the procedure, the siblings had undergone minimal preparation consisting of "a very light purgative," with a diet of fruits, vegetables, and legumes. Alva had brought them to San Andrés hospital to receive smallpox from a twenty-four-year-old *mozo* (youth) from Querétaro. Afterward they went for walks and enjoyed refreshments and were only kept inside beginning on the fourth day, when they developed fevers and pustules. María Guadalupe had fifteen over her body, Lorenzo significantly more, but all of "excellent quality."

Alva then described a household completely free of illness: "In the house it appears as if there were no sick patients, nor did [the children] consider themselves sick, moving freely throughout the room, both of them passing the time in diversion, sometimes with books, occasionally with entertainments appropriate to their gender and age, waiting impatiently for the day when they would be able to go out to Mass and the street, as they now have, with only the remedy of a light purgative remaining."[49] By demonstrating that the medical procedure might be subjugated to the ordinary routines and rhythms of the household, Alva hoped to preserve it from further public scrutiny and debate. To this end, his testimony rhetorically dissociated inoculation from the hospital, with its connotations of insecurity, vulnerability, sickness, and coercive restraint. This shift paralleled in turn a modification of policy taking place in the viceroyalty, as the government revised the rule prescribing mandatory convalescence at hospitals after it became apparent that few would volunteer for inoculation if forced into one.[50]

The notion that anecdotal evidence from a Crown attorney's home had legal bearing in this moment can only be understood within the context of the technological transition under way. His text became intermediary, in the sense that it moved between distinct communities of knowledge and domains of experience and authority to help effect this transition. Historians of science who observe that the impact of techniques depends on the format in which they are presented echo these early modern efforts to relocate the primal scene of inoculation to happier, healthier, better-lit spaces, more conducive to popular acceptance.

The sermon in Durango that opens this chapter exemplifies the way that genres morphed and medical practice incubated in domains of experience that were not strictly medical. Durango's bishop exhorted listeners to give thanks to God for favorable outcomes from inoculation, eschewing the ingratitude of the Israelites after the Red Sea parted for them, rocks quenched their thirst, and manna fell from the skies. Like these signs, inoculation signaled God's merciful hand, evident in the number who had voluntarily submitted to "a type of operation never practiced in these kingdoms and that upon first glance only appeared to be the introduction of a serious illness in a healthy body." Wishing to extend immunization to newborns, the bishop offered several metaphors to help with understanding: "Experience has shown us that inoculation is a most prudent engagement with the enemy when he is without strength, disarmed, forced to enter battle when he is still in baby blankets [*mantillas*]." His audience was then informed "that inoculation in medicine is the same, in agriculture, as cutting weeds [*las maleas*] when they are still tender, and without seeds."[51] These familial, biblical, martial, and agricultural tropes were calculated to appeal to people with other skills and references, and to render what was still foreign instead familiar, tangible, and domestic. (The printed version of the sermon included statistics as well: 39 fatalities, most of them in poor homes, of 3,824 inoculations.)

As a genre with broad applications and thematic flexibility, the sermon, along with the related pastoral letter, was well suited to facilitate the relocation and transformation of medical practice. These were oratorical occasions that strove to make better Christians and vassals of parishioners, which gave the genre significance, as one scholar has written, that "overflowed the religious or ecclesiastical spheres."[52] With the arrival of Jenner's vaccine, Oaxaca's bishop, Antonio de Bergosa y Jordán, issued a pastoral letter in compliance with royal orders that prelates support the expedition and its personnel. Following the traditional exordium wishing "parish priests, *vicarios* and other ecclesiastics, and all of the faithful" health in Christ, the letter explained that vaccine was the latest gift and sign of love by the Catholic monarch for his vassals. In the past the king had provided schools and ministers to teach Christian doctrine and supported industry, agriculture, and arts. Now he manifested his paternal love (*amor paternal*) by seeking to procure "your health, most precious good among nature's many goods, at great cost and expense to his royal treasury, eager to protect you from the contagious illness of smallpox, which tears so many innocent children from the arms of their parents, and so many adults from the center of their families." A brief history explained how the cowpox virus in Gloucester and surrounding lands had manifest in the form of pox on the cow's udders, which the "wise physician Jenner"—after observing how milkmaids contracted a mild infection—had transferred to others. Since then, a "multitude of experiments" had shown that vaccine was an effective defense against smallpox. Recast as providentially ordained, the measure was endorsed by the bishop, who directed "my beloved children" (*amados hijos mios*) to adopt it for their children and grandchildren.

As the letter circulated to the parishes in Oaxaca, parishioners in the diocese might have learned that, unlike inoculation, vaccination required no preparation, that it was available to all ages at all times of the year, that it would not spread contagion through the air, and that recovery required only good diet and regimen. (The technical instructions were accommodated, Bergosa announced, to the "limited capacities" of his audience.) The procedure itself consisted of a shallow injection of lymph, ideally on the inside of the arm with a needle (*aguja*), so lightly that "fathers, mothers, or *chichiguas* [wet nurses, from the Nahuatl, *chichihua*] can do it without fear, and with the same felicity and good effect, because in fact it is an operation more proper to women owing to the greater softness of their hands." This allowance, along with the description of the pustule on the sixth day as "the volume of a lentil," was inspired by a French medical treatise, translated into Castilian (in 1801) by the Spaniard Pedro Hernández. Bergosa's appropriation of passages from the *Orígen y descubrimiento de la vaccina* (Origin and discovery of the vaccine) helps explain why the pastoral letter's indexical practice (the manner in which audience is indicated and established) shifts in this technical section. Following it, another series of exhortations addressed parents once again, directing them not to reject the gift, because the pious and beneficent monarch, "with fatherly love," had spared no expense. Warnings and incentives were at last extended to institutionalize the practice: for priests, service on behalf of vaccination would be considered in parish reviews and promotion cases and be made obligatory in pastoral work for anyone presenting for ordination. Others were offered forty days' indulgence if they were voluntarily vaccinated or worked charitably in support of campaigns.[53]

The bland assurance by the bishop that priests and laypeople, including women, might vaccinate created problems as administrators sought to restrict the practice to trained practitioners. What impresses the reader is the range of conventions, perspectives, vocations, and assumptions that produced the so-called "facts" about immunization in these years of promotion. A kind of "administrative knowledge" that was neither strictly expert nor lay, American or European, was cobbled together from the disjointed experiences of ruling and adjudicating as agents of the colonial state.[54] A survey of twenty-four works on immunization published in Mexico between 1777 and 1840 reveals 21 percent authored by ecclesiastics, 21 percent by administrative bodies, and 58 percent by public health personnel (medical, military, or civilian), and that those with little or no medical training published proportionately more in the viceroyalty than their counterparts in Spain and Spain's other overseas territories.[55] Part of an ongoing Atlantic project to appeal to the sensibilities of governors and the general public, promotion and instruction fell to many outside of the medical profession. Yet even those works authored by professionals brimmed with extramedical imagery, symbolism, and prayer.

It warns against classifications that impose anachronistic notions of expertise on the eclectic medical culture into which vaccination entered. Drawing on medical, legal, domestic, and ecclesiastical resources, promotional texts combined statistical language with theological idioms and familial metaphors within a shared discursive field; style, content, and conventions were rearranged to produce original, genre-bending works that aimed to make abstract ideas tangible within the nonliterate habitus of colonial Mexico.[56] The intermediate, blended nature of the resulting productions mirrors the technological transition happening in the world beyond, a universe in which a proliferation of patriarchs—literal fathers but also kings, prelates, priests, and God—announced the arrival of immunization in a curiously paternalistic place. A paradigm shift, from the perspective of science, was from that of genre and ritual nothing more or less than routine.

A CAMPAIGN TO INSPIRE THE MASSES

These routines took physical form in the elaborate planning and execution of the Royal Philanthropic Vaccination Expedition. An early proposal for the expedition submitted by José Flores, royal physician and president of Guatemala's Protomedicato, is of special interest not only because Flores drew on his vast knowledge of American society and disease but because his insights into ritual were largely suppressed in the official program. As such, the text of this innovator in medical research and instruction provides an occasion to reflect on the mechanisms of Bourbon reform, whose programs were far from finished when promulgated.

In November 1803 an outbreak of smallpox in Santa Fe de Bogotá led city officials to isolate the infected in hospitals and undertake a search for cowpox on the region's haciendas. Unable to locate or acquire it beyond the viceroyalty, and with disagreement growing over funding for the isolation hospitals, Bogotá's city council wrote Spain to request remediation of segregation orders. The Council of the Indies called on the king's royal physicians for advice on whether and how to introduce Jenner's vaccine in the Indies.[57] Resident in Madrid after a tour of hospitals in the United States and Europe, Flores prefaced his proposal with an overview of the special vulnerability of the Indies to disease, the exceptional mortality of Amerindians in the Conquest, and the fact that *indios* had been accorded special civil, criminal, and ecclesiastical protections, declared "free, noble subjects, capable of all types of employment." A public health campaign to the Indies would have incalculable benefits and was the responsibility of a benevolent ruler. Because efforts to locate a viable local source of cowpox had not yielded results, Flores proposed sending it from Cádiz to the Indies in two light ships loaded with vaccinated children and cows—one destined for Puerto Rico, Trujillo, Yucatán, and Veracruz; the other for Cartagena, Bogotá, and Panama.

Flores drew on (and documented in earnest detail) his vast experience in Guatemalan epidemics to relocate vaccine from the realm of enlightened statecraft and statistics to the redemptive physical spaces of the Indies.[58] Allowing for variation by region, he proposed that with the arrival of vaccinating teams capital cities be split into *cuarteles* under the care of principal residents and one or more medical practitioners. In head towns the most expert (*hábiles*) physicians would learn the operation and issue instructions "according to their customs and adapted to the nature and care of the Indians." In pueblos and missions without Spanish or ladino physicians, priests and missionaries would vaccinate, introducing the practice at the parish level by merging vaccination with Catholic liturgy and sacramental practice: the parish priest would persuade godparents to return four to six months after baptism for a vaccinating ceremony that would include an altar boy holding a lit candle, the priest in full liturgical garb (a stole with white surplice over cassock), and blessing and prayers for the health of the child. Vaccine would be preserved between glass slides in a box in the sacristy, with the holy oils, when it could not be kept fresh by the arm-to-arm method, and even medical practitioners, when available, would vaccinate within the church. Outcomes would be recorded in a book dedicated to vaccinations and kept with other parish registers. Flores recommended that the pope be supplicated to issue a papal brief "to sanctify this practice," determine the orations to be performed by the priest, and offer indulgences, "since this good work is directed to the protection and increase of the faithful and to the prosperity of the Catholic Monarchy." Each of the *audiencias* would finally request an extract from the books of vaccination at the end of each year to compile a census, for an ambitious register (*estado general*) of all the inhabitants of the Indies.[59]

Flores saw the ceremonial considerations as the means by which appropriate gravity and esteem would be conferred on the medical technology. He advised variously to "dress it up in religious ceremony" and of the virtues of "accompanying it with religion, so that the pueblo can venerate it, appreciate it, crave it." Indeed, he sought to give preventive medicine parity with the sacraments of the Church, lending practitioners, implements, and vaccine the respect and reverence reserved for the Host. Reflecting on the mechanisms of absolutist governance, Flores in effect confirmed the views of Bourbon ministers, including Campomanes and Floridablanca, on the ideal role for the church in public life.[60] Rulers in the Age of Reason well knew "that besides it being just to give God thanks for His aid, this has been the effective route happily followed by legislators of all the ages when they have tried to introduce and establish some custom. The profound politician, the one who is obeyed and takes possession of hearts, is he who manages the heart's impulses, and prefers among them to manage skillfully the religious impulse."[61]

Despite Flores's careful design, his ideas were mostly ignored. Early on, the *fiscal* who recommended that Flores take charge of the expedition cited the royal surgeon Francisco Xavier de Balmis as another possible director.[62] This official noted that Balmis had translated Jacques-Louis Moreau de la Sarthe's treatise on vaccine (it would soon become the authoritative source on vaccination in Spanish America) and his two prior trips to New Spain, with extended residencies that signaled his knowledge of the country (*país*).[63] Perhaps experience in the all-important viceroyalty tipped things in Balmis's favor: he had served as surgeon in the Spanish army, in a battalion stationed at Veracruz beginning in 1783; as head surgeon (*cirujano mayor*) of the prestigious Amor de Dios military hospital, which specialized in syphilis cases; and upon retiring from the military as head of the syphilitic ward of San Andrés Hospital, where he studied the antisyphilitic properties of native plants, including Mexican agave (*maguey*) and begonia (samples of which he brought to Spain when he returned in 1792). Most recently he was a member of the prestigious Royal Academy of Medicine, in Madrid, where he had spent several years supervising vaccinations.

With Balmis as director, the expedition set sail from the port of La Coruña instead of Cádiz. One ship rather than two made the initial Atlantic crossing, while the ceremonial considerations deemed central by Flores, including liturgical apparatus, sacraments, vestments, ecclesiastical spaces, and indulgences, went conspicuously missing from official documents. The royal decree announcing the expedition specified only that the procedure be performed using the more reliable in vivo (arm-to-arm) method of transfer in the Americas and the Philippines, "observing the anomalies of the diversity of climate and castes."[64] The printed circular sent to administrators prescribed vaccinations in each capital, with the director and team instructing physicians and "others who may want to take advantage of this opportunity," along with the use of orphaned children to transmit vaccine fluid, where available, and glass slides for its distribution into sparsely settled regions. The document invoked the charitable dimensions of *religión* and stipulated that prelates contribute to the presentation and conservation of vaccine in their dioceses by exhorting priests and missionaries to aid the expedition and its participants, "making use of the influence that ministers of the Church regularly have over public opinion to dispel any contrary preoccupation."[65] The record is curiously silent about vaccination as the "eighth sacrament": no mention is made of association with baptism, storage of lymph in the sacristy, the priest's performance of the liturgy, or his capacity to vaccinate. Priests were good pastors for their flocks but not, in this vision, ready vaccinators.

Why were the rituals suppressed? A global expedition required simplifications. Flores had provided richly drawn and intricate scenarios tailored to the Indies, when ministers sought to vaccinate across continents and delineate the specialized functions of various administrators. If the spirit of the Chiapaneco's work was to be embodied, it would come about through local collaborations and improvisations, beginning with programmatic considerations for public spectacle as vaccine reached New Spain's cities, towns, and villages.

Shortly after arriving in Mexico City, Balmis wrote to Manuel de Flon, the intendant of Puebla and an old friend, to advise him to "entusiasmar al bajo pueblo" (inspire the common people) to embrace the king's expedition. He explained: "The ignorant commoner is only moved by imitation, as you very well know, and needs examples and aids that astonish him before being persuaded." Balmis disclosed that the Council of the Indies had consulted with the king about the fact that "vaccine would have to be received in the pueblos of America beneath a canopy, if feasible." Flon advised Balmis to write the bishop of Puebla directly: without the assistance of prelate and priests, the king's wishes would never be realized.[66]

The verb *entusiasmar* appears repeatedly in the sources from this moment. The word meant to delight and excite, to instill a state of enthusiasm, or to produce admiration, and referred especially to the unlearned masses. It became a refrain for the expedition, but the notion that Indians should be engaged by public drama was not new. A tradition of learning and unlearning through the eyes and ears had long antecedents in colonial projects of conquest and conversion. A royal ordinance on "peaceful conquests" issued in 1573 by Phillip II (and compiled in 1681 in the Laws of the Indies) recommended that preachers dress in stole and surplice and that any Spanish Christians in attendance listen with extreme respect and veneration to these holy men, "because by imitation the infidels take to being taught." The Crown recommended singing and minstrels to attract Indians and to subdue (*amansar*), pacify, and induce admiration among those otherwise disposed to wage war.[67] The same pedagogy underwrote the missionary work of Dominicans, Franciscans, Jesuits, and others, from the legendary friar Pedro de Gante on. Mendicants commented on the persuasive powers of music, made a habit of singing hymns of praise after arriving safely in towns, sometimes with converts, crosses, soldiers, and even choirs of singers in tow, and claimed that devotion entered the heart through the senses. (The last allegedly uttered by the Jesuit Juan

María de Salvatierra, who worked in the northwestern frontier missions at the beginning of the eighteenth century.)[68]

If images and pageantry transmitted Christianity's central mysteries across linguistic barriers, there were other lessons to learn during the Enlightenment. Performances staged in theaters, for instance, were endorsed to inculcate proper respect and good morals among spectators (even if the realities of a performance usually fell short of the ideal).[69] By then Mexico's visual culture included not only a flood of mechanically reproduced images of saints but also regular public acts (*demostraciones*) that placed celestial and terrestrial figures physically and symbolically at their center, including members of the royal family, images of saints and Mary, and the mystical body of Christ in lavish Corpus Christi celebrations.[70] In Silao in 1793, following the bishop's ban on Holy Week processions on the grounds that they were expensive, disorderly, and indecent, the self-described ladino Indians who served as *mayordomos* of the confraternities adopted the principle of visual learning in their protest. They defended the occasion by arguing that the senses, and particularly the stimulus of sight, opened the "doors" to the understanding of common people, for whom "living representations or images" impressed them with some idea of otherwise inaccessible, abstract mysteries of faith.[71]

Through performances in and around the church, administrators in Mexico likewise sought to embody an abstract message of salvation from disease and thereby instill a deferential and reverential stance. As the physicians, nurses, and children of the expeditions and subexpeditions approached cities and towns in 1804, royal officials, city councilmen, the clergy, prelates, and other public figures hurried to make the appropriate preparations, shuttled in and out to receive personnel, spent on illumination and fireworks, readied musical performances, composed sermons, and carefully documented these activities for their superiors and posterity.

In Puebla, where nearly twelve thousand vaccinations were recorded in the first three months of practice, the bishop received Balmis and his entourage outside of the city on September 20, 1804. He reentered Puebla in his carriage, with the dean of the cathedral chapter and the child carrier, while the intendant marched with the director and other members of the cathedral chapter to the cathedral door. Accompanied by members of the city council and a large assembly of residents, the team took the seats of honor ordinarily reserved for the cathedral clergy. From his own seat the bishop addressed the congregation in eloquent terms, urging onlookers to give thanks to God and the king for the gift that had been generously sent, and to receive it without misgivings or fear. The choir led the singing of the Te Deum Laudamus (Glory Be to God), the Catholic hymn of thanksgiving and praise (in Flon's punctilious report: "the hymn that the Church uses for this purpose"), with the congregation intoning prayers and processing outside to accompany the expedition to its lodgings. The following Sunday so many residents (more than 230) arrived for vaccination in the episcopal palace that the supply of vaccine fluid ran out. Summarizing the affair, the bishop wrote that he sought to receive vaccine "in such a way as to *entusiasmar* the pueblo," who were all the more vulnerable to smallpox due to Puebla's climate.[72] Article 11 of Puebla's vaccination regulations, which provided for subaltern vaccination boards in district seats, stipulated that the arrival of vaccine "should be advertised to the public with as many demonstrations of rejoicing and festivity as possible, so that the Indians especially understand that they are being brought a good thing, and that they should present their children to receive it, freeing themselves from the cruel scourge of smallpox."[73]

In Guadalajara, seat of an *audiencia*, the royal orders on vaccine generated confusion for city councilmen and officials. They did not know which acts were most appropriate for the occasion because the issues of the *Gazeta de México* that reported on the expedition made no mention of any in Mexico City. When the assistant director, Antonio Gutiérrez, approached Guadalajara with two boy carriers, Pedro Catani, *audiencia* president, rushed out of the city to request that Gutiérrez wait in neighboring San Pedro Tlaquepaque while preparations were completed. Two days later, they were driven in Catani's ceremonial carriage to the city entrance, where civil and religious authorities and distinguished residents joined them along with a sizable gathering of spectators in a dignified procession to the cathedral. There the infantry band struck up an overture, members of the cathedral chapter and the bishop accompanied the entourage into the church to sing the Te Deum, and soldiers performed crowd control, keeping the assembled from obstructing the path. Though these acts were delayed and apparently improvised from the memory of previous occasions, the event, it was agreed, came off successfully.[74]

Like the Inquisition's *autos de fe* in Mexico City, with their imposing shows of Catholicism's capacity for violence, *demostraciones* for vaccine drew on some less than innocent insinuations of force. It was not uncommon for militia company musicians to perform the music accompanying the issuing of official *bandos,* particularly on the northern frontier. In Celaya, to "banish those preoccupations and ideas that always accompany the *bajo pueblo*," the military corps joined the notables and officials gathered to receive Balmis and his team. From the municipal building they paraded to the parish church by foot rather than carriage, "so that it should be more visible." Council members reported the general euphoria of the crowd, with *vivas* for the royal family "mixed with general ringing of the bells and volleys of the company of grenadiers of the provincial regiment, arranged in the atrium of the church, where it remained while a Mass of thanksgiving was sung with the greatest solemnity." At the end, pealing bells and "the thunder of the military salute" accompanied another Te Deum and more *vivas*.[75] The sensory effect of volleys of gunfire and whiffs of gunpowder must have been considerable: multimedia presentations made tangible what remained abstract and literal in decrees, proposals, promotional treatises, and even sermons.

At the same time residents were treated to entertainments to help make manifest the delight (*regocijo*) with which the vaccine should be received. In Izucar, Puebla, invitations to the reception were sent to residents of the *cabecera* and surrounding Indian republics. The usual celebratory effects were poured on: bullfights featuring young bulls for two days ("siendo como son todos ellos afectos de correr toros") and, at night, music and fireworks, to attract the indigenous and black residents of surrounding estates and ranches and encourage broad participation. On Sunday, April 6, 1806, distinguished residents of the head town, haciendas, and subject pueblos were invited to witness the ceremonial entrance of vaccine. Officials in carriages received the child carriers, one Spaniard and one *mulato*, both "decently dressed and vaccinated," at the gate along the road from Puebla. The priests of the Spanish and Indian parishes (who served as presidents of the vaccination board) placed the children in separate carriages and escorted them to the former's parish church. In the procession "the indigenous population attended with their national music, which experience shows makes a great impression on them, in addition to which those from this *cabecera* embellished the act with the same music and dances in their style, as well as the leaders of each of the sixteen barrios of the *cabecera*, with their flags and bouquets of flowers." At the door of the church the children were placed prominently inside, where the pastor of the Indian parish led a solemn Te Deum, accompanied by an orchestra, with voices lifted in prayer for a successful campaign. Among the next day's thanksgiving masses, one in the Indian parish concluded "with a vast array of demonstrations of joy by the Indians, who took part according to their style in a variety of dances."[76]

As they settled in these months on culturally familiar solutions to the problem of persuasion, administrators reproduced a universe of stereotypes about learning, cultural competence, and intellect. Public acts to inspire were necessary, Balmis maintained, because unless first given some financial incentive, peasants hung back, if they were not impressed by sensuous, concrete things. His recent experience in the Canary Islands, Havana, Mérida (Yucatán) and elsewhere had convinced him that only after "a century of experience" would the commoner (*vulgo*) give a new discovery that lacked apparent financial purpose the attention it deserved. "Rustic people," he continued, require "material examples and profound demonstrations to be able to comprehend an important thing. All of them are moved by pure imitation, and the brilliant acceptance with which the people have received this expedition has made a greater impression on the common masses than that which Jenner's immortal discovery produced in all of Europe." The willingness of parents to present their children was a function of the intensity, immensity, and decorum of public demonstrations. Where these were adequate, the public flocked to churches to give thanks to God; where they were not, there was no hope of acceptance.[77]

For their part, the ecclesiastical hierarchy advocated the same methods endorsed in manuals for novice pastors, which stressed the proper reverence owed to sacred things and the conviction that devotion could be learned (and unlearned) through the priest's silent example.[78] Mexico's new archbishop, Francisco Javier de Lizana y Beaumont, proved himself an energetic supporter of Bourbon health initiatives. In 1806 he upbraided a priest in Tultitlán who had largely restricted his activities during the epidemic to hellfire sermons in the pulpit, disregarding orders to correct the erroneous ideas of parishioners about healing and speak out against "ignorant *curanderas*" and useless medicines. As he did, the archbishop spelled out the principle of imitation and education, citing biblical authority on the divine attributes of the physician:

> [I]t is necessary to labor and place oneself in front of the pueblo by example... that the public see that you receive, accompany, fete, honor, and distinguish with the greatest esteem the practitioners and whatever other persons are sent by the supreme government to that pueblo for the purpose of the sickness that afflicts it...that you exhort in public and private, by word and deed, "give the physician his place [*da locum medico*]" and "honor the physician [*honora medicum*]"; that you be vigilant in persuading those people until they are convinced, as Saint Cirilo said: "Obeying physicians as if they were ministers of God [*Medicis tanquam Ministris Dei obediendum*]." Make them recognize that the Indians' crude medications, inherited from their ancestors' ignorance, are of no effect, and perhaps entangled in certain residues of superstition; relieve them of their ideas, which are always puerile, even when their beards turn white.[79]

Giving the physician and his medicine their place meant displaying proper reverence and, as in the past, extirpating any superstitions. In the same spirit, Bishop Juan Cruz Ruiz de Cabañas reported that the aim of his sermon in Guadalajara on the occasion of the expedition's arrival had been to make the people understand that through vaccination they stood to receive a singular benefit from God, and to stimulate parish priests to inspire in heads of household, "by means of the most gentle reflections," the necessary knowledge and understanding.[80] As he put it elsewhere, "holy things should be treated in a holy manner."[81]

Members of vaccinating teams were thus joined by justices, councilmen, ecclesiastics, royal officials, prominent citizens, musicians, and performers, to consecrate preventive medicine, plant a cross for it, and make new converts out of potentially incredulous people. They touched the intellect, and body, by first touching the senses and emotions with music, sermons, fireworks, prayer, and poems. The acts of celebration centered on the most symbolically charged sites of authority in cities and villages, such as municipal buildings, the entrances and egresses, and parish churches, above all. Surviving financial records present an accountant's view of the outlay for pyrotechnics, music, singers, and the illumination of church buildings. Twenty pesos spent in Guanajuato "for the music and singers who sang the Te Deum" in the church amount to 2.3 percent of the total (878 pesos) spent on the expedition's maintenance in the city. In Sombrerete, 10.5 pesos covered pyrotechnics (pinwheels, gunpowder, and payments to workers) during the Te Deum and the reception of the expedition in the church, with another 36 pesos for illumination of church and steeple, or 5.6 percent of the total (829 pesos). (The uniforms made for children recruited for the next leg of the journey cost 135 pesos.)[82] Payments for musicians, church illumination, and preachers rivaled the cost of the most popular feast days and votive offerings sponsored by municipal councils in New Spain, including the feast of Corpus Christi, occasionally the point of reference for these celebrations.[83] From a utilitarian perspective, 46.5 pesos might have secured a practitioner to vaccinate in Sombrerete for one or two months, a sacrifice whose significance would grow in the coming years of shortage.

On the other hand, contemporaries wondered whether the population would have complied without these expenditures. Though often formulaic, beyond the rhetorical flourishes and self-congratulatory reports are administrators and physicians who believed that protocols of pageantry encouraged popular acceptance. At the head of one of the subexpeditions, Alejandro García Arboleya delayed his journey to the capital of Oaxaca when he learned that residents of Tehuacán de las Granadas, roughly halfway to his destination, were eager to take full advantage of the expedition at their doorstep. Arboleya vaccinated eighty infants (*párvulos*) there, mostly from principal families, in the presence of the subdelegate, parish priest, scribe, and a physician and surgeon. The session included enthusiastic public announcements, with a thanksgiving mass, accompanied by bell ringing and fireworks, in which the priest exhorted from the pulpit with "great energy" to give thanks to the king "for his fatherly solicitude and care in protecting his fortunate vassals." Subsequently, in Teotitlán del Camino, Arboleya reported 187 vaccinations in the district seat and surrounding towns, for which he credited the festivals in the church, masses, performances of the Te Deum for the king's health and in thanks to God, and the way parishioners had been prepared by their priests with orations in favor of the "invention."[84]

When Tenancingo's district governor, Antonio Elías Sáenz, acquired vaccine fluid from Mexico City to begin vaccinations, he likewise acknowledged the role played by its parish priest, along with those of Tecualoya and Zumpahuacan, "by the acts of joy with which they received the vaccine in their respective *doctrinas*, and because they have taken great pains to make these people understand the incomparable benefit the paternal love of our August Sovereign has provided them." Accordingly, and because no one had become ill, "the Spaniards and Indians throng with their families to be vaccinated," such that Sáenz had to regulate access to ensure a reserve of children for future sessions.[85] The report of these achievements in the October 27 issue of the gazette moved Toluca's administrator to undertake a campaign in his own district. He joined forces with the corregidor and ecclesiastical authorities to support vaccine with *demostraciones* in imitation of Sáenz, so that "these inhabitants submit with gusto." With three child carriers transported from Tenancingo, on March 2, 1805, administrators commenced vaccinating in Toluca with pomp and circumstance: after forty-two operations the official declared that with the good results and the overtures (*exordios*) of church magistrates "we will achieve my goal, banishing the fear and worries of many." He praised the viceroy for his work against "that massacring sickness that consumes robustness, beauty, and individuals."[86]

Administrators believed that a gift given by a father, his benevolence manifest in lavish public displays, would be reciprocated by enthusiastic adoption, drawing a direct causal line to the ceremonies that preceded it.[87] Outside the town of Izucar, on Raboso Hacienda, a group of young black workers, seeing that the owner intended to wait for permission before proceeding, reportedly took it upon themselves to vaccinate one another with the spines of a local plant. Glossing over the fact that the workers had broken protocol, their initiative, along with the subsequent preservation of vaccine fluid on the hacienda, was for officials proof of the effectiveness of their ceremonies, which had inspired (*entusiasmaron*) the most impassive (*estólidos*) persons.[88] Perhaps the young men really had been moved to an impatient embrace of their duty as subjects of the king. It is just as likely that they contemplated the several hundred vaccinations already performed in outlying villages. As carriages, parades, and vaccinators traversed the American landscape, they left in their wake records full of such stereotypes of culture and impressionability, and many more improvisations.

GIFTS OF COINS AND COOKIES

In these early months and years vaccination passed into a ceremonial complex built on ideas about the pervasive power of spectacle. Soon, the question of how to maintain this level of ceremony became unavoidable. Lavish public displays could not stretch out endlessly, and at some point more mundane, day-to-day patterns reasserted themselves. Administrators at the highest levels—including the viceroy, royal officials, certified physicians, and parish priests—turned to monetary incentives to compel residents to embrace vaccination. Pageantry gave way to material considerations that responded to hardship rather than the sacramental tug of the soul.

The most extensive, sustained example is from San Miguel parish in downtown Mexico City. Made up of a majority of Spanish parishioners, it became the site of the capital's most successful clinic, owing in large part to the efforts of its priest, Juan José Guereña. Records of sessions from March 1804, through 1809, when Guereña departed for a new post in Puebla's cathedral, document 11,918 vaccinations in a parish of 9,696 Spaniards, Indians, *castas*, and priests.[89] Balmis repeatedly acknowledged the pastor's work, remarking that thirty thousand people awaited vaccination in the city, and not a bit of fluid would remain for the purpose if not for the enlightened and zealous ("ilustrado y celoso") parish priest of San Miguel, the "only protector of vaccine" in Mexico City.[90]

Typical of the director's hyperbole, the statement correctly observed the battle being waged to preserve biological matter that degenerated rather easily. In the method most often employed, the active agent was propagated from person to person, which required that vaccine pustules develop properly on at least some of the children vaccinated in any session. It required also that the child and its parents return to transfer fluid from the mature pustule to the next group. The surgeon Antonio Serrano, director of the anatomical theater in the Royal Indian Hospital, reported that while briefly practicing alongside Guereña, the priest provided him with a steady supply of children for this purpose by means of his exhortations: "truth be told, if not for his care and efficiency delivering poor children to me, the fluid could have already run out." Now approaching the end of 1804, most principal residents had vaccinated their children, and the lower classes were delaying, Serrano wrote. "Only by the lively expressions of their parish priests" were they convinced of its benefit, "because it is thought that they are being tricked."[91]

Whatever his oratorical skills, Guereña's tactics to compel cooperation went beyond "lively expressions" of reassurance. He had acquired considerable technical knowledge as a vaccinator, which he displayed in correspondence with the viceroy about several proposed amendments to the regulations Balmis had issued for Mexico City. Based on nearly two years of experience, Guereña made recommendations on the continued search for cowpox, as well as its preservation, the need for attending physicians to make detailed observations of their work, and the distastefulness of segregating vaccinated patients. He advised that children regularly and punctually be drawn from each of the capital's subsectors (*cuarteles menores*) to prevent accidental loss of vaccine, proposing for this that the alcalde in charge of each provide one child for every session. But because people came "by their interest in the gift [*obsequio*]" rather than voluntarily, the priest or alcalde might "gratify each child with a half *real* and a cookie [*bizcocho*]."[92] Subsequently, a committee assembled to advise the viceregal government on how best to propagate vaccinations (comprised by practitioners Arboleya, Serrano, and García Jove) singled out Guereña's "incessant work and care" in gathering children from various poor barrios as an example to be emulated throughout the viceroyalty. Guereña spared no expense: the children acquiesced because he attracted them with a half *real*, and in this followed the example of the viceroy himself.[93]

From an early moment the viceroy's paternalism was widely publicized. In September 1804 a "notice to the public" affixed in Mexico City's public places advertised "free vaccinations" for any and all interested residents. It announced that the viceroy, aware that the poor hesitated to bring their children because it might interrupt their livelihoods, and "stimulated by love for the public under his care," had resolved that a *real* would be provided for each poor child vaccinated, in compensation for wages lost. With this he "wishes that no one for reasons of poverty or unhappiness miss this notable opportunity to free his family, by such simple and innocent means, from the cruel sickness of natural smallpox, which costs so many lives."[94] At once a reward and an incentive, it was also a policy borne of recognition of the realities of dearth and the hardship that the procedure posed for working-class parents. It was the kind of generosity expected from the king's royal figure, whose principal representative, the viceroy, was looked to for favors and alms that carried both material and symbolic value.

There were notable parallels in the conversion and pacification campaigns of frontier regions, the so-called "peaceful conquests" undertaken late in the eighteenth century, as well as other efforts to secure the cooperation of indigenous societies not yet settled or incorporated into Spain's dominion. A 1777 royal *cédula* to the viceroy of La Plata referred to gifts as "the real means to bring about conversions," while indigenous collaborators in scientific expeditions were compensated for their work as informants, translators, and allies during Malaspina's artifact-gathering expedition through the Americas (1789–1791). "Our peaceful contact with the natives had put down solid roots at that time, even at the cost of various gifts," the explorer and naval officer reflected, "[and] a steady contribution of biscuits [*galletas*]."[95] A few years later, in a public vaccinating session in Mexico City, its barrios, and surrounding villages,

Arboleya observed viceroys provide patients with a *real* (or two) from their personal accounts whenever they were present.[96]

Balmis disdained these monetary gestures.[97] After Charles IV had graciously offered to educate and care for the children taken to the Philippines as carriers upon their return to Mexico, parents in Celaya and Querétaro had consistently preferred a single payment up front, instead of the royal education. (Not one for subtlety, Balmis wrote: "the distrustful and stupid character of these natives makes them prefer and more highly esteem a single pecuniary reward in exchange for the voluntary loan of their children.") It seemed to him crass and unfortunate, yet by his own admission, he had distributed innumerable *pesetas* (2-*real* coins) to persuade Indians to assent to vaccinations ("para que se dejasen vacunar"), and toys for the entertainment of the children embarked on the journey.[98]

Apparently it was the price of admission to this world, where tokens of generosity, extended by powerful patrons to their dependents, were the norm. Formally, the practice was codified in vaccination regulations. Durango's stipulated that while principal families were to continue to set an example by presenting their children at the public vaccination house (*casa de vacunación*), experience had shown it necessary to attract many with alms (*limosnas*), the term invoking charitable acts as conceived within Catholic cultures of salvation. In the future each of the vaccinated poor would receive a *real* in relief or aid. Guadalajara's regulations likewise stipulated gratuities or rewards for *miserables* and the "solemn poor"—a distinction that derived from centuries of thinking about the moral predisposition that marked the recipient's worthiness of charity.[99]

As a practical matter, administrators in the provinces routinely incorporated these tokens into sessions: whether construed as alms, gifts, rewards, incentives, or payments, evidence indicates that they flowed readily. From the old mining frontier of the near north of New Spain, the vaccination committee formed in Zacatecas reported, in August 1805, that its twelve members had contributed 525 pesos, with another 368 solicited from "zealots and patriots" in the city. With this they had managed sessions almost weekly (an average of 151 vaccinations a month since December). In addition to a porter and *maestro sangrador* (a licensed phlebotomist), who were paid 10 and 30 pesos a month, the funds went toward gratifications for the children, each of whom received a half *real* after the incision, "to attract them to the good they receive and begin to obliterate the preoccupations and fears that the lower classes [*pueblo ínfimo*] form with new and strange enterprises."[100]

At the end of 1804, vaccine arrived from Zacatecas in neighboring San Luis Potosí. In Real de Santa María de los Ramos, where 1,653 children were vaccinated, parents were persuaded "with the incentive [*aliciente*] of a half *real* for each of the vaccinated, whose effect has not been insignificant, especially among the common people here [*en la gente común del Pueblo*]."[101] In Chalco, southeast of Mexico City, the administrator expended more than 800 *pesetas* for such incentives in 1806. He observed that once they stopped, "parents did not return to deliver their children, the lymph was lost, and vaccination ceased." Two years later, as he prepared to resume vaccinations, he asked whether he should also continue payments, which he deemed indispensable to ensure the return trip.[102] Among the administrators and practitioners who stepped forward with their own resources was Querétaro's corregidor, Miguel Domínguez, who assisted the vaccinator-surgeon by "giving from my pocket one or another small gratuity to some of the parents of the children" so that they would look after them and bring them back when their pustules were ready for use. With his wife, Domínguez soon became an active advocate for Mexican independence. At the time the creole official characterized all of the activity in his jurisdiction—parents freely presenting their children for vaccination, the surgeon patriotically vaccinating without pay, and his own voluntary donations—as service rendered to the king.[103] If a meaningful demonstration of goodwill and loyalty, it also, in the eyes of many, improved the likelihood of a successful outcome.

Meanwhile, some with a taste for efficiency looked ahead to preserve and regularize these practical and principled transactions. Reporting successful vaccinations in Michoacán in 1808, the intendant, Phelipe Díaz de Hortega, observed in a note that "la plebe" made up the majority of inhabitants in city and countryside, "of such a low type that only self-interest, and the most careful vigilance by salaried persons assigned to the task, has sufficed to make vaccination effective." Assistant director Antonio Gutiérrez had opted to reward both vaccine porters and the vaccinated for their cooperation. Although the official favored this approach, the costs generated if repeated annually were excessive (vaccinations in Valladolid had ceased the previous year with the depletion of municipal funds). He proposed an alternate plan, in which surplus funds from communal income and rents (*bienes de comunidad y propios*) would be amassed and spent by district governors and priests every three to four years on gratuities for custodians of vaccine and patients. Primarily those born since the previous campaign would be targeted, to manage the nonimmune population, along with costs.[104] Thus entering into an ongoing debate over the benefits and burdens of preventive medicine, his solution—intended in part to avoid dependence on the whims of charitable patrons and colonial benefactors—identified a source that would become even more irregular in the coming years of insurgency.

CONCLUSION

On New Year's Day, 1805, the *Gazeta de México* reported on receptions of vaccine in Aguascalientes, Celaya, and Durango. In Celaya, whose population had been hit hard in the previous smallpox epidemic, the comportment of the director and the *demostraciones* sponsored by the *ayuntamiento* stirred up a commotion "not easily made visible by means of the pen," but that reportedly moved the plebe to adopt a procedure previously unknown. Residents were "wordlessly called" by the example of distinguished persons who offered their own children, whose "silent eloquence" attracted all classes "in such manner that from then until now the Indians have presented their children for the beneficial operation."[105] Insisting on docility and compliance, the passage highlighted the model of the upper classes and imputed motives for the behaviors of the lower classes. What made reporters so certain? What anthropological insight or cultural depth did such assessments contain?

It was not the first time that science was made spectacle in colonial Mexico. Public demonstrations featuring lightning rods, air balloons, dissected cadavers, and various instruments, common in Europe, were not unknown there.[106] These too were sensuous affairs, meant to capture the amassed energy of a curious audience and, by means of entertainment and wonder, convert it into the driving steam of utility. In popularizing immunization, promoters sponsored "demonstrations" that had a particular meaning: they were religious, ceremonial, and charitable, as often as experimental. The idea that knowledge was affective and penetrated the intellect by means of the senses was not novel in the Enlightenment, but germane to the pedagogy of Christian missionary practice in Spanish America, which appealed to the eyes, ears, and feeling. Reformers adapted this culture within clinical spaces, where it became the means by which preventive technologies might be applied.

In other ways promoters sought to harness the force of religion to move the masses to embrace their designs. Vaccination programs can be seen as a late manifestation of a mode of governance that revived religion's special role in advancing a variety of colonial projects. Beginning with the promotional works and proposals of physicians, royal attorneys, American prelates, and priests, in the indulgences proffered in pastoral letters and sermons, and through the vast coordination of expeditions and early years of practice, administrators came together to "give medicine its place" by connecting smallpox vaccine to the sacred realm—its buildings, ceremonial accouterments, rituals of thanksgiving, economy of salvation (an indulgence wiped away sin), and mystical substances—as part of a concerted effort to legitimize and consecrate its agents, instruments, and material. The descriptions do little justice to the experience, in which choreographed performances were intended as sensory lessons in the vaccine's import in relation to a wider moral universe.

Not all entrances were so grand, not all audiences rapturously attentive, not all spiritual incentives compelling for those populations that could not afford the luxury of state pageantry. From the beginning, ceremonial considerations were supplemented by others, including gifted coins, which responded to material hardship, and cookies, a savory delight. These gestures contained an element of noblesse oblige: as French sociologist Marcel Mauss wrote about the mechanisms of a gift, alms to children and the poor carry special symbolic force as a result of ideas about the generosity that underpins the ruler's right to rule. "Alms are the fruits of a moral notion of the gift and of fortune on the one hand, and of a notion of sacrifice, on the other. Generosity is an obligation," Mauss observed. "This is the ancient morality of the gift, which has become a principle of justice."[107] In colonial Mexico such obligatory gifts were not to go unrequited. A gift given and received was not the terminus but rather incited an interminable chain of considerations and reciprocities, directing sacrifices up and down the colonial hierarchy, instead of scattering them, anonymously and impersonally, throughout a body politic whose members were equally responsible for mass immunity against disease. Charity was redistributive and salvific but also politically effective: the administrator who boasted of his efforts in service to the king expected his name to appear in public papers, his family to acquire fame, his position in the colonial hierarchy to improve, and his charges to assume their role as dutiful, grateful subjects.

Tracking these "sacrifices" through the documentary record, with hymns of praise, showy parades, sugary treats, and shiny coins, leads to the realization that the colonial state, as its representatives looked to introduce foreign matter into children's bodies, relied on the repertoire of persuasive techniques that inhered in sacred and secular relations of dependency. Without the option of legal compulsion, the importation of so-called Western medical practices drew not just on statistics but on cultural resources, colonial discourses, and customary practice, including ritualized ties of paternalistic benevolence and mutual obligation between *patrón* and dependent, priest and parishioner, or *hacendado* and worker. These ties were as easily broken by selfish neglect as bolstered by shows of generosity. In August 1810 the physician in charge of weekly sessions in Mexico City's four departments reported that vaccine fluid had finally run out in San Miguel parish, just months after Juan José Guereña departed, because the children needed to propagate it were unavailable. The new priest was unwilling to continue the work of his predecessor: he only compensated the vaccinator, not the schoolteachers who delivered children, "nor the children with a *bizcocho*, as until now was custom [*se tiene de costumbre*] and was considered an effective attraction."[108]

The dilemma at the center of this study is the relative lack of testimony from those most affected—namely the lower classes, their households, and children. Vaccination campaigns did not ordinarily lead to lawsuits or criminal investigations, and as a result one common route to finding out the words, perceptions, or beliefs of laypeople is unavailable to us. If contemporaries insisted that this paternalistic universe enabled practice, registers full of quantitative data are stubbornly silent on the reasons that parents and communities opted to vaccinate. Here we have traced a path around this obstacle by considering elite notions about peasant or plebeian culture, but there are clear interpretive risks in following official commentary. Like "missionaries" of medicine and civilization elsewhere, those who helped to introduce immunization sought to transform subject populations often construed as backward, uncivilized, stubborn, or impressionable, which only intensified discourse about their capacity to adopt reform and reasons for acting.

What comes into focus is the personalism of colonial rule, expressed here as a gifting economy in which preventive medicine began to acquire its meanings and stability, in which underlying principles of redistribution and paternal indulgence were designed to structure people's interactions with public health programs. From calculated attempts to impinge on the senses in the public spectacle and festivities, to payments made to parents, to other kinds of domestication, literal and figurative, in promotional works, these strategies ran the gamut of possible solutions and reveal authorities tacking between perceptions of cultural sensitivity and susceptibility to rituals of rule—the "childlike-ness" of Indian parishioners, the simple obedience of black estate workers—and the socioeconomic hardships and anxieties that formed part of the daily realities of these groups. Somewhere between the symbolic and the material, the ornamental and the instrumental, the emotional and statistical, an unworldly gift grasped at by spectators and benefactors was made earthbound and efficacious, if only for the length of a hymn.

CHAPTER 5

Republics of Vaccinators

Everyday Expertise through the Insurgency

The vaccine porters will instruct in how to identify the pustule, the correct moment for its use, and the simple act of inoculating. For further instruction I am including three copies of a printed work that contains everything leading to the use of this excellent discovery, even though to learn it, it is enough to see it done.

—Bernardo Bonavía, intendant governor of Durango, 1804

In order to vaccinate, someone had to identify a viable source of vaccine, manipulate an instrument, make an incision, and observe symptoms. Who possessed the ability to do these things? What kind of labor was it, and how would it be compensated? Much ink would be spilled over these matters in the months before and after the Royal Philanthropic Vaccination Expedition. Appearing as a supplement to the May 26, 1804, issue of the *Gazeta de México*, a French guide and history of vaccine insisted on the procedure's accessibility: "Fathers, mothers, and caretakers or wet nurses [*amas de cría* o *nodrizas*] can practice it with the same utility and good success" as medical practitioners did.[1] Soon after, the bishop of Oaxaca composed a pastoral letter for his diocese in which he announced the availability of *punzones* (steel or flint tools) for parish priests, *vicarios* (assistant pastors), and other aficionados in medicine who wished to vaccinate. The incision was so simple, made so lightly in the skin, that "it can be done without fear and with the same felicity and good effect by fathers, mothers, or *chichiguas* [wet nurses]," he wrote, "and in fact it is an operation more proper to women for their softer hands." Glossing the Spanish *nodriza* (wet nurse) with the Nahuatl equivalent, the *carta* asserted that women possessed equal and even greater ability to vaccinate owing to their manual dexterity.[2]

Simultaneously, the regulations being written for the propagation of vaccine in New Spain insisted that only those specially approved by vaccination officials would have access to a lancet. Learning that the Crown intended to restrict practice to authorized persons, Bishop Bergosa wrote to Madrid in alarm, wondering whether he had countermanded royal wishes by interpreting practice more broadly. The letter produced a minor crisis in the Secretaría de Estado, Charles IV's executive arm, whose ministers could not at first make sense of the matter. After learning that regulations were being issued in the provinces that did in fact restrict practice, ministers split on the matter of practice. An official of the assembly (*mesa*) pronounced it prudent to limit vaccination initially to experts (*peritos*) who might instruct others and distinguish between viable and spurious vaccine. He recommended that the bishop be charged with ensuring that clergy "abstain for now from vaccinating by themselves" and instead focus on "exhorting the public to admit this admirable preservative." A second minister disagreed, noting the simplicity of the procedure. He recommended that it be made "popular y común," so that even mothers might practice it once a simple instruction was available, "as is done in many parts." Separate orders to this effect went to the bishop of Oaxaca and New Spain's viceroy two weeks later, ordering that the method be popularized in pueblos without practitioners, and even in those with them, once a simple instruction for practice was available.[3]

Scholars have located the institutionalization of modern medicine and expansion of state power in the introduction of vaccine and the juntas established to coordinate practice in Spanish America. According to this view, these institutions subjected more Spanish subjects over a greater geographic terrain than ever before to the will of the Crown in matters of public health.[4] How, when, and why to employ the new technology—and at whose hands—were matters that were seemingly more carefully delineated and controlled by virtue of having been set down on paper. As disagreement over the scope and requirements of practice suggest, however, institutionalization was a more complicated affair. Decrees and instructions that aimed to restrict the technique to trained practitioners, ostensibly to control the quality of the vaccine being disseminated, were countered by those who thought that only the most rudimentary knowledge or skill was required. From debates on the ability of mothers to vaccinate, to the proper role of amateur healers, to payment for associated costs, and the responsibility of religious corporations for public health, much of preventive medicine's meaning and practice remained open.

The realities of Mexico's political crisis only prolonged debate about who was qualified to vaccinate, and at what cost. One of the ironies of this history is that the Bourbons undertook an ambitious attempt to make vaccine universally available in the Americas just a few years before Napoleon invaded the Iberian Peninsula and toppled the Spanish monarch. The imperial crisis catalyzed movements for self-rule and independence, during which violence and economic depression engulfed New Spain's cities and countryside. Military campaigns were accompanied by recurring subsistence crises, a plunge in real wages, the occupation of towns by troops and bandits, sacked archives and vandalized buildings, drained coffers, periodic stoppages of transport, and breakdowns in communication.[5] One effect of insurrection was to make vaccine fluid unavailable in many regions and encourage practitioners to inoculate with human smallpox.[6] Judgments of immunization's worth and the emergence of routines for practice become inseparable from this setting of warfare, penury, material deprivation, and political instability.

Following a detour through Oaxaca, where difficulties funding the endeavor were especially pronounced, this chapter offers a synoptic account of the personnel who propagated vaccine as technicians, assistants, carriers, translators, and operators. Many were rendered anonymous or invisible owing to the low esteem in which their contributions were held at the time, and the ways that expertise and experimental knowledge have been evaluated since.[7] Frequently those who signed their names to registers as practitioners, certified campaigns, or sponsored sessions were assigned "authorship," rendering the identities and the nature of work of other "technicians" difficult to reconstruct. Other sources nevertheless make clear that ongoing struggles with epidemic disease, perennial shortages of funds, and the tense relationship between city practitioners and rural populations ensured that the fragmenting state depended on other healers, including bleeders, *curanderos*, and priests, for reasons of availability, affordability, and more. The capillary system by which vaccine arrived in towns and villages thus pulled more actors into the ambit of state-sponsored public health programs, in major and minor roles. The debate over qualification and access was hardly resolved in the king's executive chamber in the summer of 1805; in many ways, it reverberated in towns and villages for decades to come.

"THE RICH AND NEEDY HAVE THE SAME RIGHT"

Smallpox vaccine accorded well with the enlightened sensibilities of Puebla's intendant, Manuel de Flon. An avid reader of Europe's gazettes, from which he learned of Edward Jenner's discovery, Flon vaccinated all nine of his children at home, with vaccine fluid acquired from Louisiana via the port of Veracruz, as an example for the populace. He subsequently proved an enthusiastic supporter of the Royal Vaccination Expedition. "Distribution should be done without stipend, as a gesture of goodwill,"

Flon declared. "Nobles and plebeians, the rich and needy have the same right to it."[8] In championing these universalist precepts in Puebla, Flon furthered the objective of the Spanish state to make immunizations available to even the most socially marginal and destitute of Spain's subjects.

At the level of physical geography, this required transporting organic virus material, often in the body of a child, through harsh terrain and variable climates. The solution was to perpetuate vaccinating chains in major cities and regional centers, by means of which fluid might be kept and periodically distributed to the countryside. Juntas or committees to coordinate vaccines and vaccination were sporadically established in New Spain for this purpose. Puebla's statutes provided for a vaccination junta in each *cabecera*: district seats, it was reasoned, possessed the necessary royal administrator, priest, tax official, and residents of means to constitute committees and support vaccinations. A position was reserved for a physician, surgeon, "or inquisitive *curandero*, who never lack in the villages." This expert practitioner (*perito*), "or others who will learn to execute the operation in the *cabecera*," was to make trips to subject villages, accompanied by members of the committee, and thereby facilitate operations without having to ask burdened villagers (*aquellos infelices*) to travel to head towns. Otherwise progress would slow, "because they will resist the journey on the pretext of their need to always be employed in their jobs."[9]

Records on the establishment of subaltern juntas in Puebla's *cabeceras* document their coordination of several dozen or several hundred vaccinations each month through 1805 and 1806 (see map 4). In some cases the parish priest took responsibility for establishing the junta, as in Huauchinango. In Cholula, juntas in the *cabecera* and four outlying pueblos each had a *cura propio* (parish priest), in one instance a *cura interino* (substitute priest), as president. In Izucar the two priests (one for Spaniards and one for the majority Indian population) alternated as head, alongside the subdelegate. It was an ideal arrangement in which the clergy might not only encourage parishioners to be vaccinated but also, with their access to baptismal registers, track vaccinations against births (as stipulated in regulations) and keep records of sessions.[10] The elaborate ceremony for the establishment of Santiago Tecali's junta included the reading of statutes out loud by the subdelegate, an exegesis of the practice by the parish priest (accommodated to the audience's "limited understanding"), and communal prayers of thanksgiving.[11]

This activity was so extensive that in 1807 don José Francisco López Gamboa, *cura* of Tlaxcala, complained that subaltern juntas had been established everywhere else in the bishopric but there. As a result, nothing had been accomplished and his parishioners had not benefited from the generosity of Spain's monarch, his repeated efforts notwithstanding. Gamboa requested instructions with which physicians might vaccinate,

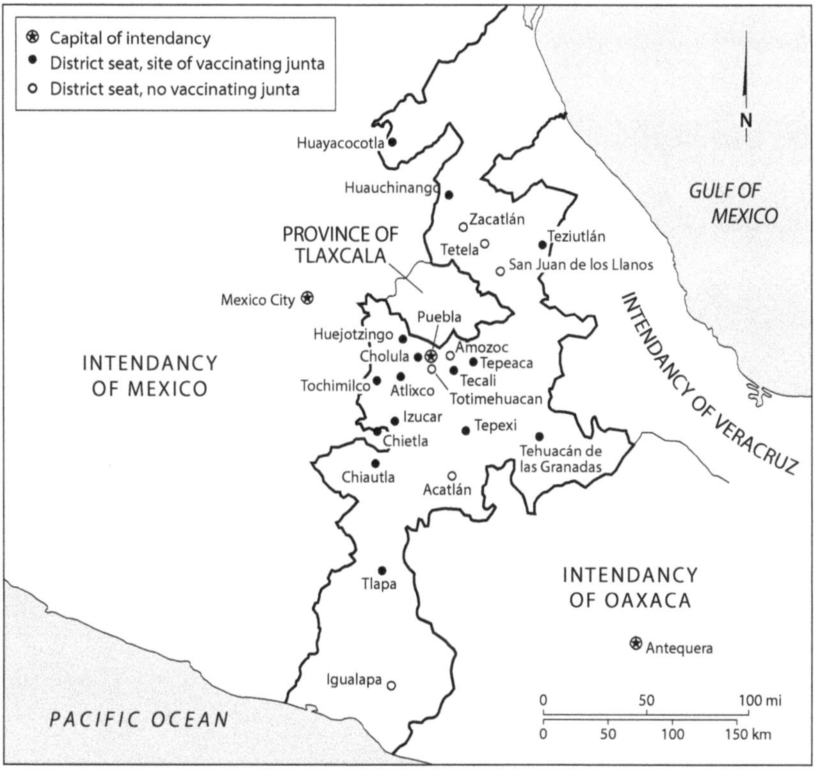

Map 4. Subaltern vaccination juntas in Puebla, 1805–1806.

offering his home and resources to cover costs. In response members of Puebla's Junta Central thanked him for his zeal and forwarded the statutes of the juntas so that he might establish one for Tlaxcala, in consultation with the district governor.[12] Thus vaccination in Puebla, under the royal administration of an avowed man of science and with dozens of priests to collect and oversee vital statistics, was partially institutionalized, if not everywhere. Documentation for several *cabeceras* is conspicuously absent; while some of the districts were small, the forty-five thousand Indian tributaries in Zacatlán and the forty-three thousand in San Juan de los Llanos apparently went without the operation for the time being.[13]

Elsewhere vaccination was practiced without these institutions by means of periodic campaigns in the countryside. In New Mexico, one of the most inaccessible provinces in the viceroyalty, army surgeon Cristóbal María Larrañaga acquired live vaccine from the commander of the Interior Provinces of New Spain in the winter of 1805 and used it to oversee

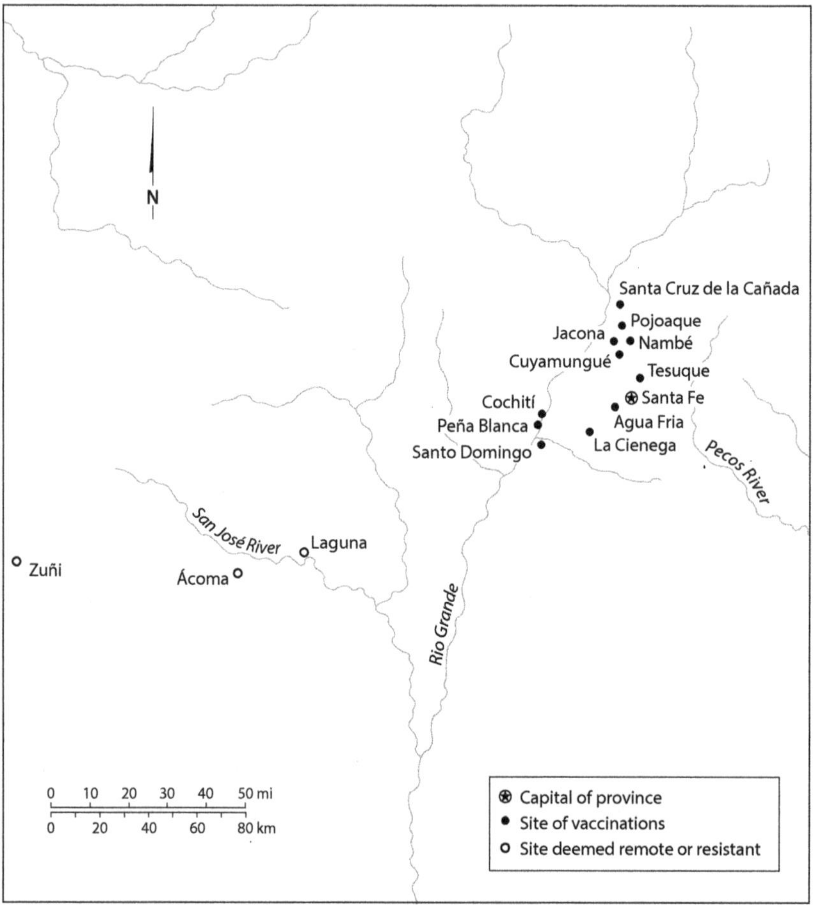

Map 5. Vaccination sessions in Santa Fe and vicinity, 1815.

some 3,610 operations. New Mexico's governor claimed success everywhere in the province, except for the Ácoma, Laguna, and Zuñi populations, as a result of their remoteness and alleged resistance to the practice. Paid for with sales tax revenue and donations, vaccinations took place yearly through 1810, followed by an interruption of several years that coincided with a period in which resources everywhere were redirected toward Spain's war efforts.[14] José Larrañaga, likely the son of the army surgeon who first introduced vaccination, took over in 1815 as practicing vaccinator. Larrañaga conducted sessions in the presidios and outlying *partidos* of the Spanish capital of Santa Fe, traveled to the southwest for

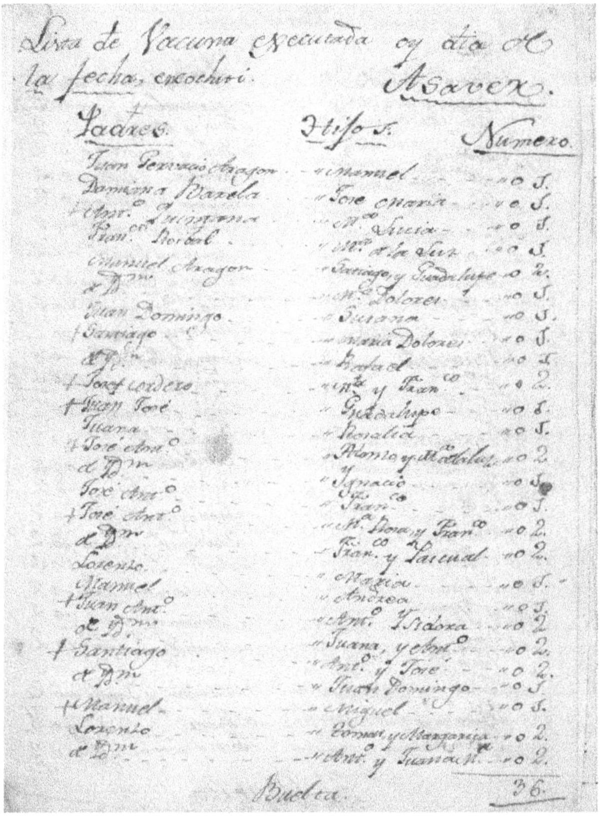

Figure 5.1 An 1815 register of vaccinations in Cochití, a Pueblo village in New Mexico. Crosses beside parents' names here and in other registers from the region probably designated affiliates of the missions, persons who had taken communion and confessed.

SOURCE: Huntington mssRI 70, box 3.
Courtesy of the Huntington Library, San Marino, California.

sessions in several mission communities and villages, and circled back north to target additional settlements in the Rio Grande river valley (see map 5).

Census records allow calculation of approximate statistics for the settlements through which Larrañaga passed. In mission San Buenaventura de Cochití, for example, 172 children were vaccinated out of some 1,310 residents (701 registered as *indios*), around 13 percent of the population; in Santo Domingo pueblo, another missionary center, 189 children represented around 16 percent of a mixed population of 1,208 (726 *indios*).[15] A high proportion of these recipients of the vaccine were Pueblo, as indicated by the absence of surnames among the parents (figure 5.1). Those vaccinated in previous sessions or infected by human smallpox were not as a rule vaccinated during campaigns, having already acquired immunity.[16] Assuming that this left only a small percentage of children available for vaccination, the percentages seen during the 1815 campaign in Santa Fe represent near-universal practice.[17] Again, however, despite regular coordination of campaigns, outcomes varied by region: those populations farther to the west of Santa Fe were apparently overlooked once more.

Yet another picture emerges in a third region, the central-western intendancy of Michoacán. In May 1808, Phelipe Díaz de Hortega reported some 25,000 total vaccinations in a jurisdiction of approximately 150,000 Indian tributaries (table 5.1).[18] Many sessions took place in the wealthier, more densely populated regions around Valladolid, the capital and seat of the bishopric; in the Purépecha basin of Pátzcuaro; and to the east in and around the villas of Tlalpujahua and Zitácuaro, whose Mazahua and Otomí speakers were some 150 kilometers from the capital (see map 6). The latter district seats were still well within the orbit of the mining economy, among the most demographically and economically important in Michoacán, in fact, as indicated by their possession of the title *villa*.[19] The registers also show that these campaigns, despite the aversion Michoacán's administrator, depended on the largesse of charitable patrons (*algunas personas caritativas*); with the drying up of alms, practice had already ceased in many places.

Meanwhile, the districts of Huetamo and Coahuayana, even more distant from Valladolid, in the poorer cotton-producing *tierra caliente* regions along the coast, lacked access to any vaccine and had been entirely neglected. The intendant confirmed that vaccination had not even been attempted there, "despite having received orders for it, because of its remoteness from this capital, extremely hot temperatures, and lack of resources."[20] Also neglected were the Tarascan speakers in outlying Pénjamo's haciendas and villages, in a more sparsely settled region of the diocese of Michoacán and equidistant from the major distribution centers in Celaya, Guanajuato, and Valladolid. Not until the summer of 1819 did an impending epidemic move its district governor to set up a provisional hospital and request permission to vaccinate, "given that residents of this district have never acquired this benefit as a result of the current rebellion." After more than a decade, a disease outbreak finally provided the impetus to immunize Pénjamo's children.[21]

Evidence from campaigns reveals variation in practice across regions but also the ways in which material, economic, and geographic factors might vary the experience within. In Michoacán, the Mazahua, Otomí, Purépecha, and Spanish communities with access to vaccination at an

Table 5.1 Vaccinations by district with population estimates in Michoacán, through May 1808.

District	*Number vaccinated*	*Indian population*
Valladolid	4,250	
*Apatzingán and outlying pueblos	471	1,848
*Ario and outlying	811	2,530
*Charo	179	2,183
Coahuayana	0	1,760[a]
Cuitzeo de la Laguna and outlying	2,210	6,887
Huaniqueo and outlying	406	2,156
Huetamo	0	9,058
*Jiquilpan and outlying	1,213	11,364
*Paracho and outlying	112	6,521
*Pátzcuaro and outlying	2,893	13,815[b]
*Puruándiro and outlying	2,978	12,218[c]
*Tacámbaro	201	680
*Taretan	75	1,532
Tiripetío and outlying	402	3,020
*Tlalpujahua and outlying	1,027	3,546
*Tlazazalca and outlying	2,314	97,44
*Uruapan and outlying	278	6,844
Zamora and outlying	1,840	5,842
*Zinapécuaro and outlying	678	7,488
*Zitácuaro and outlying	2,651	25,746
Total vaccinated to date (May 1808)	24,989	~150,000

Asterisks (*) denote places where funds were exhausted and vaccinations ceased.
Notes: a. Population of Motines substituted here, presuming that the intendant's report refers to this district.
b. Population statistics for Pátzcuaro aggregated with neighboring Erongarícuaro and Santa Clara, unaccounted for in the intendant's report.
c. Population statistics for Puruándiro aggregated with neighboring Angamacutiro, Chucándiro, Cocupao, and Huango, unaccounted for in the intendant's report.
SOURCE: AHDF 3678 exp. 17, Valladolid, May 13, 1808; and Tanck de Estrada, *Atlas ilustrado de los pueblos de indios*, 126.

early date were more populous, wealthier, and physically closer to commercial centers. Evidence is too irregular to allow generalization for all of New Spain, but it is suggestive on two points. First, in many places the majority of vulnerable populations of children were injected with vaccine matter (if not necessarily at the time expeditions passed through New

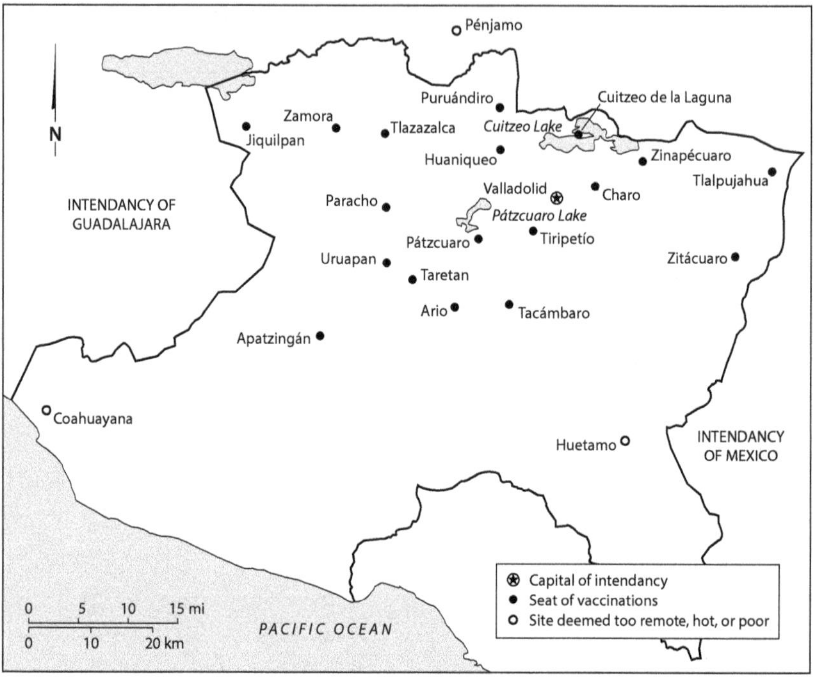

Map 6. Vaccinations in Michoacán, through 1808.

Spain in 1805 and 1806). Second, populations farthest from centers of distribution and nodes of economic activity were neglected, while smaller pueblos and villages fell off the radar after initial enthusiasm or the passing of acute disease episodes. The global aspirations of Flon and other promoters of modern medical practice were occasionally achieved, often by virtue of their efforts, but also considerably tempered in the crucible of practice.

One reason was that the preferred method of transport was costly and dangerous. Days of travel might be required along the frontier in places that were plagued by skirmishes, and the imminent dangers multiplied once the violence of insurgency engulfed the countryside. In the first year of practice, surgeons and administrators in San Miguel parish (in Mexico City), along the northern frontier of New Spain, and elsewhere were experimenting with a method reported in the *Gazeta de Madrid* in which the dried scabs of vaccinated patients were substituted for human carriers. Upon arrival at a vaccination site, the material was pulverized and rehydrated with a few drops of water and injected into the patient. Physicians and administrators found that this compared favorably with the arm-to-arm method and recommended it as a cost-saving measure to transport vaccine to the provinces and the more dispersed populations of the frontier.[22] If this solution limited costs and the danger of travel, results were mixed—administrators often struggled to reactivate the material and ended up seeking out live carriers anyway.

Vaccine's caretakers nevertheless insisted on transportation, because asking agriculturalists to journey to district seats or other administrative centers imposed too great an inconvenience. In 1807, with Mexico City's surroundings in a state of epidemic, the physician who had been commissioned to vaccinate in Texcoco sent an update to Ciriaco González Carvajal, who presided over the Junta de Sanidad, the committee established in the capital to coordinate public health response. The doctor reported 2,621 vaccinations and stressed that he had worked diligently, suffering inconveniences in his travels from pueblo to pueblo. The practice had not propagated as quickly as he wished because the Indians were not receiving it well; he noted days when only five or six had been presented to him for vaccination. Yet he saw no alternative: "consider if they had instead been called to this head town of Texcoco, inconvenienced by being made to depart their pueblos, leave their homes?" With assistance from the priest, the physician wrote, "and the reasons I give them in their manner of understanding, I manage occasionally to see a great number presented to me." For eight months of work he received 250 pesos, or 31 pesos a month, at the recommendation of the Protomedicato.[23]

If transport to the countryside was necessary, this was an extravagant cost, as officials noted in the coming years. Faced with difficult terrain and cultural, technical, and linguistic complications, administrators disagreed over the kind of expertise that was most appropriate for the task. Whether funds would come from community resources (*bienes de comunidad*) and municipal income or from another source required additional clarification at the viceregal level, but for years this too was beyond a government ensnared in insurgency movements. In the meantime, expenses mounted and administrators deliberated over the nature of the technology and the kinds of experts who might support it.

THE BURDENS OF PREVENTION: A TECHNICAL INTERLUDE

In December 1804 the city physician José Bermúdez found himself in Jamiltepec, in the cotton-producing region along Oaxaca's coast. Using vaccine brought from Juquila he began vaccinating in the district's oppressive heat, where the fluid seemed to deteriorate even more quickly. In an agreement with the district governor, Bermúdez had vaccinated in the first three of the district's fifty-seven pueblos without payment in exchange for compensation for the remainder. In January Oaxaca's intendant bragged to the viceroy that vaccinations had already been extended to pueblos adjacent to the capital, parts of Villa Alta, and a considerable portion of Jamiltepec "without incurring a single expense." In June, after 2,003 operations, Bermúdez stopped vaccinating when he received no response from the Junta Central about compensation.[24] Meanwhile vaccination's costs continued to mount. The surgeon Santiago Coda received a commission to propagate vaccine in the Mixteca Baja, the arid lowland bordering Puebla. According to Antonio María Izquierdo, the royal legal assessor, Oaxaca's vaccination junta had recommended for Coda an honorarium of 3 pesos daily, the least that might be offered in consideration of the region's difficult terrain, few provisions, and inadequate transport. With scarce municipal revenues, alternatives were discussed, including whether to solicit donations from citizens of means or pay the expense from village income. The vaccination committee had decided that communal coffers (*cajas de comunidad*) were most appropriate, reasoning that these were established for the general welfare of *indios* and that there was no good more worthy than vaccine. As for private citizens who might finance such an undertaking, "merchants cannot be considered invested in the fate of distant pueblos."[25] Through the end of 1805 Coda reported 16,983 vaccinations, and requested payment of his honorarium. Junta officials were eager to know whether the viceroy had approved the use of village funds for this and other expenses.[26]

In January 1807 the government's response arrived. It declared that communities that benefited from the propagation and conservation of vaccine should cover costs from communal properties and coffers.[27] But it left open the salary and type of practitioner, which might mean considerable expenses for communities already facing revenue shortfalls. The president of Antequera's junta, the Spanish merchant Diego de Villasante, clarified that while he and other members (*vocales*) had been underwriting vaccinations in the capital, it was not possible to collect adequate funds to transport vaccine to distant parts, thus absolving the committee of any financial commitment or responsibility.[28] In September 1808 the city's physicians and surgeons were invited by the intendant to weigh in on the matter of distribution and instruction. They advised that one of them should be sent with child carriers to each of the district seats, where he would stay to vaccinate and instruct for a month, "so that the barbers remain instructed, or whatever other practitioners are judged apt to communicate it to other pueblos." For their services they recommended a salary of 200 pesos monthly, factoring in the rough terrain (*fragoso*) and related expenses, including an assistant, pack and riding animals, and food. Izquierdo supported this plan, stressing that none of the physicians cared to leave the city for anything less.[29]

From the countryside, where poverty and variable harvests constrained the ability to support expensive professional services, these deliberations would have seemed fantastical. Reports on the status of vaccination around this time referenced the difficulty of terrain and remoteness of pueblos, the extreme poverty of rural communities, and the general recalcitrance or apathy of Indian residents. In Teozacualco district only some pueblos had been previously vaccinated owing to remoteness and high transportation costs. Teococuilco's pueblos were so far removed from the main roads that "it would have been necessary to assign its own practitioner for this purpose." Villa de Oaxaca's administrator observed that a physician could not be maintained in the pueblos because of the limited understanding (*cortas facultades*) of Indians. Despite opposition to "remedies and customs of the Spaniards," however, "they can be obligated to observe them because the result is to their benefit." After Santiago Coda passed through to vaccinate in Teposcolula, fluid had reportedly been lost in the district owing to the great apathy (*suma desidia*) of the natives, which would persist "even if a subject is once again commissioned for this interesting operation."[30] These and other assessments about geography, culture, and civilization construed the urban practitioner as impractical. Tehuantepec's official, overseeing populations too small and poor to finance the trip by tapping communal funds, instead proposed vaccinations at the expense of the royal treasury, to which *indios* in his district contributed, he stressed, as tributaries.[31]

Francisco Xavier de Balmis, who returned to New Spain in the summer of 1810 to oversee vaccinations and standardize practice, had other plans. He issued new regulations, in eighteen articles, that pursued ambitious goals: free vaccinations for all, an improved store of knowledge about vaccination by means of better recordkeeping, and weekly vaccinations in urban centers. The statutes allowed that barbers or other practitioners might transport vaccinated children from vaccination centers to outlying pueblos for propagation, with prior approval (Article 7). Nevertheless, while vaccination was so "simple and easy" that mothers might perform it themselves with greater familiarity, so benign that it could not really be considered an illness (Article 13), the new plan also insisted once again that the "most distinguished professors" be selected for official commissions.[32]

Any hardship imposed by this rule was easily resolved, according to Balmis. In provincial capitals he recommended that cathedral chapters (*cabildos eclesiásticos*), in coordination with bishops, cover costs that amounted to a small portion of the alms otherwise distributed to parishioners. In cities without these, such as Guanajuato, San Luis Potosí, and Zacatecas, mining representatives should allocate funds. Balmis reasoned that these corporations maintained a stake in public happiness (*felicidad pública*) and "will take much satisfaction in doing this good service to the King and the Patria." Additional costs incurred by annual campaigns in rural pueblos would come from rents and communal coffers; where these did not exist, subdelegates would propose whatever source was available.[33] Noting the regularity with which vaccination had been practiced in Yucatán, Balmis recommended that both Alejo Dancourt and Ciprian Blanco, practitioners in Mérida and Campeche, be commissioned for vaccinations in perpetuity, with an annual salary of 200 pesos each. Balmis proposed the same arrangement for each of the provinces of Mexico, excepting the more populous viceregal capital. (In Mexico City, Antonio Serrano, director and surgeon of the Royal Indian Hospital, and surgeon Miguel María Muñoz, were selected, with yearly salaries of 400 and 300 pesos, respectively.)[34]

With their provision for two trained *facultativos* (plus an amanuensis to keep a list of vaccinations), the new regulations, implemented by viceregal order on December 12, 1810, generated considerable expenses that appeared unnecessary and produced an immediate backlash. Mexico City's cathedral chapter informed the archbishop that its donations for the year had already been set, adding that for the past two years it had made considerable contributions to the war effort against France, and suggested as an alternative that a portion of tithes designated for hospitals be redirected toward the costs of vaccination, as practiced in Madrid.[35] The archbishop insisted that as a prelate he could not privilege alms for vaccination over many other urgent and regular needs, amounting to more than 2,000 pesos monthly.[36] Oaxaca's bishop stressed his previous efforts to introduce vaccine—a worthy endeavor, in his mind—but maintained that current hardships ruled out his financial support. (He nevertheless managed to reallocate 200 pesos originally destined for a presidio and other public works for vaccinations in the capital, refusing any further commitment or responsibility.)[37] From San Luis Potosí, José María Gómez, member of the cathedral chapter and future bishop of Michoacán, painted a vivid picture of the sacking of the city by insurgents the previous fall. They had emptied royal coffers of the little remaining silver along with the contents of the *arca de minería*, trashed the homes of Europeans, and in some instances kidnapped their inhabitants. Now, with no one willing to purchase silver, commerce was at a standstill, and the poorest of the city's miners, according to Gómez, lacked food. He would contribute from new revenue, leaving open the matter of when such contributions would be forthcoming.[38]

By 1811 imperial warfare and American insurgency provided ready-made reasons for corporate bodies to decline to cover public health costs. Manuel Abad y Queipo, Michoacán's eminent bishop, argued instead that the costs in the new plan were simply unnecessary. A supporter of liberal reforms on behalf of the poor and marginalized, Abad was also a medical savant, having read treatises on vaccination and searched for cowpox in New Spain. This placed him at odds with Balmis beginning in 1804, when the surgeon arrived in Valladolid to search for a source of vaccine among cows on the surrounding haciendas. Abad thought that Balmis had not done enough to locate a source at the time and insisted that the primary purpose of Balmis's subsequent commission in Mexico was to complete the search. The bishop repeatedly cast doubt on his work and finally delayed Balmis's departure from New Spain after the director reportedly questioned the loyalty to Spain of Abad and others in Valladolid, demanding that Balmis account for his statements.[39]

Technical disagreements about medical practice were not mere pretext for these political animosities. In their dispute Abad had the advantage of half a decade of experience with vaccination in New Spain, which he wielded mercilessly. He noted that he had established vaccinations in Valladolid prior to the director's arrival and that, when vaccine had expired on two previous occasions, he personally had acquired a new source from Guanajuato.[40] "And finally," Abad disclosed, "I myself suggested to Señor Balmis the notion that the most illustrious prelates and *cabildos* could be resorted to for the costs of vaccination in their respective capitals, but following a method much simpler, and less costly, than the one he proposes now. Although not as complicated as the one he advocated in the year 1804, it is still too complicated to be fulfilled and have permanent effect." To illustrate this, the bishop performed a calculation. Hiring the two best medical practitioners to vaccinate meant paying each 300 pesos, with an additional 100 pesos to secure the services of an extra operator, "because *facultativos* do not as a rule of thumb know how to handle a lancet," he observed, and "when one does know, he disdains the method, considering it the work of a barber bleeder [*barbero sangrador*]." Factoring in an extra 100 pesos each for the amanuensis and for incentives (*alicientes*) to entice the return visit to drain the pustule, Abad arrived at a hypothetical 900 pesos. This simply could not be sustained: "it would be paid once or twice at the outset and then forever abandoned, as has happened with the extravagant system of the first [vaccination] juntas, which survived only a few months."

By contrast, success in Michoacán boiled down to cost-consciousness. "Vaccine has been maintained here for the last five years by the simple method of entrusting it to the barber Pedro Eustaquio, with the minor cost of 100 pesos paid him, some 70 or 80 spent for a man charged with collecting the vaccinated, and gratuities for the latter."[41] In effect, this system circumvented expensive professionals (whose expertise Abad considered of little relevance anyway) and more realistically matched the technical requirements of vaccination with the skills of a practitioner.

The effect was to reduce yearly costs from nearly 1,000 pesos to less than 200. By relying on less expensive *sangradores* or *barberos* (the terms used interchangeably to refer to common bleeders), provincial capitals were able to maintain vaccine with a similarly modest budget. Anything more, Abad concluded, was an obstacle to practice.

It appears that a similar arrangement obtained in Oaxaca until the occupation of its capital. In November of 1812 insurgents arrived, and for the next sixteen months the priest José María Morelos and his rebel army ruled the city. The occupation forced the flight of officials, destroyed documents in the archive (including many of those on vaccination), and redirected municipal funds, which had supported Antequera's only vaccinating physician. (Eight months into the occupation he stopped working when it became clear that he would not receive payment.) Only in 1815, with a lull in fighting and the prospect of another epidemic, did authorities revive the conversation on public health.

Presented with a *cédula* issued by Viceroy Francisco Xavier Venegas, which resolved that bishops and cathedral chapters pay the costs of practitioners in vaccination campaigns, Oaxaca's cathedral chapter, city council, and bishop all declined to cover the expense. If these parties had not seen fit to expend a portion of rents or income prior to the arrival of the insurgents, it was less likely now owing to considerable financial hardship in the province.[42] When a viceregal decree revived vaccinations, the royalist commander and acting intendant of Oaxaca, Melchor Álvarez, found himself in an awkward position. In correspondence with Viceroy Calleja he requested a new supply of vaccine, explaining that it had been sorely needed in the previous year's smallpox epidemic, and related the difficulties he faced in securing payment.[43]

Still in exile, Bishop Bergosa objected vehemently when the royal attorney proposed drawing on revenue from confraternities to cover the costs, reasoning that they were established to care for the sick. Oaxaca's confraternities could not assume responsibility for public health (*salubridad pública*), Bergosa countered, because their concerns were more specific and the resources of even the wealthiest stretched to the limit after months of occupation and forced loans to defend the province and capital against insurgents.[44] Bergosa proposed municipal funds, as in Mexico City and Spain, where hardly a villa did not use them to retain a physician or surgeon, and complained that the request to support a physician had been made without indicating his salary or class. The prelate observed that there was an "enormous difference between maintaining a phlebotomist [*facultativo sangrador y barbero*] with 8 pesos monthly, as the bishop-elect of Valladolid [Abad] proposed, and maintaining a learned physician [*médico sabio*], as the *señor* Director of Vaccination [Balmis] proposed; for the first considerable sums of money would not be necessary, while for the second, they would." In a rare description of practice in these years, Bergosa related how in 1812 he had reestablished the vaccination junta after reading of the efforts of Puebla's bishop in the gazette. Arranging for the priests of Huautla and Tamazulapa parishes, on the border with Puebla, to bring *muchachos* to San Andrés Chalchicomula to be vaccinated, fluid was subsequently propagated by means of the *punzones* that Bergosa again distributed for vaccination, and "a great number of persons were vaccinated perfectly." Unlike Mexico City, Oaxaca did not abound in certified physicians: its faculty had been reduced to three, plus two surgeons, who were committed to vaccinating in the capital and its immediate vicinity. This meant that for distant places (*parajes distantes*) in Villa Alta and Tehuantepec they relied on the best *barberos sangradores* to vaccinate, with a surgeon designated for the Mixteca. Roaming from pueblo to pueblo, these mobile vaccinators had been maintained by parish priests, with food and shelter; by Indian *repúblicas*, with mules for transport; and by the city of Antequera, with stipends.[45] By this arrangement the province had managed to avoid the exorbitant costs that were still being needlessly imposed.

The central government implicitly endorsed this arrangement when it rejected the proposal of Antequera's city council, which declined to commit its funds to support a physician and recommended instead shifting the burden of public health onto communities by drawing from *bienes de comunidad*. Councilmen reasoned that everyone stood to benefit from ongoing vaccinations in the capital when vaccine was subsequently propagated beyond and that communal support might encourage practitioners to oversee its implementation in each district.[46] The official of the accounts office (*contaduría general*) thought it impractical to expect a single practitioner to extend care and personal assistance to all in the intendancy of Oaxaca. With its numerous villages it was simply too large to ask communities to pay for a benefit they might never see. Furthermore, anything remaining in communal coffers was destined "for the urgencies that follow seed shortages, the repair of prisons, viceregal buildings, communal edifices, churches, bridges, and other public works, and in treating epidemics [*curación de epidemias*]." While expenditures on vaccine could in theory be included in the last category, the economic method employed before—"designating two *barberos sangradores* paid by communal funds"—might be followed without needlessly burdening communities with the cost of city physicians. Villagers could not in good conscience be compelled to contribute if it meant neglecting pressing needs, and "there is no reason to make them contribute to maintaining in the capital a good that they will not enjoy."[47]

The inability to designate scarce public funds to support vaccination went to the heart of the limitations of public health in this period. From one perspective, communities should be made to spend resources on a predetermined good to prevent future disaster. At the start of 1817 the royal attorney for Indian affairs (*fiscal protector de naturales*), reviewing Oaxaca's case, noted the king's wishes for timely propagation of vaccine and recommended that the main records on its administration be appended to the dossier, indicating that propagation should continue even absent an epidemic.[48] But how much would this cost, and who would pay? From the beginning, the Crown had left open the matter, and it generated no end of headaches for Balmis. In his ongoing feud with Michoacán's bishop-elect, Balmis insisted that Abad had interfered in business about which he knew nothing; the prelate had maintained that a barber was capable of overseeing vaccine, which Balmis pronounced impossible.[49] A certain kind of administrator sought to restrict the number and type of person who might manipulate a lancet, transport vaccinated children, or otherwise toil on its behalf, in large part to control for the unpredictable effects of human bodies interacting with organic material in variable conditions.

As a result, residents were sometimes unprepared when an epidemic arrived because preparations would have incurred hardships for farmers, artisans, day laborers, and Indian *repúblicas*. Rural inhabitants were spared the inconvenience of having to travel to *cabeceras*, but they often paid indirectly, as members of corporate villages. Vaccination was in theory a legitimate use of communal resources, but in these tumultuous times it was in everyone's interest, including those responsible for the interests of the Crown, to limit the strain on finances by pursuing more economical alternatives.[50] Faced with this reality, officials at multiple levels saw fit to tackle the problem when the time came, with less expensive personnel, and through a combination of charitable donations, parish priests, and municipal governments, the solution that Spanish American prelates had favored and endorsed for years.

In 1817 Oaxaca's new intendant had yet to hear from his superiors on the matter, and the province remained in a holding pattern, merely maintaining vaccine lymph through periodic sessions. He blamed the entrance of the "rebel leader [*cabecilla*] Morelos" for the waning practice, noting that when insurgents took charge of the archive, the province had lost copies of printed regulations and of "the work published by Gener [*sic*], inoculator of vaccine, in quarto volume," which left only the slim instruction published by order of Viceroy Calleja in 1814.[51] The physicians there were generally useless, "subjects of few faculties" who required hefty salaries to vaccinate. The intendant proposed an informal vaccinating junta in Tehuantepec, to intercept disease outbreaks arriving from Guatemala, and that in other *cabeceras* a commissioned practitioner instruct "some barber" in the arm-to-arm method for propagation elsewhere.[52]

With the arrival of relative political stability, administrators in Antequera at last revived general sessions: 666 vaccinations in 1818, 417 in 1819, and 813 in 1820, according to the junta's records. In June 1819 the group of previously vaccinated children appeared with their arms scabbed over, however, "because some had torn off the mature pustule, and others, owing to their poverty, scratched their arms on the mats on which they sleep," thus ruining the vaccine and halting vaccinations for three months while it was reacquired from Puebla.[53] Might a more expensive, regular route have avoided this and other misfires?[54] Even the experts, looking to make vaccination viable across diverse geographic and linguistic terrain beyond Mexico's wealthiest cities, did not agree. While administrators at the highest ranks debated matters of skill and proficiency, similar assessments were being made on the ground, in campaigns that reflected local conditions and considered alternate sources of labor. To see how the chaos and cacophony of these years might yield an adequate and even elegant practice requires understanding these accommodations.

COLONIAL HEALERS

Taking stock of the different members of society who participated as healers, technicians, and caretakers clarifies, at a basic level, how the colonial system addressed a perennial problem of funding and personnel in a moment when the European/creole medical expert—an ideal practitioner, in the eyes of some—was simply not available, practical, or desirable. Many administrators drew on a coterie of local vaccinators instead, including barber-bleeders, parish priests, and a diverse group of amateurs who dabbled in medicine, collectively referred to as *aficionados*. At another level this focus shows what unlicensed practitioners contributed once they became involved as coparticipants in the provision of preventive medicine. Frugal authorities in Michoacán, Oaxaca, Puebla, or Zacatecas who turned to these persons not only cut costs, they made immunization feasible for their communities. These choices would have consequences for the propagation of the technique, by avoiding costs deemed unnecessary, shielding communities from potentially disruptive outside intervention, and otherwise shaping the experience of campaigns.

Physicians and Surgeons, "Most Distinguished Professors"

In spite of vocal objections, Spain's medical imperium undoubtedly relied on *facultativos*, licensed practitioners, particularly in major cities and their environs. These were "regular" practitioners not because they subscribed to any standard medical practice but because they had undertaken formal study and examination that gained them legal recognition. More often than their "irregular" counterparts, these practitioners dedicated themselves to the medical profession full-time, as the high price of admission demanded. To the extent that they monopolized vaccinations in places like Mexico City (for example, during outbreaks of smallpox in 1814), this was largely an effect of the Protomedicato's jurisdiction over professional practice there and hardly true across the viceroyalty.

The methods of regular healers did not always depart from those of the irregulars, nor did they agree with one another on the practice and introduction of vaccination. Professional rivalries and disputes manifested repeatedly, beginning in the months before Balmis and the vaccinating team arrived, when administrators in New Spain sought to propagate vaccine lymph on the basis of news in gazettes and correspondence. In May 1804 the *ayuntamiento* of Veracruz commissioned licensed surgeon Miguel José Monzón to bring a supply of fluid to Campeche. Soon after, Monzón attributed waning interest in the city and barrios to one Carlos Escofiet, a surgeon who assisted in the search for vaccine as a member of Mérida's advisory board. Escofiet was allegedly spreading the opinion that Monzón's supply was spurious (perhaps having seen a letter from Balmis arguing the same). Mérida's captain general issued a reprimand in which he reminded Escofiet that officials in Veracruz had already examined the sample and that his opinion was not required, "and much less the spread of rumors that dissuade people from being vaccinated and make them despise an operation so useful to humanity." Monzón referred to Escofiet as a "cirujano romancista"—pointedly using the term for a lower class of surgeon—and rebuked his undermining remarks ("seductivas conversaciones anti-vacunales"). He noted that Escofiet had arrived in the province from overseas before Jenner's discovery and therefore could not possibly possess real or practical knowledge ("conocimiento práctico"), never having actually seen cowpox. Meanwhile, in Campeche, "already the other practitioners of this plaza, without excluding the barbers, possess more than enough *knowledge* [*conocimientos*] to administer and propagate vaccine without need of other instructions."[55]

Possibly Escofiet was the victim of national prejudices, but it is worth noting the medical nature of their disagreement, along with remarks about what kind of knowledge counted as valuable and practical and how it was acquired.[56] The status of surgeons had risen in the final third of the eighteenth century after improved training in surgical schools, the professionalization of royal armies, and the arrival of peninsular surgeons from Spain. Yet for many, some overlap with barber-bleeders remained economically advantageous, a way for surgeons to supplement income when bleeding patients was still a popular and remunerative therapy.[57] Their involvement accorded with the contemporary view that vaccination's practice was less theoretical or erudite than it was manual and visual. As Ramón de Castro, the governor of Puerto Rico, noted in a heated exchange with Director Balmis over the efficacy of early vaccinations on the island: "here they have been very good and very beautiful, because no more science is necessary to recognize it than to have eyes."[58] This visual order rendered practice suitable, according to some, to the kind of apprenticeship that imparted instant *conocimientos*, as was standard in most medical training at the time.

These early years of humanitarian service, medical breakthroughs, and patriotic feeling occasionally moved city physicians dispatched to heal and vaccinate during emergencies to exercise their vow to treat the poor for free. When in January 1805 Tala's parish priest informed authorities in Guadalajara of an outbreak of smallpox, José María Jaramillo, certified physician, embarked with two vaccinated boys on the arduous journey to the town. The next day Tala's magistrate, informed of orders to vaccinate, issued a *bando* announcing the reasons for the group's arrival. A vaccination session was convoked at three in the afternoon at the *cura*'s home, where in the span of half an hour Jaramillo vaccinated forty of the town's children. The following morning the magistrate convened the community at the priest's home. He lauded the intendant for his generous interest in their health, conveyed the wishes of the priest that all those who had not previously contracted smallpox avoid infection by means of vaccination, and thanked the physician for working without salary or gratuity. Jaramillo took the floor to praise the beneficence of the king in sending vaccine, the vigilant response of the intendant, and the advantages and simplicity of the procedure. The next day Jaramillo returned to Guadalajara, as he wrote, "with the comfort of having fulfilled as much as I have been able the duties imposed on me by vassalage, humanity, and patria."[59] Physicians expressed these humanitarian sentiments as part of their view that vaccine was a significant medical advancement in humankind's battle against disease.[60]

More often they were compensated for their labors. In the province of Yucatán certified practitioners oversaw vaccinations for years without interruption and helped propagate vaccine to dozens of Indian pueblos in what amounted to marathon sessions. In the summer of 1806, Alejo Dancourt requested 20 pesos monthly in compensation for his work in Mérida and surrounding communities. Treasury officials opted to pay him from *propios* and *el común de indios* and set future compensation at 30 pesos monthly (the additional sum drawn from the latter source). This was justified by the fact that Indians "make up the greater part of the population, not just in this city, but rather in all of the surrounding pueblos and the rest of this province." Ciprian Blanco, vaccinating in and around Campeche, received the same, from the same sources.[61] In 1811 their salaries were moderated to 200 pesos annually, still a considerable hit to communal revenue that can be explained by the fact that Yucatán was far enough from the fighting of the insurgency years to be spared its colossal economic and political disruptions, and to override a cumbersome legal apparatus to designate funds.[62] When propagating vaccine to more distant villages in the region, the same practice was adopted. In 1817 Mérida's royal governor, citing the fact that Indians did not wish to pay the vaccinator, proposed appropriating a half *real* for every two vaccinations from communal coffers (any non-Indians would pay the same fee from their pockets).[63] When José Sebastián María González received his commission to vaccinate in the Costa Alta and Baja, he received a half *real* for each of the 8,800 *indios* vaccinated from December 23, 1817, to May 8, 1818, totaling 550 pesos.[64] Perhaps only in a region undisturbed by the vagaries of banditry and warfare could such high payments in the countryside have been sustained.

Coordinated campaigns more typically highlighted the shortage of these practitioners. In the first major drive to vaccinate in the intendancy of Mexico following the Balmis expedition, the viceroy directed local governors to cover costs for vaccinators from communal coffers in Indian villages, while non-Indians (*de razón*) and other castes would pay themselves (*de su bolsillo*).[65] Administrators in more populous centers—including Chalco, Coyoacán, Cuernavaca, Querétaro, and Tacuba (but also Chilapa, Guerrero's market center)—pledged compliance, apparently able to secure and pay a practitioner without difficulties worthy of note (Taxco boasted a physician and surgeon). At most, responses inquired into the source of vaccine or, as in Chalco and Texcoco, the salary the vaccinators were to be paid.[66]

In many instances practitioners were unavailable or deemed prohibitively expensive. The district seat of Tecpam (Guerrero), fifty kilometers up the coast from Acapulco, lacked physicians for many leagues around, and bringing one would incur exorbitant costs that erratic sources of income could not defray. There and in nearby Atoyac the health of communal coffers depended on cotton harvests, which were "so completely contingent that one cannot dictate any decisions for the reestablishment of vaccination until one comes to terms with whether or not the harvests can manage it, which will not be verified until February of next year." Also in Guerrero, Tlalchapa's official reported no medical personnel in the region ("estos países") or nearby, remarking on the great rusticity of Indians and other castes.[67] North of Mexico City, Ecatepec's official observed that it would not be easy to put vaccination into practice because there was no *facultativo* in Zumpango de la Laguna district, or any instruction in the archive. Lacking its own in Santiago Tianquistenco, a physician was brought from Toluca to vaccinate part of the European population as an example for Indian residents (who reportedly declined anyway). From the Huasteca, a region overlooked by the expedition, Yahualica's administrator reported no *facultativo* there or "in all of the Huasteca" and thought none would come from the capital "without a very large fixed salary." Without a drugstore or medications, "some old women make exclusive use of herbs from the land, to which can be added that the common food of these natives is beans, chile, and tortilla alone." He proposed that a practitioner be shared between Yahualica and surrounding districts to mitigate costs, given scarce communal resources. Nearby, Huejutla's subdelegate doubted that communal funds (amounting to slightly more than 300 pesos) would cover the cost of a practitioner from the capital. There were few residents "de razón" available to supplement, moreover, although they would be asked to contribute.[68]

While the fees actually commanded by city doctors depended on training, class, distance traveled, and market size, the expense was generally feared and studiously avoided if possible.[69] When Esteban Melgar, still administering the weaving village of Teotitlán del Valle, suggested that a physician might be sent to propagate vaccine, he specified that he leave without delay and additional expense, "because in this district seat there is a designated *barbero* who will shortly be informed of *inoculación* [*sic*], of its effects, and of the method that should be followed, and this individual can be paid at a far lower rate [*con mucho menos interés*]."[70] Others imagined that because medical practitioners specialized in matters of the body, they were unfit for the symbolic and persuasive aspects of the work. Medical officials in Mexico City advised that vaccine would not last if placed solely under the care of doctors, because "the character of *facultativos* is insufficient to move the masses, particularly those from the outskirts," even when assisted by alcaldes and other officials.[71]

Barber-Bleeders

Colonial *barberos*, or *sangradores* if they limited their work to bleeding, are invoked repeatedly in the sources on vaccination. They worked in some capacity with blood and veins, while also dabbling in tooth extraction, the application of caustics, and hair cutting. On the whole, phlebotomists were less educated, wealthy, or subject to oversight by the Protomedicato than physicians and surgeons, and less inclined to travel to Mexico City to pay 50 pesos or more for a license that would allow them to practice what many did anyway. Owing to the popularity of bleeding as a therapeutic practice and the fact that they typically charged less than their licensed counterparts, these figures provided indispensable service to people of all social classes and backgrounds.[72]

A role for the colonial barber was written into the earliest statutes for vaccination, particularly in the less populated peripheries of New Spain. Durango's regulations ordered *barberos* named by physicians to attend vaccinating sessions for instruction, so that they might transmit fluid to other pueblos ("instructing in them others of their profession"). This was because the only physicians in the province were in the capital or the military hospital of Chihuahua.[73] In Nueva Vizcaya the commander of Interior Provinces remarked on the "absolute lack of physicians and surgeons" as the principal obstacle to propagating vaccine in other towns, villages, haciendas, and ranches. He ordered the military surgeon in Chihuahua's hospital to train (*adiestrar*) not only its practitioners but also "the bleeders and barbers" there and in the presidios of Nueva Vizcaya.[74] According to one study, those entrusted with vaccine belonged almost exclusively to the personnel of the military hospital. If so, this would explain why, between 1804 and 1809, the thousands vaccinated in Nueva Vizcaya concentrated in and around the most important *ayuntamientos* of Parral and Chihuahua, while carriers sent beyond Chihuahua attended primarily to the populations of military presidios and ignored the indigenous sierra to the west.[75]

Administrators elsewhere came to similar conclusions about the usefulness of barbers and called on them to transport and vaccinate in places deemed distant. By the summer of 1807 vaccine still had not arrived in Huajuapan, a commercial hub in Oaxaca's Mixteca Baja, which encouraged its district governor, together with its priest, to pay for a bleeder and four children to bring vaccine from Chila, in neighboring Acatlán (Guerrero), and operate in the district's four *doctrinas*. The official clarified that "we have been vaccinating with our own hands," but with numerous other duties he and the priest simply could not preserve vaccine in the town. The practice was to be renewed yearly, presumably by relying on bleeders again in the future.[76] In Celaya, where several towns managed to pay a physician or surgeon to acquire and propagate vaccine, Acámbaro's district governor instead paid a barber named Pedro Camargo to travel to Celaya, roughly twenty miles away. Apparently the majority of parents were unwilling to compel their reluctant children to submit to vaccinations, and the pueblo lacked the funds necessary to continue the operation.[77]

In the summer of 1807 an outbreak of *fiebres pútridas* in the valley of Tacuba struck Tecamachalco, a pueblo of Indians ("de puros indios") two rough, insurmountable leagues from the district seat, as described by the district governor. Ciriaco González Carvajal, as head of the central vaccination committee, ordered vaccinations in imitation of those recently implemented in nearby Cuautitlán, and noted the many barbers in the region available to take one or two child carriers to vaccinate in surrounding villages.[78] In effect, one from Tacuba arrived at Mexico City's San

Miguel parish on July 13, 1807, to coordinate the transportation of children, and the following week four barbers in the district received commissions to vaccinate. Tacuba's administrator described the arrangement: "I have offered to compensate [*gratificarles*] the four *barberos* who will leave from various villages next Monday for each hundred vaccinated, in spite of my scant resources, which is the best proof of my effort." How much he did not disclose, but presumably less than a certified physician would have needed to perform such demanding work.[79]

During months of insurgency, as vaccination fell into neglect and disuse, multiple healers worked in tandem to revive it.[80] The struggle in Valladolid (Michoacán) was especially prolonged. According to intendant Manuel Merino, fluid ran out in 1811 when insurrection cut communication with Mexico City. Vaccine was reacquired in August 1814, when the spreading epidemic compelled Merino to resort first to inoculation, then vaccination with fluid obtained from a village in the Bajío. On this occasion Francisco Córdoba, a licensed surgeon, injected the vaccine, assisted by several *barberos* and the 1810 regulations composed by Balmis—the only guidelines available owing to the archive's disarray. In March 1817, spurred by Viceroy Apodaca's revival of monthly vaccinations, Merino wrote Mexico City to request a fresh supply, which arrived in vitro rather than in the arms of child carriers. In Merino's home vaccinations overseen once again by Córdoba used up all six vials without indication of success. After another was depleted with the same result, Merino requested a new supply but indicated that this time he would have "distinct subjects" perform the operation, in case failure was the fault of the two certified vaccinators he had used. "Although those I am thinking of making use of are not *facultativos*, but rather *barberos*," he disclosed, "who administered inoculation and vaccination in former periods with good effect. Here there are no more of the first than the two who have been vaccinating." This time the vaccinations took, and on November 15 two boys were brought from Zinapécuaro, thirty miles east of Valladolid, to continue propagation in that direction. Merino vowed to do his best to bring it to those places where insurgents were not in control (at the end of the month the last batch of vaccinated children returned with their pustules destroyed, and vaccine was lost again).[81]

Many circumstances were out of the control of these officials and practitioners. It was thought, for instance, that the vaccine material dripped into vials or coated onto glass slides might be vitiated, its virtues depleted, in hot climates or seasons.[82] As in Valladolid, this led administrators to consider proper technique, with barbers and surgeons thought to possess special dexterity as a result of their manipulation of surgical instruments. The former were sometimes casually classified with the latter, as when in 1807 the district governor of Huamelula (Oaxaca) lamented that nothing had yet been achieved owing to lack of "cirujano, barbero, ni otra persona útil" in his jurisdiction to oversee vaccinations.[83] The correlative was that some commanded fees as high as their more prestigious counterparts, particularly when they had far to travel. In 1807 Villa Alta's administrator specifically invoked a phlebotomist ("maestro barbero u otro facultativo") from the provincial capital to transport child carriers, which would hardly have been inexpensive.[84] In 1806 the vaccination committee in Zacatecas reported that 2,448 vaccinations performed by a licensed bleeder earning 20 pesos monthly had exhausted municipal funds (another 10 pesos monthly were paid for the porter).[85] These persons were sometimes as esteemed and costly as their more prestigious colleagues, which necessitated other less expensive, if not necessarily less desirable, practitioners.

Curanderos *and Aficionados*

Stark racial and caste divisions, strict blood purity requirements, and the high cost of licensing in the viceroyalty meant that most who healed in the countryside never secured authorization to do so via any state mechanism. In the conventional interpretation the medical establishment tolerated informally trained and unlicensed healers because it lacked the ability and will to enforce regulations in Indian towns and villages. Sometimes the Protomedicato even profited from collecting fines generated as these healers plied their trade.[86] Rural residents did not in any case have the means to afford the services of university-trained and licensed practitioners, who typically preferred to reside in cities. Instead they looked to a large cadre of irregular healers and empirics, often trusted members of communities, esteemed to extract a tooth, birth a child, set a broken bone, or cure a cold without gouging the patient in the process.

The records of Mexico's Inquisition, charged with stamping out unorthodoxies in practice, confirm that these figures belonged to social networks whose therapies were verified by reference to shared norms and expectations, even if the source provides few clues about the roles they assumed in public health campaigns.[87] The enlightened journalist and physician José Ignacio Bartolache, a frequent collaborator with the viceregal state on matters of disease control, indicated the importance of kinship when complaining about the influence of lay healers on his patients: "Those who would abhor a medication prescribed by a learned physician consume the most absurd and unwise concoctions by order and hand of their *comadres* [godmothers], no matter the cost."[88] If the homespun methods of these women lacked formal training, the term *comadre* evoked a relationship that could not be learned or reproduced through books. The distinction between "ontological" and "prudential" expertise, suggested by the historian of science Steven Shapin, illuminates the kind of trust they enjoyed. The learning of physicians, who formed notions about the underlying order of sickness and health from theories of ultimate causes or qualities, was bookish; it carried a whiff of prestige for those who recognized such expertise as authoritative but might nevertheless seem "unreliable and unverifiable" to their patients.[89] Irregular healers, on the other hand, possessed expertise that stemmed from accumulated experience, sound judgment, and practical action on sick bodies, and it did not hurt that they were like family.

In epidemics, irregular healers were valued mediators and experts, not merely tolerated or overlooked. In 1796 Tehuantepec's district governor, Pedro Fessar, dispatched one Faustina Baleria, resident of the district seat, to heal in the smallpox outbreak in Tequisistlan, in the Chontal region to the east. He described her as of good comportment and in possession of "the singular gift to heal smallpox," citing her previous work healing and inoculating children in Santiago Lachiguiri pueblo, "as well as those she inoculated in this Villa, under the direction of the captain don Luis Joseph de Ribas." The Zapotec inhabitants of Lachiguiri were said to have received inoculation compliantly; for her work there alongside its schoolmaster, Cipriano Villalobos, Baleria was compensated 32 pesos. In Tequisistlan, where more than forty children were inoculated daily, Baleria was joined by another woman from the district seat, a doña named Ramona de Cuebas, who had previously inoculated in Santa María Guenagati (also in the Sierra Zapoteca).[90]

When the gazette reported on the campaign in Villa de Tehuantepec, the article credited only Joseph de Ribas, a Spanish merchant and prominent citizen. He became the "author" of its success, and Baleria's contributions were rendered invisible. Such erasures complicate our perception and understanding of these unlicensed healers, who clearly brought technical expertise and healing knowledge to outbreaks and whom officials deemed qualified and able to inoculate. Suggestive of their importance in Tehuantepec, for instance, is the way that inoculation elsewhere ran up against repeated difficulties. In San Juan Guichicobi the schoolteacher and administrator of taxes, Rafael Melo, attempted inoculations with the parish priest and his *teniente*. When residents reportedly closed their doors to Melo and left with their children for an outlying settlement, Fessar cited the *rusticidad* of its Mixe Indians, and not so much the men as the women, who "do not socialize with others and rarely leave their village and as such are immune to reason [*son incombencibles a la razón*]."[91] Following this logic, in which women were more closed off to the outside world and impervious to the model of schoolteacher, priest, and Indian governors, scholars have adduced differences in ethnicity and economic activity to explain varied dispositions toward inoculation: the fact that many Zapotecos of the sierra, including residents of Guenagati and Lachiguiri, produced and trafficked in cochineal (red dyestuff) meant relatively more exposure to trade and to the cosmopolitan world beyond.[92]

Though more distant, the Mixe of Guichicobi also traveled to the Villa de Tehuantepec and were not in any case decisively opposed to immunization. After another resident of the district seat experienced a similarly violent rejection when he arrived to inoculate, Juan de Iriarte, a *teniente de milicias*, prevailed. Perhaps it was because he embodied military authority or, as Fessar reported, because "he went supplied with various simples [medications], to show them that he had them, and with this incentive incline them to allow themselves to be healed and inoculated."[93] In Iriarte's account, after some negotiation he was allowed to send for *curanderas* from an unnamed barrio to heal and persuade others to be inoculated. Not otherwise identified, these women healers were deemed indispensable in converting Guichicobi's villagers—not after all as closed-off, closed-minded, or uncosmopolitan as some insisted.[94]

Evidence that practical knowledge of smallpox and its cure was indigenous to Mexico by this time comes from a report from San Antonio de Oquitoa Mission in the Pimería Alta, Sonora (published in the gazette in 1799), which boasted that inoculation in smallpox outbreaks "is so ancient in these missions that it can be considered immemorial." Elderly residents told of having been saved by the procedure or performing it, alongside *gentes de razón*, by injecting it—"inserting smallpox [*metiéndolas*] (that is how they put it)"—into the legs of the immunized.[95] By then, several guides to practice were available in the colony, including copies of the instructions prepared by José Flores for "rustic people," which turned up in rural places.[96] The simple instruction authored by the Protomedicato in 1797 appeared not only in the pages of the gazette but arrived in pamphlet form in nearly every parish of the archbishopric of Mexico, terminating some two hundred miles away at Pánuco. After directing priests to request God's mercy with prayers, Archbishop Núñez de Haro drew their attention to the printed instruction. The largest parishes were to keep a copy in the archive, while others were to record the text in the parish books so that they might instruct themselves and "exhort and persuade" parishioners to practice. In a few parishes the circular arrived without a copy of the instruction, while not all pastors were sanguine about the procedure's introduction. One referred to "abusos, tonteras, etc." among parishioners (San Pedro Actopan), another to ancient customs (San Gregorio Atlapulco), as likely obstacles. These exceptional comments were likely inspired by Milpa Alta's pastor, Rafael Valencia, who described an earlier attempt to implement the healing method endorsed by Dr. Bartolache, only to find that his flock continued "following the orders of their *curanderos* and taking herbs" instead.[97]

While there was skepticism, the contents of the instruction can be read as evidence of what some medical and religious authorities thought possible in matters of public health in the less administratively central places where vaccine eventually arrived.[98] At just under seven pages the pamphlet was, as its authors stressed, a grossly simplified version of medical practice, translated for the layperson on the basis of a simple premise: there were communities in New Spain that lacked even the basic skills of an unlicensed bleeder or the knowledge of aficionados or *curiosos*, who had acquired sufficient understanding to inoculate by studying the "many common works [*opúsculos vulgares*]" in circulation. Informed by a humoral view of the body, the text addressed the proper preparation of children, the use of a lancet or needle to inject smallpox superficially into the hollow between the first and second fingers of each hand, and the importance of allowing the ensuing mild infection to run its course.[99]

As elsewhere, simplifications in technique and shortened preparation times encouraged reliance on a broader swathe of society, including amateur inoculators and even parents, to take up an instrument and perform the required maneuvers.[100] Resembling the 1797 method in tone, the French work on the "origin and discovery of vaccine," appearing in Spanish translation in Mexico's gazette, informed readers that vaccination was a major safety improvement over inoculation. Published before the expedition's arrival, it instructed in the depth and location of the incisions on the arms, how to insert the fluid, and how to identify viable pustules. An *estampa* at the end transposed these instructions into a visual register (figure 5.2). The print illustrated the shape and width of the needle to be used—a needle being preferable to a lancet because it was less likely to scare the children—and distinguished the correct appearance of pustules (*granos*) from a spurious case. Instructions were being made available in the gazette "with the aim of conveying this news to the entire Kingdom," the prologue announced, and in conclusion offered a digest of frequently asked questions.[101] Portions of the text were reproduced in the pastoral letter remitted to parishes in Oaxaca's diocese.

More expensive volumes arrived with the expedition. Five hundred copies of Jacques-Louis Moreau de la Sarthe's *Tratado histórico y práctico de la vacuna* (Historical and practical treatise on vaccination), translated by Balmis, were distributed in the Canary Islands, Asia, and Spanish America. In 1810 an additional 389 copies were printed and distributed to New Spain's thirteen intendancies. The new regulations on vaccination endorsed the work, to "make uniform" the instruction and practice of vaccinators (Article 8). Mexico's intendant passed his sixty-four copies to subdelegates with orders that in places without a practicing physician or surgeon they be placed in the archive and made available to parish priests

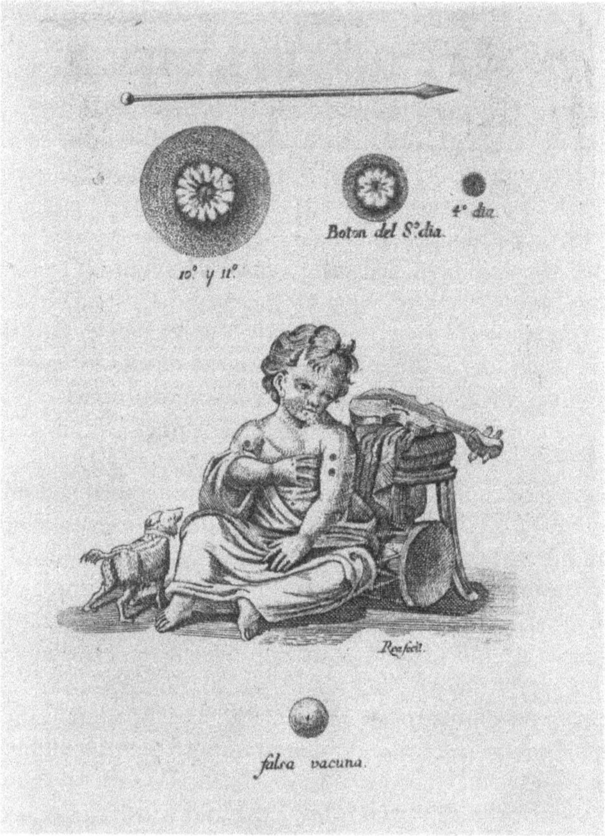

Figure 5.2 Engraving of vaccinated child with illustrations of needle and pustules. This illustration appeared in the May 26, 1804, issue of the *Gazeta de México*, showing the correct appearance of vaccine pustules on days four, eight, and ten/eleven as well as a spurious case.
SOURCE: Courtesy of the Huntington Library, San Marino, California.

and residents of learning, who might use them to advise the pueblo of vaccination's benefits.[102]

The statutes of Puebla's Junta Central stipulated that that each subaltern junta receive a copy of the *Tratado histórico*, as part of a mission to inform elected officials and elders of pueblos about the nature of vaccination so that they might help to persuade their communities to participate. Not only would the treatise provide the necessary knowledge of vaccination to communal leaders, the *estampa* following the author's

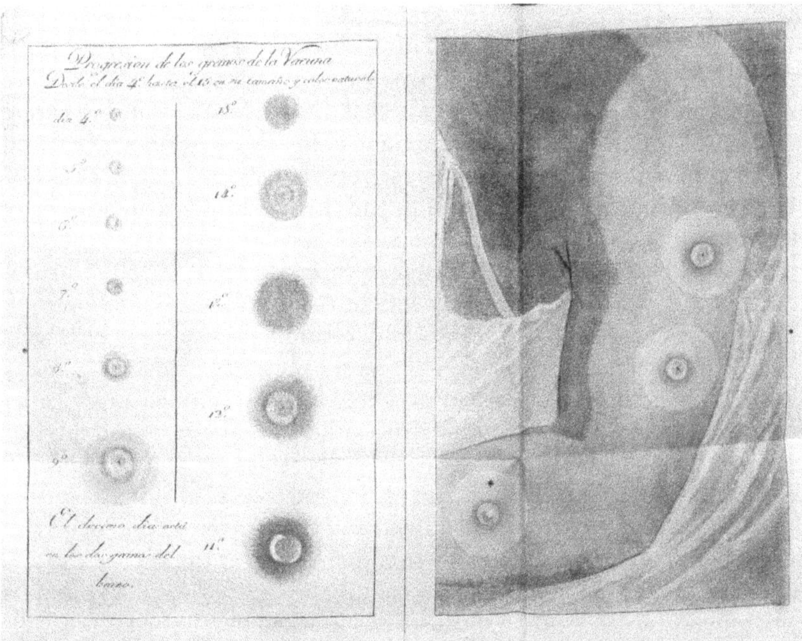

Figure 5.3 Color diagram of the progression of pustules. This 1803 illustration appeared as a foldout in Moreau de la Sarthe's *Tratado histórico y práctico de la vacuna.* Hundreds of copies of the volume were distributed in New Spain, apparently used as a guide to practice or to encourage parents, or stored in district archives.
SOURCE: Courtesy of the John Crerar Library of Medicine, University of Chicago.

prologue—referring to the fold-out color illustration—was called an "instrument" by which to demonstrate to *indios* both the small size of pustules and the minimal inconvenience to which they would subject their children (figure 5.3). The book was to circulate for viewing and be placed in the district archive for safekeeping.[103]

Also probably referring to the *Tratado histórico,* in August 1804 Bernardo Bonavía, Durango's intendant, sent provincial officials three copies each of a printed work on vaccination with orders announcing the arrival of vaccine carriers. Although it sufficed to observe the procedure to learn it, Bonavía noted, the work might provide further instruction. One copy was to be placed in the archive after it was read aloud in a meeting of residents, the other two distributed between the priest and principal residents. The intendant went on to refer to the numerous female healers who charitably applied their homemade remedies (*remedios caseros*) to the sick poor. He hoped they would do the same "in the application of this preservative" and be rewarded for their work by those with means.[104] Whether he wanted these women to observe and practice the procedure as well is ambiguous; possibly he expected them to work as nurses, caring for children once they had been vaccinated. In any case Bonavía believed that people without any formal education, including women, would be involved through an apprenticeship, and that written instructions were largely superfluous for the undertaking.

Practical experience in this visual culture was often acquired by observing other practitioners: to the extent that medical instruction took place far from anatomical theaters and lecture halls, vaccinators largely followed this pattern. Physicians in general campaigns made use of many assistants, whether they were in principle open to popular practice, as geography dictated the need to instruct others to take responsibility for the procedure beyond cities and district seats. This was acknowledged in disparaging comments about the vices, incompetence, or unreliability of these healers, who were quickly trained and from lower on the social ladder. In Ixmiquilpan, the surgeon wrote the viceroy at the end of 1804 to report on the grave necessity of vaccination in light of the many infants (*parvulitos*) recently born in the district. He asked that he be granted sole responsibility for vaccination, because in three years he had witnessed the excesses committed by various practitioners, "some for their lack practice and studies and others for their compete lack of knowledge of the climate." The surgeon feared further infection if anyone besides him operated.[105]

Charges of incompetence were leveled at so-called aficionados especially, a term that sometimes suggested a dilettante approach believed to be inappropriate to medical practice. In Miahuatlán, Oaxaca, between the coast and the provincial capital, the district governor reported 6,753 vaccinations over the summer of 1810 with the help of certified phlebotomist José Nestor Cortés (more than 1,100 in the district seat, the rest by Cortés in surrounding villages). Things had gone to plan, for which the official credited the care he had personally taken to see that the operation was performed by "a trained [*práctico*] and intelligent man like the expressed Cortés, and not by one of these aficionados who, making the incision too deep, spurt blood so that the lymph comes out, or who have the pus on their finger when they press the incision. And in sum because they are not trained in it they make many involuntary mistakes."[106] Licensed phlebotomists like Cortés were less likely than physicians or surgeons to be of "legitimate" birth, pure racial ancestry, or literate (when Cortés was examined and licensed in 1805, one of the three witnesses identified his parents, both orphans, as reputed *mulatos*).[107] In comparison, the practitioners condemned in the report were even more likely to reflect the mixed racial composition and low literacy levels of colonial Mexico.

If criticized as deficient in experience, training, or skill, they were often indispensable figures of medical authority. Regulations for Puebla stipulated that in those provinces in which governors were ladino (referring to acculturated Indians) and "expertos," they would be given places on the subaltern juntas and allowed to vote. The document referred specifically to Cholula, Huejotzingo, Tehuacán, and other unnamed districts and added that the same could be done in less civilized (*menos civilizados*) pueblos according to circumstances. In an exceptional case one subaltern junta in Puebla listed, in addition to the parish priest and subdelegate, the Indian governor, Julian de la Luz, in the role of *piadoso y curioso curandero* (pious and inquisitive healer). Also called an "aficionado" in medicine, he would have been a prominent community member whose healing experience qualified him to look after *salud pública*, which entailed vaccination in this moment.[108] Disease episodes further helped administrators to forget that restrictions had been placed on practice. In 1814, Mexico City's *ayuntamiento*, trying to forestall smallpox, notified the viceroy that it would increase vaccination's frequency and that it had advised surrounding municipal councils to send children for the procedure. The capital's vaccination junta would oversee it, along with instruction of "the subject who brings them in the manner of performing the operation," so that they might immunize their pueblos as well.[109]

The inquisitive healers selected for training and propagation were nevertheless among the most acculturated, considered already part of the Spanish world. When the government propagated vaccine beyond Mérida in the spring of 1817, *mozos inteligentes* (learned young men) arrived in the capital to train under Alejo Dancourt. A rare acknowledgment of his technical assistants (who were still not named), they performed the procedure in his presence, received advice and instruction, and returned to their villages to vaccinate.[110] Who were they? What did they think of their commission? Many trained physicians saw themselves as missionaries of medicine, but like even the most precocious polyglots of the religious orders they lacked sufficient time, resources, or patience to travel personally to places in need or acquire local dialects beyond superficial forays. They relied instead on people better versed in languages and politics, such as these *mozos* and Indian governors, to manipulate vaccine and transmit the technique by the influence they were assumed to wield in their communities.

These ongoing campaigns raise a category quandary in respect to the ideal types that appear most often in the sources. The meeting minutes of Puebla's Junta de Sanidad in the pestilential years of 1812, 1813, and 1814 are a record of frustrations with apothecaries for reportedly filling prescriptions haphazardly or dispensing the wrong drugs and an array of anonymous *curanderos* for healing without prior training, certification, or permission.[111] The label *curandero* might refer generally to someone who healed but also denote more specifically an indigenous or *casta* healer or even some other aficionado—a creole tailor or merchant, for example—who lacked formal medical training. In Tecali, Puebla, the two individuals appointed to serve on the vaccination junta, both carrying the title "don," were first announced as phlebotomists who worked as surgeons ("maestros barberos que hacen oficio de cirujano"). Later they appear as *curiosos aficionados*.[112] Whatever their title, some prior experience wielding a surgical needle most likely qualified the men for the post. Meanwhile, the "poor" physicians or surgeons invoked in sources probably did not have the means for a license. These and other considerations cast into doubt the boundaries of the categories in common but imprecise use. Some of the distance between licensed and unlicensed (and allegedly subversive) healers is closed in these struggles with disease prevention, when shared functions and acquired training not only complicated the available terminology but helps explain how vaccine infiltrated so far—and also why discernment of these ostensibly distinct categories is so difficult in retrospect.[113]

For reasons that were economic, geographic, and cultural, the colonial system drew on a considerable range of local proficiency to make viable its utopian project. In light of this observation, a body of literature arguing that New Spain's licensing practices and professionalization had the effect of excluding or restricting the sphere of action available to midwives, *curanderos*, bleeders, and indigenous healers requires modification.[114] Attempts to prosecute unlicensed practitioners, especially in cities, abound in Mexico, and often followed Bartolache in casting aspersions on the abilities of *comadres* and other undocumented prescribers. But these healers, who so often become visible to us in Inquisition records—wielding peyote, crosses, Catholic prayers, and liturgical paraphernalia—were not only persecuted as subversive, superstitious, or heterodox. To the extent that public health programs drew on their skill and labor, suppression, marginalization, and mere tolerance is only part of the picture. Unlicensed practitioners remained relevant, not because regulatory institutions lacked the resources to fully police and silence these threats but because they were not always seen as such.

Priests: "Curanderos *Closest at Hand*"

In Acayucan, Oaxaca, the Parisian surgeon Francisco de la Barrera was denounced to the Inquisition for blasphemy in 1760 by two of his clerical competitors: a friar who was said to covet the surgeon's medicine chest, and a diocesan priest who had been refused a supply of opium by the surgeon for his own medical practice.[115] The colonial priest's dual functions as caretaker of body and soul were inscribed in colonial healing manuals that associated religious men with charitable healing of the body, in hospitals and on the frontiers.[116] In the eighteenth century, convent hospitals in Guadalajara, Mexico City, Puebla, Valladolid, and other cities and towns remained staffed with friars from the religious orders, usually assisted by a small team of nurses and the occasional physician. The mission of the order of San Juan de Dios actually committed friars to heal the poor and travel beyond the convent's walls in search of alms and patients. In response to reports from Izucar that Pedro Paez, a friar with a history of insubordination, had undermined the hospital's prelate, Joseph Benavides, *comisario* of San Juan de Dios in Mexico City, tried to have the wayward Paez transferred on grounds that he did not have even minimal knowledge of medicine. Izucar's subdelegate opposed the transfer and defended Paez as an indispensable healer. Benavides consented to allow Paez to remain in the role of nurse on the pretext that a friar who practiced medicine without authorization would bring Benavides into conflict with the Protomedicato.[117] The subdelegate's response is telling: "we must realize that necessity lacks norms [*Ley*], and that in this place there is much necessity as a result of not having in the entire jurisdiction a single physician, or even a surgeon. This obliges one to make use of the *curandero* who is closest at hand, as the padres of San Juan de Dios regularly are." Their mere inclination toward charity, he thought, qualified some of these friars to meet the demand.[118]

Alonso de la Peña Montenegro's *Itinerario para párrocos de indios*, the widely read manual for pastors of Indian parishes, makes no mention of immunization, which was not widespread at the time of its final (1771) edition. Its focus was on the practice and meaning of the sacraments and the role of the parish priest, who was cast as judge, teacher, and physician (*médico*). The last referred primarily to his capacity as healer of ailing souls, a duty that was sacramental, with penance according to one's sins prescribed as the remedy.[119] Nevertheless, the manual instructed the *cura* to place himself at the center of everyday affairs, to "govern his subjects not only in spiritual matters but also in the temporal, and everything that leads toward the welfare and benefit of their souls."[120] In the 1760s, Bourbon reformers sought to challenge the priest's intermediary position between communities and higher secular authorities, through rules about parish fees and administrative restructuring to expand the sphere of the secular state and circumscribe sacerdotal functions. The reformist view envisioned priests in their parishes as teachers but not judges, an activity reserved for royal or secular courts.[121] "Especially in emergencies," however, as historian William Taylor has noted in his study of eighteenth-century parish life, "the curas were called back toward their traditional roles by royal governors and prelates."[122]

They were recalled as healers of bodies on a massive scale during the 1785 epidemic and food shortage in Mexico. On that occasion Valladolid's bishop prepared loans of 1,000 pesos to distribute by means of priests to poor parishioners to plant maize. "In one word," he admonished in a circular, "you are by your example as parish priest Father of your Parishioners, their Tutor and Protector."[123] Months of famine, epidemic, and drought saw priests in their parishes making seeds available for planting, establishing hospices for the sick or poor, and other acts of charity and care.[124] In the 1797 smallpox outbreak, when the viceroy reestablished the Junta de Caridad to collect and distribute alms for the poor and destitute, he distinguished between parishioners whose ailments required only spiritual care, and those who required also temporal care; the spiritual came first, but priests were to assume responsibility for both.[125] In the frontier town of Monterrey, a settlement of some four thousand inhabitants, the governor put Franciscan friar Antonio de la Vera in charge of the hospital established for the poor in 1798. Referred to, in a *relación de méritos* (report of merits) submitted by the city's *cabildo* to the king following the epidemic, as sole medical practitioner ("único facultativo de medicina"), the friar purchased remaining medications for his own pharmacy (for 46 pesos) when the provisional hospital was disbanded.[126] If priests did not exercise medical authority exclusively, in their performance of sacramental duties—above all baptisms, last rites, and burials—sickness and healing remained unavoidable experiences, even as their position in public life changed.

Given his perceived influence, it is hardly surprising that the priest was written into public health measures. The plan for a vaccinating expedition to the Indies designed by Guatemala's *protomédico* placed priests, the church building, and Catholic liturgy at the center, as the means by which appropriate gravity and esteem would be transferred to vaccine and vaccinators.[127] In his 1804 pastoral letter, Puebla's new bishop addressed *curas* on "the influence that your words and example have on public opinion" and sermonized that these would help fulfill the king's wishes to propagate vaccine.[128] The prelate stipulated, however, that in the event that Indians resisted vaccination, or subjects capable of the procedure should not be found, "priests and ministers have to practice it themselves, in the same way that they perform and are obligated to perform Caesarean sections, though [in the latter] owing to the more specific obligation imposed by the spiritual life of the young [*prole*]."[129] Oaxaca's bishop espoused a similarly expansive interpretation of pastoral duties, making available instruments for vaccination and exhorting the clergy not to ignore the value of this "precious discovery" and "sure remedy" against smallpox for the physical and spiritual health of their parishioners. "God would not allow among you one so indolent to believe himself not obligated," he wrote, "and to dare to say crudely that he is physician of souls, and not of bodies, because he would prove his ignorance and lack of charity." Like all humankind, the priest was created to protect the life of his neighbor, and "he would not be a good spiritual physician of souls, who so easily able did not try to conserve the bodily life of his parishioners."[130]

These injunctions, and the institutional culture of which they were part, did not always line up with the proposals, decrees, and instructions formally issued for vaccination, as Oaxaca's bishop soon realized. In practice, priests nevertheless followed their instincts, their training, or local custom. At the end of 1804, Tehuacán's pastor lamented that of twenty thousand souls in the district, not even two hundred had been vaccinated during Alejandro García Arboleya's jaunt through the region before vaccine was carelessly lost. Seeking to discharge his duties as *sacerdote* for the public good, the priest located a supply nearby and requested that the viceroy commission physician José Mariano Castro, or another resident, to transport it, and recommended the prior of the Convento del Carmen, certain that the friar could manage the operation.[131] Before Oaxaca's bishop ordered it, Juan Nepomucena, Teotitlán del Camino's pastor, took charge of vaccinations himself. After inspecting Arboleya's 187 operations, Nepomucena identified and revaccinated seven unsuccessful cases and performed another twenty-five, according to the district governor. The priests of Huehuetlan and Huautla parishes arrived in the district seat to bring vaccine by means of two boys to their own parishes. Three years later, Nepomucena informed the newly installed district governor that he had continued vaccinations in Teotitlán, Huehuetlan, and Huautla, but that because the practice had not been extended to adjoining jurisdictions, "the seed [*el Germen*] ran out once there were no more children capable of receiving it." The implication was that all susceptible children there had been vaccinated—a feat that largely depended on the activity of a single vaccinator-priest, who now vowed to request vaccine from Oaxaca's junta to revive the practice.[132]

Parish priests were cultural mediators as well. When Toluca's surgeon wrote the viceroy for permission to propagate vaccine to villages in and beyond the district in the summer of 1807, he reminded him of the need of assistance from justices and parish priests in each village. To this end, the surgeon requested a decree to the effect that he be provided with the necessary help in territories he traversed to persuade and obligate the parents and caretakers to submit, "because otherwise it will not be possible to uproot the false impressions that the masses have received."[133] At the same time the district governor of Zoyaltepec, Oaxaca, lamented that vaccine was still unknown there and suggested several reasons: villages in his jurisdiction were distant (*lejanos*), situated in hot, mountainous country, and uncouth (*incultas*), "entirely of Indians and difficult and diverse languages." To address these matters, the governor requested a knowledgeable vaccinator, with "parish priests and *vicarios* assisting so that they manage to induce and persuade them in their own language."[134] Geographic, social, and cultural distances were powerfully felt if not insurmountable: in the administrator's view villagers required both a capable practitioner and a priest to translate.

By the insurgency years, priests were in the habit of listing their work in support of vaccinations in their professional résumés (*relaciones de méritos y servicios*) for promotion. Among the merits of don José Francisco Arroyo (verified by the commander-general and intendant of Nueva Galicia) was having established in the parish buildings of Guadalupe, Guadalajara, a "dispensary" for vaccine when pestilential fevers threatened in 1814, which he subsequently transported to the parish of Haltenango when he relocated.[135] Summaries of these reports in the archive of Mexico's archbishopric provide a pointillist picture of pastoral work during the insurgency. Although most entries concern repairs of church buildings, enhancement of divine *culto* (devotional objects), and the occasional contribution to the education of youth—or vaguely refer to "many services"—several *curas* left no doubt that they understood pastoral work to include labors on behalf of vaccine. Among these vaccinator-priests was the *cura* of San Gregorio Çuautzingo, who listed, in addition to expenditures for the church building, vaccination of the entire village by his influence ("a su influxo"). In the same district, Chalco's *cura interino*, who absented himself for two years of a four-year appointment to attend the national congress as a deputy, reported conserving vaccine lymph at his own expense. (He claimed that as a result of these efforts only nine parishioners died in the subsequent epidemic.) José Rafael Malgarejo, fluent in Otomí, served Atitalaquía parish (Hidalgo) as *vicario* and *cura interino* for some twenty-three years, during which time he counted among his merits the implementation of vaccination, maintained at his expense. When the former *cura interino* of Tenancingo sought promotion, he listed his work on behalf of vaccine, in addition to schools and contributions to the splendor of worship. José Crecencio Villegas, who served in various parishes in central Mexico, including Tláhuac and Temascaltepec, claimed that the government had officially acknowledged his work in maintaining vaccine and preventing the death of scores of parishioners. Also passing through several parishes, including Zumpahuacan (in the state of Mexico), Manuel Cruz Manjarres labored on behalf of primary schools and "la bacuna."[136]

Pastoral résumés are self-serving records, far from transparent. That priests came to include as a routine matter their service on behalf of preventive medicine tells us mostly about their self-understanding and about changing conceptions of pastoral work. At same time they at least suggest how the technique became embedded in rural life through the parish in these years, where the spiritual and medical were intertwined. After Independence, when the republican government sought to revive campaigns in response to an outbreak in Mexico City, priests remained entangled in these efforts. In 1829 Oaxaca's vaccination junta opined that general propagation would succeed only if priests took to the pulpit to exhort villagers and performed vaccinations themselves.[137] In the same epidemic, a circular letter from José Miguel Gordoa, governor (*vicario capitular*) and soon to be consecrated bishop of the vacant diocese of Guadalajara, similarly charged the clergy of its 136 parishes with assisting the secular government's renewed vaccination campaign. Echoing his colonial predecessors, Gordoa's letter cited "the influence that *párrocos* and other ecclesiastics exercise, principally among indigenous families," and was accompanied by a pamphlet containing a remedy against infection and a prayer that entreated God to free the faithful from the *peste*. ("In your hands, God, I place my spirit, my heart, and my body.") Guadalajara's priests were kept busy in the epidemic, owing to a shortage of personnel and the fact that vaccination was still not universally practiced. Prayers invoking the power of the cross to banish "demons, vitiated air, and *peste*" ("los demonios, el aire corruptible, y la peste") were not incompatible with vaccination, which became the instrument by which God himself expelled smallpox "from this place and from my body."[138]

Given Enlightenment currents that sought modifications to the public role of priests, their presence in medical campaigns is noteworthy. Bourbon ministers attempting to substitute the military for the church as an instrument of governance, through *fueros* (special legal privileges) that raised the status of the former, came to appreciate in the course of prolonged and ineffectual military campaigns the usefulness of ecclesiastical mediators, for reasons having to do with costs and the preferences of people on the ground as much as any guiding ideology.[139] In emergencies and preventive campaigns contemporaries likewise continued to reserve for these figures principal moral, ceremonial, medical, and political functions, although the tendency among historians to overstate the influence of priests on Indian parishioners, particularly in the context of Mexican Independence, can be misleading. Indians did not simply fall in line, or kneel before him, as royal judge Baltasar Ladrón de Guevara had observed in the streets of Mexico City. Parishioners had multiple options for action, distinct goals that frequently broke with those of their pastor, and were often embroiled in political conflicts over water, taxes, tithes, and customary arrangements that either did not involve their pastors or involved them in antagonistic ways.[140]

Nevertheless, the recall of parish priests to traditional roles can be said to have been more regular than exceptional and to have shouldered them with new technical responsibilities that many, judging by their résumés, readily assumed. This meant that through vaccine's introduction, Christianity's personnel and idioms, unlike in France, were readily available, if not uniformly in all times and places, to assist in the education and conversion implied in such transformation.

District Governors

Disease threatened healthy populations, labor, and revenue, so that public health efforts typically enlisted secular officials to coordinate efforts, persuade civilians, and even practice medicine during vaccination campaigns. From the viceroy to royal governors to local administrators, these figures provided models, often by volunteering their children. "Knowing that in the majority of these inhabitants there reigns much preoccupation concerning any novelty," the acting intendant of Oaxaca wrote, he had his young son vaccinated first when Dr. Arboleya passed through in October 1804. A year later, when interest flagged, the senior councilman Diego de Villasante, who had provided the second floor of his home in the city center for vaccinations, speculated that it was either because residents considered the danger from smallpox to be remote "or because the lure of novelty has already worn off."[141]

The patriotic sentiment that evolved from service on behalf of vaccine found a ready outlet in Mexico City's newspapers. Some practitioners and administrators hoped that their names and efforts would appear in their pages.[142] Tenancingo's subdelegate, Antonio Elías Sáenz, last seen praising the persuasive efforts of the district's priests, responded to royal orders by requesting from the viceroy permission to send children to bring the vaccine in vivo to his district. Sáenz stressed in correspondence that as a public servant, he had poured energies into work on behalf of *industria*: breeding silkworms, building roadways to handle carriage traffic, laying pipes to divert water, and establishing reserves for schools. He viewed the most recent public health effort as among these many services for Spain. The viceroy not only approved the request, he ordered the administrator's "sentiment of loyalty and patriotism" announced to the public in the *Gazeta de México*.[143] A benefactor who saw little in the way of monetary remuneration might expect this type of publicity, which confirmed his honor and worth.[144]

These announcements, meant to advertise and enhance in others feelings of piety or patriotic responsibility, were exceptional. Through years of insurgency, a more likely motivator was the potentially devastating results of inaction in the face of disease, or the prospect that a hastily executed immunization campaign might leave villagers fleeing for the hills, with priests and administrators left to deal with the fallout. For these reasons administrators kept in sight both the government's public health mandates and the local material, political, and cultural conditions that might constrain practice. A cache of correspondence generated during a final general vaccination campaign illustrates this role and helps fill in the lacuna produced by military campaigns and bureaucratic disorder in the preceding years of insurgency.

Conducting a pastoral review of the church buildings and baptismal and marriage books in the Sierra and Huasteca regions, Mexico's archbishop witnessed the great destruction inflicted by smallpox in the scarred faces of the young. It was a regrettable situation, he remarked in correspondence with Ramón Gutiérrez del Mazo, the intendant of Mexico, and all the more so in light of the fact that Spain's monarchs had made vaccine, "certain" preservative against smallpox, available in New Spain, which had apparently not protected these children. The prelate had already commissioned and compensated a medical practitioner to vaccinate in the "nations" he had visited since February 1820 and would continue to cover the expense for six months. Now he requested the assistance of the intendant in obtaining the cooperation of other administrators, "without the formalities of juntas and sessions," the archbishop stressed, "which would in my judgment only lead to displays that I wish to avoid as I apply myself solely to the benefit of those worthy pueblos."[145] In ideal circumstances these administrative bodies, established to coordinate and institutionalize vaccinations, might have functioned to make the practice universal, but circumstances had been anything but ideal. The solution, in the face of perceived need, was to revive vaccinations summarily.

The next day Gutiérrez del Mazo circulated copies of the archbishop's letter to district governors, perhaps to amplify the moral authority of the enterprise, and echoed in his own cover the need to reestablish vaccination.[146] Responses pledged compliance, noted difficulties, and occasionally described current and past experiences, producing a snapshot of vaccination's practice in Mexico on the eve of Independence. In those districts where the archbishop had met with administrators, including Yahualica and Metztitlán, the initiative was under way. The latter's official responded that, once the archbishop had expressed his resolve to propagate vaccine, he had designated one day a week for sessions in the district seat, and many had been vaccinated in his presence.[147] In Actopan, where the official was apprised of the campaign from the archbishop's letter, eleven children were vaccinated on the day he received a fresh supply of vaccine.[148] In these places the initiative corrected neglect; in others it was redundant and unnecessary. Some fifteen years after spearheading vaccinations in Tenancingo, the energetic Elías Sáenz reported from Texcoco that vaccination had been introduced with such good effect in the district "that many parents have diligently brought their children to that capital [Mexico City] when vaccine lymph has run short here."[149] In Cadereyta, hundreds of miles north of Mexico City (near Monterrey), the administrator was informed by residents that "said *vaguna* [*sic*]" had been established since 1814, when smallpox last struck; the report referred simply to success in "all those children" vaccinated.[150]

Elsewhere the new initiative revived patterns of the previous decade. Toluca's administrator did not know vaccination's history in his jurisdiction, but the primary physician of the military hospital informed him that since 1813 and up until just two years before, he, Casimiro Liceaga, and Ignacio Garcés, along with "various other practitioners," had overseen vaccinations in five distinct periods. As a result, only those born in the time elapsed remained to be vaccinated, for which a fresh supply of vaccine was requested from the capital.[151] Toluca's arrangement approximated the ideal: periodic campaigns to immunize an ever-growing population of susceptible children. With certified practitioners, a military hospital, and proximity to a supply in Mexico City, Toluca was better endowed than neighboring Lerma, in Toluca's greater valley. Yet a similar arrangement obtained there: vaccinations had been carried out before, "because for the operation there are two *barberos* who have executed it with the greatest perfection on other occasions, and the results have been very favorable." They now lacked only vaccine, which would be obtained from Mexico City or Toluca.[152]

In places with fewer means, effective disease prevention remained a struggle. Otumba's administrator reported that he had been overseeing vaccinations since receiving the intendant's order, referring vaguely to difficulties ("aunque con algún trabajo"), with thirty-two vaccinations, and more to come.[153] Several responses requested a supply of vaccine or offered to send a child (*muchacho*) to the capital to be vaccinated as human carrier. Cuernavaca's official proposed sending two *muchachos* by carriage ("en una litera"), a precaution to ensure that the fluid would be preserved on their return; from there he intended to remit vaccine to Tetecala, Tlaquiltenango, Xocanate, and Yantepec districts.[154] Huichapan boasted two surgeons, with whom Manuel de la Hoz was conferring after receiving the order for vaccination. A supply of vaccine was needed because it could not be found in those parts "until the rains come and the necessary inspection can be made of the few cattle [*ganado bacuno*] there are on the haciendas." He added that the surgeons, though prepared to perform their duty in all the pueblos, haciendas, and ranches, were poor and responsible for their own families. He requested permission to compensate them one half *real* for each vaccinated Indian from communal coffers, while non-Indians would pay twice this (*con doble peculio*), the solemn poor nothing.[155] Here the administrator had a sense of who might be vaccinated with communal funds and who for free. On the same point, Cuautitlán's district governor, who had been reporting magnificent treatments of ulcers and other ailments with vaccine, expressed uncertainty. He referred to unanswered letters informing the intendant that the physician vaccinating in the district seat had pressed him for payment to go out to "pueblos distant from this *cabecera*." The official wondered what source he should use to cover the costly journey.[156]

Finally, there were places where vaccination's practice was improbable, although administrators pledged support. Fifty kilometers north of Mexico City, the district of Zumpango was in a miserable state owing to a serious dearth of maize, "of first necessity," with two consecutive years of shortfall. José Horabuena did not think vaccination likely in such a place, by which he meant both the rusticity of its population and the enormous struggle each year merely to grow sufficient quantities of food. Apparently vaccine was a luxury the community could not afford.[157] On the coast of Veracruz, Zempoala's official similarly offered mixed assurances: he would do what he could, but within nine leagues there was no certified practitioner, medical or surgical, and there was apparently no one else who might perform the operation.[158] Also in Veracruz, Rafael Zevallos wrote from Coatepec to say that in his jurisdiction there were no physicians to practice, nor did he have a source of vaccine. He assured the intendant that if both were provided, "certainly much benefit would redound to these miserable folk." Zevallos then struck upon inspiration, adding that the operation seemed simple ("me parece sencilla") and that if the intendant sent "an easy instruction and the *semilla* [fluid, seed], without doubt there will appear a subject to perform the operation, and if all else fails, I myself, as a gift to humanity...will do whatever my limited abilities allow me."[159]

As we continue to grasp the paths by which public health programs became reality, it should not surprise that a middle-tier administrator, the lever of a colonial system that worked through local adjustments and customary arrangements, would note the ease of the procedure and think to carry it out himself. For his part, Gutiérrez del Mazo, a veteran administrator, would not have marveled at the variation described in the reports, which confirms what we have seen for Michoacán, Oaxaca, the northern mining frontiers, and even Puebla. Experience varied according to geography, climate, population size, distance from vaccination hubs, harvests, and the zeal of administrators, who came to rely officially and extra-officially on a constellation of practitioners in the face of inadequate resources—and dearth was salient for most everyone involved.

Behind the latest effort was the archbishop, whose moral authority, technical knowledge, and administrative fluency guided his determined intervention. When the perception of physical suffering and deformity compelled him to action, he enlisted local authorities, observing that too much pomp and circumstance in pursuit of making uniform, regular, orderly, and fixed might be as detrimental to campaigns as too little preparation. In reviving vaccination, the archbishop opted for a timelier, more spontaneous, salvific outpouring of charitable aid, inconsistent rather than systematic, in a language of suffering and sacrifice that many still spoke.

CONCLUSION

By the end of Spanish rule, vaccination was no longer a novelty. From the flat limestone shelves of Yucatán, to the port of Acapulco, to the mining centers of the north, few administrators receiving orders claimed ignorance, even if some did not see how to sustain the practice. Through repeated losses of vaccine, prolonged insurgency, and three major vaccinating cycles (coinciding with impending epidemics, as in 1813 and 1814), reports in the waning years of the colony show communities coordinating across regions to preserve a source. Requests for "unos vidrios de pus" (vials or glass plates of fluid) came from everywhere, often fulfilled by administrators in Mexico City, Puebla, Toluca, and Zacatecas (the last, to Aguascalientes, Fresnillo, and San Luis Potosí).[160] In 1820 Mérida's intendant reported an adequate supply for the province and declined an offer to send more.[161] Acapulco's destitute public health committee, by contrast, tried repeatedly without success to bring vaccine there in vitro; the appearance of a child with smallpox in the port on February 12, 1821, spurred members to propose to the viceroy chain vaccinations (in vivo) from Mexico City, with the cost of transport covered by *ayuntamientos* along the way whose populations were in need of fluid.[162] Public lashings, village uprisings, and persecuted *curanderos* make for better drama, but the insinuation of vaccine into the routines of the viceroyalty was a more mundane affair that played out over years.

Much attention, then and since, has nevertheless focused on the Royal Vaccination Expedition, which made fluid available in dozens of polities in New Spain. Almost without exception, studies of vaccine's introduction end with the expedition's departure, leaving us to wonder what happened once governmental support became sporadic or nonexistent.[163] Whatever its considerable accolades, the undertaking was less definitive in several important respects. The program was not self-sustaining after 1805: children in many regions were first vaccinated years later, often spurred by the onset of disease; many of the vaccinating juntas prescribed in regulations were never established, soon ceased to function, or were dysfunctional from the start; the eventful return of Balmis to Mexico was inconclusive or counterproductive; and funding shortages and warfare threatened to derail campaigns in even the most important centers. As sources show, disease outbreaks and military campaigns especially impacted vaccination's practice: generally, sessions become more consistent when the vagaries of warfare ease.

It is no surprise that campaigns ebbed and flowed depending on local conditions. But we have also seen the extent to which matters of personnel, expertise, and finance remained unresolved with the passing of the expedition. Not only a question of politics and identity, immunization occasioned fundamental confusion and disagreement over the nature of the technology and the role of the colonial government in supporting it. On the one hand, the period saw both physicians and surgeons undergoing an overall improvement in status as a result of reforms in training and anatomical instruction, the premium placed on medicine and the healing arts as practical tools of governance, the entrance of medical topics into public discourse, and the professionalization of the Spanish army.[164] On the other, despite their self-regard, certified practitioners were either largely unavailable outside of cities and towns or, paradoxically, rendered unfit by their costly training to introduce vaccine in Mexico's impoverished countryside, at least in the eyes of local administrators and communities. Because of this the medical establishment did not control the movement of the technology, whose use adhered to other rhythms, patterns, and needs. This fact directs our attention away from professional squabbles and self-representations and toward the assessments of other groups, along with pragmatic considerations and arrangements that often departed from what was prescribed.

Tools and techniques were placed in the hands of priests, *hacendados*, Indian governors, Spanish administrators, and many more healers with experience in rural healing, surgical instrumentation, venesection, indigenous languages, and regional topography and climate. Lay healers, unlike diocesan priests, rarely produced résumés of their own, but the nature of their expertise can be gleaned from legal cases that document the work of *curanderos* into the first decades of the Mexican republic. Throughout the 1830s and 1840s, Oaxaca's legal system relied on dozens of informally trained practitioners to provide expert testimony in criminal cases. Though their judgment was not always decisive, magistrates in Huajuapan, Ejutla, and Ocotlán (in Oaxaca's central valleys) called on tailors, hatters, shoemakers, tanners, bakers, barbers, and other aficionados to inspect wounds in homicides, tend to injured victims, and visit sick prisoners in holding cells. In 1834 one Josefa Juliana González, a fifty-year-old widow from Huajuapan, issued her opinion in a criminal case involving an unmarried woman who had been wounded by a cutting instrument. González prognosticated correctly that the "cancer" induced by the wound would eventually kill the woman, and though she was unable to sign, being illiterate, she spoke "with experience, because she has been a healer of wounds [*curandera de heridos*] for a long time, as her husband, the late don Manuel Robles, a practitioner of medicine, instructed her and commissioned her to heal." The attorney of the accused sought a mistrial on the technical grounds that González had failed to measure the width and gravity of the wound, and because the two witnesses required to certify the forensic review had been absent.[165] Female healers were not simply ignored: in thirteen of fourteen cases of sexual violence tried between 1756 and 1831 the judge's decision followed the opinions offered by the midwives called in to review the victim.[166]

Through the unlettered participation of these healers, their uncertified procedures and approaches acquired institutional ramifications. The nature of colonial power comes to look more diffuse, the meanings of public health campaigns and medical technologies less fixed, once we consider the variety of people enrolled to transport, inject, elaborate, and judge. Like the crushed scabs used in vaccinating campaigns, medical authority, skill, and knowledge were ground up, suspended in liquid flowing through multiple domains and jurisdictions, rendering preventive medicine legitimate, accessible, and viable. Along the way communities of laypeople were involved as well to assess the skill, cultural aptitude, reputation, virtues, and trustworthiness of these occasional agents of immunity.

CHAPTER 6

Medicine's Malcontents

An Oral History

> Some say that with the incisions the vaccinators mark them to remove them from this Kingdom and relocate them to old Spain; others that they are signs enlisting in the militia those who bear them; others that it is my own design, to increase the number of deceased and profit from burial fees (no matter that there has not been an example of anyone dying as a result).
>
> —Father Nicolás Junguera, Santa María Tlatlauquitepec, 1806

Words counted in colonial Mexico. In prayers for relief, rituals of shaming and disrespect, disputes over communal property and the appropriate care of children, recitations of the Te Deum, *boleros* and pasquinades, pastoral letters and sermons, and murmurs of death from botched operations, words were influential in the resolution of disease and the perception of reform. Emergencies and public health campaigns that brought diverse groups together in cities, towns, and villages to address illness, repeat news, and negotiate more suitable arrangements only drew further attention to the import of nonliterate cultures, communities, and ways of knowing. In January 1805, Francisco Xavier de Balmis was forced to reckon with this reality in the port of Acapulco. While he and his retinue of nurses and children labored to vaccinate residents before departing on the next leg of the journey, administrators caught wind of reports that any child handed over for vaccination would be forcibly taken to the Philippines with the team. Apparently facing the prospect of kidnapping, parents in Acapulco were concealing their children from practitioners and officials, and Balmis was momentarily able to do little more than set about creating a junta for future practice.[1]

Histories of medicine have long aspired to follow the views and participation of laypeople. For colonial Mexico, they have largely depended on Inquisition documents, rather than diaries, journals, and letters, which few inhabitants left behind. Inquisitorial records have been used effectively to address matters of race, gender, and the plural healing cultures of New Spain, but they are mostly silent in the matter of Bourbon medical programs, to say nothing of the political action that these frequently provoked.[2] Records of epidemic outbreaks and immunization campaigns provide a different evidentiary seam from which to reconstruct these cultures and experiences. Beginning in the 1770s, *pueblos de indios* in the vicinity of Mexico City struck by disease were periodically subjected to secular and ecclesiastical measures to provide care, contain infection, and introduce more hygienic, enlightened practices among Indian subjects. In the course of these interventions, Spanish nurses, city physicians, administrators, and rural priests in barrios, villages, and homes healed and pronounced on matters of morality, propriety, and civilization. Their social position, combined with the learning, skills, and training some acquired in a hospital or university, moved them to police what they construed as excesses in ways that sometimes betrayed limited understandings of local practices.[3]

These campaigns of disease control illustrate how trust at the communal level might be secured, or betrayed, in the decades leading up to the arrival of Jennerian vaccine. More than a science, medical practice was a performance, a ritualized interaction between patient and practitioner, in which success was rarely judged "solely in terms of technical proficiency, scientific breakthroughs and cure-rates."[4] While success rates might be striking, healers and experts demonstrated their relevance and efficacy in other ways. Among the therapeutic practices that drew official attention in these years were *temascales*, where local empirics and family members bled, sweat, and purged their patients with plants and heady foods and beverages. "Yesterday an *india* coming down with smallpox died in the barrio of Santa Anita," an official in Orizaba reported in the 1797 epidemic, "and seeking the cause I learned that she had been bathed in *temascale* [*sic*], which they use for every sickness and with much harm to their health. I found it advisable to order its alcalde to tear all of them down."[5] Rural and urban populations considered these baths essential to good health, but medical theories of contagion and a more diffuse constellation of ideas about temperance and propriety recast them as incubators of infection and sin.

For reforms to have effect, administrators could not simply override codes of behavior, modes of governance, or healing rituals. Indian tributaries had somehow to verify that the outsiders possessed the tools and common sense to make them and their children well. Rumors can be especially helpful when trying to discern the deliberations and insights that facilitated the relocation of medical protocols, therapeutics, techniques, and expertise to places with complex healing repertoires of their own. Following the arrival of Jennerian vaccine, charges of kidnapping, enslavement, sorcery, and compulsory enlistment in the king's armies surfaced in multiple rural communities, most of which had no prior experience with immunization. These reports suggest politicized conversations, criticisms, and interpretations that were informed by other kinds of experience and knowledge.[6] Partial and highly mediated, oral culture helped to make sense of change in these early years of preventive practice.

Rumors pose considerable methodological and interpretive challenges for historians. Because the vast majority of Mexico's rural population did not write, their words were recorded and reported by non-Indians, often called *gente de razón*, including priests, scribes, attorneys, administrators, and physicians. Commentary filtered through the pens of Mexico's upper and middle sectors recalls the predicament identified by subaltern studies scholars, who asked how texts produced by and for society's elite can be read to recover the voices of the poor and illiterate.[7] Even if the documents relate roughly what some people said and did, reported in good faith, they are a far cry from what all people said and did all of the time. Reports typically elide distinctions of gender, generation, ethnicity, and occupation, and most of the nonverbal aspects—including gestures, inflection, intonation, and even setting—are lost once words are set down on paper. This casts into doubt even the most basic matters, including whether the intent of the utterance was figurative or literal. Did parents in Acapulco *actually believe* that their offspring would be kidnapped? And what persons repeated the rumor?

Elite reporters occasionally dismissed charges of kidnapping, branding, witchcraft, and compulsory enlistment as nonsense, but there is ample reason to try to understand the ways that sentiment articulated verbally worked in public health initiatives. As medications, healing personnel, and medical technologies moved across viceregal space, *pública voz y fama*, or opinion verified in some sense by virtue of being held in common, might derail the vaccinating machinery. Speech was a source of considerable anxiety for administrators, who were less quick to dismiss a rumor that might spiral out of hand. Apparent failures and setbacks—moments when theories, healing regimens, and instruments were not easily adopted—can therefore be as illuminating of political process, communal norms, and the reasons for success. To the extent that speech conveyed information and framed skepticism and dissent, its study can suggest how laypeople explained and interpreted change, in irreducibly political ways. Scholars have argued that a segmented public sphere in modern Mexico has seen political ritual and gossip stand in for a fully developed arena of debate and dissent. Often gendered, and dismissed as "women's talk," gossip nevertheless continues to make intelligible the opinion taking shape within communities.[8] In rumors as in other ephemeral cultural productions, we are left agreeing with Claude Lévi-Strauss, who in his study of South American myths noted that behind each recorded instance are many unknown, and "we are only too pleased with the samples and scraps at our disposal."[9]

PURGING THERAPIES

In October 1773, while collecting tribute in Santa Marta village, in Mexicaltzingo, southwest of Mexico City, the district governor accidentally happened upon the devastation inflicted by a regional outbreak of *matlazahuatl.* He requested a priest to dispense "spiritual medications" and surmised in correspondence with the viceroy that the outbreak had not been discovered sooner because the village lacked a pastor: it was too distant from Ixtapalapa's *doctrina*, whose interim priest did not in any case speak Nahuatl.[10] Soon after the discovery, Miguel Dávila Galindo, experienced *vicario de idioma* (ordained because of his fluency in an indigenous language), arrived to confess the sick. Galindo determined that over the previous year some 218 out of 685 Indian tributaries had died in Santa Marta and its adjacent barrios, with similar mortality rates in neighboring Reyes.[11]

From Mexico City the second physician of the Royal Indian Hospital, Manuel Gómez, was dispatched to heal, along with one of the institution's barber-surgeons, after some discussion of the utility of medical personnel in a place without the necessary support.[12] Gómez requested from the hospital emetics, an opiate, and febrifuges; straw mats and blankets (*fresadas*) to cover his patients; and two nurses, male and female, to help administer medications and carry out his instructions. He offered typical explanations for the magnitude of devastation: the village's proximity to Lake Texcoco, whose state of desiccation was releasing harmful miasmas; the lack of suitable shelter for residents; the reuse of clothing from the sick and deceased; poor water quality; and the dietary habits of the sick, who "sustain themselves with unripe prickly pear fruit [*tunas*] and much chile."[13]

With a team in place to combat infection and bad habits, the priest wrote approvingly of the physician's healing method and dietary regimen: daily rations of bread, *caldos* (broths) for the sick, stewed mutton for the convalescing, and clean water for cooking and boiling herbs (transported in barrels from a spring two leagues away), along with an assortment of botanicals from the capital.[14] The problem was that few observed the prescribed regimen, and many were dying as a result of "desarreglos y excesos," eating what they pleased in their homes. Only if a guard policed each dwelling or a temporary isolation hospital was established, Galindo concluded, would the method be enforced. In his short time there he had witnessed the sick eating poorly cooked squash, the fleshy fruit of prickly pear, and *frijoles*—all detrimental, he thought, to their health. The parade of officials through the village included Mexico City's corregidor and two licensed physicians, whose inspection led them to agree that the epidemic had turned fatal there "because of the neglect [*desidia*] and distraction of the miserable *indios*," who in their meager huts feverishly rejected blankets and refused to eat the good foods provided them.[15]

It was a time of change in the administration of rural villages that transgressed spiritual, economic, and cultural boundaries. Five years before the intervention in Santa Marta, Francisco Antonio de Lorenzana, archbishop of Mexico (tenure from 1766 to 1771), promulgated a pastoral letter, at once a manifesto and set of rules for reform, to pastors of Indian parishes. Known as the "Exhortation to parish priests to take care that the natives know and practice the indicated rules," it was the overture for Lorenzana's major initiatives: to complete the secularization of parishes, promote agriculture and industry, and acculturate the indigenous populations of Mexico, largely by introducing schools for instruction of Christian doctrine in Spanish. By means of full indoctrination into the cultural norms and habits of Spanish Catholicism one not only learned the maxims of divine and natural law but also "casts off idleness, achieves cleanliness and purity, banishes ignorance and idolatry, and becomes a Christian citizen, useful to society, head of family, and good republican. And though we will not reap the fruit in just a few years, we can be sure that in times to come the harvest will be abundant."[16]

Of the fourteen rules (*reglas*) promulgated to priests, four addressed matters of health and hygiene alluded to in the prologue. In addition to the need to raise chickens and livestock, be gainfully employed, learn and use the Spanish language, and construct homes sturdily and near the parish church, parishioners were to ensure that the beds or *tapestles* (reed mats, in Nahuatl) on which they and their children slept were clean and raised, "because they contract many grave illnesses from sleeping in humid areas or right on the ground," and avoid *embriaguezes* (bouts of drinking to intoxication), "which are the cause of their poverty, idleness, and sins, as well as many illnesses and *pestes*." When an Indian parishioner fell sick, others were to assist with a "bird, tortillas, or eggs," or whatever he or she was able so that no one died for want of care or the sacraments. Parishioners were not to go about without clothing or in a state of filth, which deprived them of "modesty and health, and because many children die for lack of cleanliness, the stench killing old and young alike, and especially if they use cotton clothing, which is not as healthy as linen, or hemp."[17] The *reglas* made three general observations pertaining to health: that clothing, sleeping arrangements, the environment, and consumption of alcohol all had immediate effects on physical well-being; that Indian parishioners were generally but not hopelessly negligent in looking after themselves and others; and that neglect in these matters was a function of excessive cultural and linguistic diversity (or inadequate acculturation). The rules were to be read and explained twice monthly in parishes, so that their lessons would sink in.[18]

Enlightened reformers worked within a matrix of ideas and symbols whose domains were medical, social, and religious. Medical practice had its own references but often focused the idiom by which distinctions in orderly and disorderly customs were routinely made. Physicians who conceived of disease as nature's way of expelling corrupted humors, for instance, prescribed restraint and moderation above all: according to the widely disseminated instruction for preventing and treating smallpox by Dr. Bartolache, the worst the healer could do was interfere with nature's remedy, by using too many medications or varying them daily, "giving in to interested parties who prefer it, especially women."[19] Theories of moderation came to dominate thinking about health among the elite, a philosophy imbibed by priests as well as physicians and other administrators, who were irregularly conversant in local practices but reflexively skeptical of their effects.

Given their distance from the *doctrina*, villagers in Santa Marta were likely spared the assault on indigenous languages that was in the interim pursued by Archbishop Lorenzana. Instead they experienced the acculturating force that he championed in the form of an assault on their healing practices. As religious, medical, and secular officials campaigned against these, the same people left observations that point toward their underlying logic. Residents insisted, the *vicario de idioma* complained, on substituting their own healing repertoire, "eating bitter *tunas* and using them as unctions, sucking on limes, and bathing in *temascales*, all because of that moment when, in their thought, they experience instinctual relief [*alivio*]." They were prone to "place themselves in the sun when they feel chills from the fever [and] change places without covering themselves or protecting against the air, not preparing for the convulsions that could result."[20] The district governor elaborated: "the sick Indians lie down before and against their doors so that the wind blows on them, or remain beside their wood burner [*fogón de leña*], which they call *tlecuile* [*sic: tecuile*] and which makes their blood boil." Families caring for patients in drafty, tiny spaces, as he described them, provided pulque and *aguardiente*, "even when they are breathing their last breath."[21] The Protomedicato, whose members described residents of Mexico City's barrios similarly gathered around the hearths of homes (see Chapter 2), reiterated that residents of Santa Marta were "bleeding themselves six times, spreading tomato and chile all over their body, and not forsaking the use of pulque, *aguardiente*, *tunas*, etc."[22] Reports thus identified therapies with a perceptible physiological effect: consumption of foods and intoxicating beverages with known hot or cold properties; bleeding and sweating; and regulating bodily temperature by relocating patients according to their state.[23] In these ways residents apparently pursued what the priest dismissively called *alivio* (relief).

Within a humoral model, *sangrías*, *purgas*, and *sudores* comprised the "Holy Trinity" of early modern therapeutics: the extraction of some substance from the body—blood, food, sweat—signified that one had been successfully healed, or protected.[24] Insofar as bodily symptoms were salient, healers across class, age, and caste looked to physiology and a precarious bodily and environmental balance to explain and restore health. When José de Gálvez, as visitor-general of New Spain, fell ill in September 1770 during military campaigns against the Seris and Pimas in Sonora, the troop surgeon prescribed for him bathing in temperate waters, and no fewer than five *sangrías*.[25] A licensed physician's endorsement of thermal waters a league outside Mexico City trumpeted their therapeutic virtues, renowned among laypeople, secular authorities, and physicians alike as "casi milagrosos."[26] Still within this framework, elite reformers and caretakers expressed and encouraged enlightened attitudes by advising moderation in healing, eating, drinking, and recreating, targeting especially the domestic conditions of the lower classes. The Mexican experience seems to confirm the observation that when it came to medicine before the twentieth century, practice "changed a good deal less than the rhetoric surrounding it would suggest."[27]

For villagers besieged by disease, insistence on moderation in diet and healing might appear useless, and even dangerous. The seemingly arbitrary regulation of bleeding and other therapies in Santa Marta in 1773 created difficulties for villagers, who eventually lost their patience. They refused to follow Gómez's orders, only reluctantly allowed him even to take their pulse, and, as they informed the priest in confessions, neglected to call him when they took ill "because he did not heal them to their satisfaction." Few came when the bell rang announcing the distribution of his medications, which were said to kill patients. "They also allege that he does not rub oil on them," Galindo specified, "or apply plasters, and especially, that he does not bleed them." When he pressed them on the last point, "they explained to me, and even begged in tears, that they should be bled, because they are, as they say, accustomed to it."[28] Now villagers refused even to be purged, and residents from neighboring Santa María, who had been transporting the sick on horseback for *purgas*, no longer arrived.[29] After a failed attempt to acquire horses, presumably to pay visits to those who no longer came, Gómez retreated to Mexico City in a feverish state, debilitated by the illness he had labored to cure.[30]

No fewer than three certified physicians from Mexico City arrived in Santa Marta in the course of the outbreak, a situation that, observers noted, served communities poorly and meant a great deal of lost experience.[31] The only indication of success reportedly came when residents prevailed upon the priest to be bled; the bleeder-surgeon who stayed behind had time for little else in visits to dispersed villages and barrios than extracting blood, a transformative substance in early modern healing rituals.[32] Not only had authorities persecuted (or misrecognized) a familiar repertoire of extractive techniques on the body—salves of cool fruit and hot chile, spells in cool doorways or beside the hot brazier, and bleedings—they had failed to discern or avail themselves of any local authority figure, finally opting to construct two infirmaries, with nurses and porters stationed to prevent the entrance of prohibited food and drink.[33] Looking more like retaining cells than places of convalescence, mechanisms of persuasion had failed, and with it any possibility for reform.

These scenarios became more common after the promulgation of the anticontagion program. During Viceroy Revillagigedo's tenure, reports of smallpox in Campeche, Mexico City, Tabasco, and Veracruz spurred inspections of neighborhoods and homes and measures to contain infection. Most turned out to be false alarms, but even the most minor signs were magnified as a result of the government's vigilance.[34] In 1793, for instance, an outbreak in the *cabecera* of Tlalnepantla (district of Tacuba) placed the alcaldes and *repúblicas* of subject villages on alert. Deeming a single infirmary in which to separate patients too disruptive—according to officials, the measure would send parents fleeing with their children—residents were ordered by the *vicario* and subdelegate to build small huts (*xacalillos*) of hay and shingles on their properties. With these orders indigenous officials received supplies of borage and poppy (*amapola*), "which is what the Indians are accustomed to and what they use to heal [*alivian*], without need of a physician or pharmacy."[35] Esteban Morel, onetime promoter of inoculation, was selected for his expertise to inspect patients in San Pedro Azcapotzaltongo, the apparent epicenter. He diagnosed an outbreak of spurious or fatuous (*fatuas*) pox, perhaps chicken pox, and not smallpox. But even he had difficulty diagnosing the cases, speculating during another inspection about "a third order of pox [*viruelas*] not described by the authors." He had not seen it before: "Perhaps it is singular to the Indians." Morel had not been able to inspect all of the sick and described a mother fleeing with her son in her arms "despite the calm and kindness that I had shown and ordered in administering the measure."[36] He recommended that villagers be excused from any further anticontagion measures, and eventually they were, but not before many were forced by threat of imprisonment to construct the *xacalillos* that had been ordered.[37] The likelihood of flight to forests (*bosques*) and ravines was real, the *vicario* stressed in his report. He had known his Indian parishioners (in thirty-nine years of experience) to be opposed to healing with the medicines of Spaniards ("son enemigos de curarse con medicinas de que usan los españoles"), and villagers were so poor that before they had time to fully convalesce they returned to producing the linen, shingles ("tabletas de taxamanil"), and coal that they sold in Mexico City.[38]

Reports from outbreaks suggest that Jenner's vaccine arrived at a particularly inauspicious time for establishing trust. Following a succession of emergency measures imposed in the 1797 smallpox epidemic, an outbreak of mysterious fevers in the region north of Mexico City in 1805 attracted further administrative attention. As royal officials dispatched teams of medical practitioners to infected villages, the archbishop sent missives to Cuautitlán, Ecatepec, Tacuba, Tizayuca, and Tultitlán parishes instructing priests to cooperate with physicians and disabuse their parishioners of the use of "ignorant *curanderas* or ineffective medicines" (and to remind them to confess fully and not sin again, for the outbreak was surely punishment from God).[39] An especially virulent outbreak in San Bartolomé Cuautlalpan, northeast of Mexico City, moved Tizayuca's priest, Dr. José Rafael Valdés de Anaya, to extemporize on the reasons for the infection, which had been festering in the region for the past seven years. Fourteen years as a minister had taught Valdés that in spite of the time that elapsed since their conquest, and various sage laws legislated to protect them, the moral and political instruction of the *indios* of New Spain had advanced hardly at all. He extolled the virtues of Archbishop Lorenzana, who had endeavored to change this. Nevertheless, Indians continued to live like domestic animals ("fieras domésticas"), easily given to vices of drunkenness and idolatry and inclined to theft of cattle, rapine, and pillaging.

The unavoidable result was the current epidemic disaster. Residents were "steeped in all manners of superstition, particularly with respect to medications," while the "barbaric" use of *temascales*, an "infernal bath," disposed the healthy to infection, exacerbated the condition of the sick, and caused those who had recovered to relapse. Despite attempts to care for them, there was little that could be done. The Indians lived and died in a drunken state, they despised and looked with horror on "our medicines," and they persisted in their customs: *friegas* (massages) and infusions of the ground-up leaves and dark red berries of the "poisonous" *árbol del Perú* (pepper plant, often used as a diuretic, analgesic, digestive, purgative, or stimulant), or from another tree villagers called *colorines* (perhaps the deciduous naked coral tree), boiled in pulque or urine. Their refusal to burn the straw mats and clothing used by patients was founded in a "crude superstition": "they believe and are persuaded that with this precaution 'the sickness gets angry,' becomes obstinate, and pursues them."[40] Valdés divulged in a postscript that recent news of two women found deceased in a *temascal* in San Marco Yxtlahuaca (in Pachuca), clinging to one another, had moved him to try to collect the sick in a makeshift hospital, where villagers might be better supervised by a *curandero* from neighboring Zumpango.

The plan was sidelined when Anastasio Bustamante, certified physician and future president of the Republic of Mexico, arrived from Mexico City with two nurses to provide medical treatment.[41] The Junta de Sanidad (Public Health Board), which met regularly in the capital to oversee management of the outbreak, had identified San Bartolomé as the epicenter, in consultation with the Protomedicato, and promptly dispatched Bustamante. Twenty-five years old at the time, Bustamante had been baptized in the reformist spirit of New Spain's professional classes and possessed all the convictions of youth. He immediately set to work: as he informed the Protomedicato's president, the illness indicated the use of mild evacuants, "and bleeding, once," he stressed, done "with proper circumspection." He requested small dosages of tartaric emetic, to induce vomiting; enemas; "antiseptics" to fight putrefaction, including quinine (used for fevers and pain), *serpentaria*, or canker weed (a stimulant, diaphoretic, or digestive, producing nausea and vomiting in sufficient doses), and solutions of alkaline salts and wine; and a tincture of the aromatic Winter's bark (*drimis de Winter*), mixed into oil for massages.[42]

In its physiological effects, Bustamante's regimen shared affinities with that of his patients: emetics, sudorifics, massages with oils and aromatic herbs, foot rubs (*pediluvios*), blistering plasters (*vejigatorios*) applied to the neck, arms, or legs, an infusion of tamarind, and lime in *caldo*, along with occasional, moderate bleedings. Any similarities were lost on Bustamante, who explained the infection's propagation by identifying—in addition to three atmospheric causes (miasmas exhaled from the surrounding lakes and swamps, frequent changes in atmospheric temperature, and irregular winds blowing from the southwest and southeast)—four factors related to lifestyle: the poor protection offered by villagers' huts; crude and unwholesome foods; lack of hygiene in homes and dress; and "drunkenness and abuses of *temascales* and of berries from the *árbol del Pirú* [*sic*]."[43] He emphasized the last category, hoping to stamp out the excesses he had witnessed.

Residents thus found themselves in the care of two unsympathetic authorities who blamed, assaulted, or dismissed their healing practices. Almost immediately, Bustamante complained bitterly in repeated dispatches about an apparent breakdown of authority. One official, a *regidor*, likely elected by the *común* of male villagers, proved to be less than helpful.[44] Desperate reports emphasized that villagers did not recognize Bustamante's authority, or any, as far as he could see. In a rage about delays in putting his orders into effect, Bustamante singled out for blame one Vicente Ramón Jaen, the individual commissioned to serve in place of an ailing subdelegate. Among other tasks, Jaen had been instructed to prohibit use of *temascales* by the sick and convalescent in infected villages, "destroying them if necessary," but as Jaen reported he had only prohibited their use, not needing to destroy them "by virtue of not having known any violators." Bustamante thought that Jaen had good intentions but was young and overburdened by the duties of the district. He deemed the Indian governor equally unfit, "because the sons [of the village] neither obey nor respect him." Bustamante requested that the government deputize someone with sufficient authority to accompany him on rounds, and "in this manner I will manage to get them to bring the sick to me on time and not leave for other villages, or remain hidden in their homes, with the risk of spreading infection." With this person's help, the *temascal* baths, "theaters of impurities and various abuses that are as harmful to the soul as the body," might finally be demolished.[45]

Inadvertently, the young doctor provided the best explanation for the disregard he had been shown. In partnership with the parish priest, Bustamante had revived the assault on sweat baths, seeking to destroy them along with poorly constructed, contaminated homes; attacked what he perceived as excesses in consumption of alcohol and *tunas*; and sought to dissuade mourners, "who were going blindly to contract infection by embracing the cadavers to bid their farewells (a harm that neither the parish priest nor I have been able to remedy)."[46] Almost half of San Bartolomé's eight hundred residents were supposed to have perished in the previous year, and plagued villagers in search of relief apparently ignored, to the extent they were able, the aggravating intrusions of outsiders.

Elsewhere in the zone of infection, this commitment to enlightened principles complicated the experience of vaccine's introduction. At the end of 1806, José Osorio was commissioned to heal in San Pablo Tlaquilpan (Zempoala district), where the epidemic of *fiebres* had raged for months. After some initial cooperation, residents refused to enter the infirmary he had established, reportedly insisting that no one was being healed there, and ignored his dietary prescriptions. Instead, they requested blankets and other kinds of support to care for the sick in their homes, at the hospital's expense, and bombarded the physician with contrary opinions about his methods. In the matter of vaccination, however, residents were more cooperative. An absentee district governor claimed that he had "corrected" the excesses of Indian villagers, who in considerable numbers sought out the physician for the procedure. No mere boast, two months after arriving, Osorio reported 548 vaccinations, which continued after the neglected infirmary was closed. The relieved physician declared the campaign a success, even as he admitted that the operation's effect in about a third of cases was unknown because the patients never returned for inspection: "although I visit the homes I can daily and order the officials of the *república* to summon them, I learn nothing." Prescribing that the vaccinated bathe once or twice to keep the incision clean, Osorio had stipulated that it not be done in a *temascal*, and residents had refused to comply.[47] A seemingly insurmountable breach in relations between the outsider and the community had been overcome with the timely intervention of a local authority, yet Osorio continued to pursue his medical agenda by dictating the terms of washing.

Months later villagers of neighboring San Juan Temamatla (Chalco district) ejected the same Osorio from their village. Its pastor, accompanying Osorio's replacement on rounds of infected villages, managed to elicit a plausible explanation. After some seventy people in the head village perished, the thirty infected villagers who remained refused admission to the hospital, noting "that all who entered it died." They recounted a disturbing incident: that the nurse, "brother of Dr. Osorio," had perished from the same affliction. Residents reportedly concluded: "'if the physician could not heal the Spaniard, much less could he heal the Indian.'"[48] In this assessment, healers were aided in their work by cultural, racial, or social familiarity; a Spanish physician interested in the health of his kin should possess the expertise necessary to save his life. The outcome had left villagers to wonder whether the medical expert had any chance of healing them. How would he know what counted as normal, or anticipate and control the effects of drugs and therapies? Bookish learning did not preclude common sense, but neither did villagers assume it. Refusing to enter the hospital where the physician presided, they passed judgment on his abilities from without.

In Juanico pueblo, nearer the capital, in the jurisdiction of Guadalupe's shrine, residents similarly assessed the commissioned physician on the basis of information gleaned through preliminary interactions. Pedro Ramírez arrived on December 3, 1806, and joined with Antonio María Campos, *teniente* and *prebendo* (member of the cathedral chapter), in implementing precautions in burials and fumigations with vinegar, as ordered by Mexico City's health board. Ramírez helped raise a provisional infirmary after an inspection of houses by Campos revealed more than seventy sick and thirty deceased Indian villagers. Officials in Mexico City settled on a course of vaccination as the best measure, which the physician would oversee. But by the end of the month Ramírez had been replaced. According to Campos, residents had received him poorly: the condition of only ten of the twenty-nine patients treated in the hospital had improved, and as a result others would not go near it, or even allow treatment in their homes. Plausibly, a dismal survival rate in the first few weeks under the physician's care, combined with resentment over his assignment to the community without their consent, had generated discontent. "In attending to the matter, I proposed to the Indians that they choose the physician to whom they would like to be brought," Campos related, "and they agreed that it should be don Diego Cansinos, who since the thirty-first of the last month has been attending to them."[49]

How villagers arrived at Cansinos as a suitable replacement is unclear; officials requested a description of his preferred healing method, but there is no sign that it arrived. From other reports, one can surmise that it involved much of the sweating, purging, and rubbing typical of the time. In addition to wine, vinegar, *aguardiente*, and foods prescribed for their healing properties, medicinal specifics included quinine, ipecac, and opium, when available, along with sudorifics, purgatives, and laxatives. One administrator healing in the epidemic proclaimed fumigations with aromatic substances, cleanliness, abundant use of quality vinegar, and early consumption of cooling acids like vinaigrette the rule of thumb ("regla cierta") in achieving the end of *pestes* among Indians and other plebes.[50] Expenses generated to run infirmaries in the countryside provide another glimpse of care. Tesoyuca's costs included the salaries of personnel (inspector [*interventor*], nurse, and physician, including his transport from Mexico City), preparation of meals (bread, meat, lard, corn, sugar, chocolate, beans, chickens, eggs, and fuel for cooking), and clothing and bedding (*fresadas*, *petates*, and blankets). With the exception of large sums spent to acquire barrels of vinegar for disinfection, this was typical. Accounting records suggest, in other words, that these were more innocuous endeavors than the vitriol spewed in reports, even if treatment did nothing to improve mortality rates (in Tesoyuca the majority of patients who entered its hospital perished, with 142 deaths, against 26 recoveries).[51] In Juanico residents changed their opinion of the infirmary with the substitution of personnel. As a result, the sick and their families, who previously refused care, went voluntarily, with twenty-three new patients in the week since Cansinos arrived, and the majority faring well.[52] There the complaint was not with hospitals in general or outside intervention per se: villagers embraced the intervention and aid of a university-trained doctor once they found, with the priest's intervention, the right person and appropriate manner to dispense it.

Deliberations in which villagers discerned medical expertise and efficacy belie simplistic portrayals of nonconformity or negligence scattered throughout the archival record. This process was no less important in evaluating claims to efficacy made for vaccination, where people had good reason to be skeptical. In the summer of 1807, the administrator of Tochimilco (Puebla) sent a girl to neighboring Atlixco to be vaccinated. She returned deathly ill, "her body so full of pox that she appeared in the arms of death." Instead of propagating vaccine, this first attempt "propagated horror and fear," leaving an especially strong impression on the Indian population, according to the report, which the administrator labored long to undo.[53] Medical practice, knowledge, and medications might appear in many guises, as in the shape of an incapacitated, recently vaccinated girl, or an abusive or dogmatic vaccinator. Villagers looked beyond statistical proofs to what was salient within the context of practice and employed criteria of ethnicity, culture, kinship, and physical effects to pass judgment.[54]

Instead, as in an echo chamber, portrayals of stubborn nonconformity, backwardness, and excess were amplified in 1805 and 1806. Members of the health board—*oidor* Ciriaco González Carvajal, two royal attorneys, and several elite physicians—regularly gathered in the judge's home during these pestilential months to read reports and coordinate policy. Impressionistic correspondence from Tultitlán, for example, described Indians fleeing the infirmary en masse amid general decimation. Sent to the archbishop in defense of a priest accused of impeding the physician's work, the report neatly shifted blame to residents, whose fear of the administered remedies caused them to "hide and deny their sickness, healing themselves privately in their manner and performing other remedies that look more like those of brutes than rational beings, like bleeding themselves from their temples until they spill a considerable amount of blood, for which the current priest has acridly admonished them."[55] The accused clergyman might well have encouraged flight and rejection of the physician to temper what he took to be rash public health interventions in his jurisdiction. The friars of the convent-hospital of San Juan de Dios, dispatched to Ecatepec by order of the health board to persuade Indian residents to allow themselves to be healed, were instead, according to Tizayuca's opinionated priest José Rafael Valdés (Lorenzana's outspoken protégé), responsible for the sick fleeing the infirmary. The friars had allegedly "encouraged the ideas of the Indians" by "condemning in their presence the healing method that the practitioner observes with the Junta de Sanidad's approval."[56]

Eliding political struggles and disagreement over treatment, the unmistakable impression was of Indians rejecting the ministrations of trained healers in irrational and inexplicable manner. This view informed missives leaving the capital, which warned that the reasons for the propagation of fevers included primarily "the wretched constitution of the Indians, their poor nourishment, and worse inclination in being healed...and what is more, once they become victims they are bled according to their manner, and they go inside their *temascales*, whose excesses add more fuel to the fire."[57] It was also promulgated in pastoral letters, medical instructions, and administrative reports; as credible discursive formations their influence on cross-cultural and cross-class interactions during disease emergencies is not easily dismissed.[58] In them the countryside becomes a place of chaos and rusticity—a montage of fearful Indians refusing to approach a hospital and spilling excessive quantities of blood.

If medicine in this period seems ineffectual to modern eyes, many young physicians and surgeons who traveled to the countryside to heal were confident in their preparation, assured of their powers of observation, and set on assimilating communities to their way of healing. Brash young creoles who invoked famous European physicians to validate their regimens—Sydenham, Boerhaave, Huxham, de Haen—converged in the belief that the lower classes were too prone to excesses and that, if they would only heed their sage advice, epidemic destruction might be avoided. These personalities came to the fore in calamities, but in matters of propriety and medical *policía* the boundaries were less clearly drawn, and many more weighed in on the proper treatment and containment of disease.

Examining the ways in which communities evaluated this medicine in critical periods reveals the discretionary capacities and practices that elite commentators often denied the underclasses.[59] With a shift in perspective, objection no longer appears as blanket resistance to Spanish practitioners, medications, or sensibilities, but rather it emerges from concerns about the perceived success of the healer, his relation to the community's political hierarchy, and his willingness to step beyond the realm of theoretical learning and philosophical bromides to treat residents with dignity. In the midst of suffering, no one did not want to get better, despite the frequent insistence of frustrated observers. Good medicine, as Mexican anthropologist and physician Gonzalo Aguirre Beltrán wrote, "is what provides security to society; bad, that which raises anxiety."[60] Villagers were intent on getting good medicine and took cues from political and social realities as they attempted to discern in what form it would arrive.

SPEECH ACTS AND VACCINATION'S FACTS

In Tlatlauquitepec parish, in Puebla's Sierra Norte, certain parishioners allegedly believed that the vaccine being introduced would harm their children. The previous week, parents in Santiago Yaonahuac had refused to hand their children over to the Indian governor when they learned the purpose, and many had departed with their families, thinking vaccination a reckless endeavor ("cosa mui temeraria"). Village elders reasoned that force would only frighten the children further, and the governor agreed, declining to compel parents. The *cura*, Nicolás Junguera, marveled that the antivaccinators had declared in *cabildo* meetings and drinking sessions that they would present themselves before the bishop to request that he order the priest to desist from bothering them about vaccine. Otherwise, they would convince him to substitute a more accommodating pastor. Junguera asked the bishop to consider the thoughts these "crude natives" (*rudos naturales*) had about vaccine, including concerns about kidnapping, forced enlistment in the militia, and the priest's selfish pursuit of revenue, "because it goes far toward an understanding of their distinguishing character." These were "ridiculous worries," their repetition in his report even indecent. But the notions were tenaciously defended, "as if they were evident truths."[61]

Dispatches from this parish are preceded and followed by many more that confirm, in quantitative and qualitative terms, the successful adoption of vaccination. Evidence that entire villages compliantly submitted their children, despite unevenness in programs and decades of oppressive hardship, is so convincing that perhaps episodes of noncompliance should be dismissed, as the priest proposed, as fanciful aberrations, hardly reflective of the prevailing outcomes. If dubious distortions of reality, disparaging remarks about vaccine, vaccination, and vaccinators nevertheless made ripples. Lacking a developed print culture, newsworthy information in New Spain took shape in oral form, in face-to-face encounters in such places of sociability as the parish church and shrines, in knots of people at the edges of a plaza or market, in meetings of elders, and during bouts of drinking—the *embriagueces* to which the priest alluded. Elite actors might characterize the rumors that emerged as ignorant or intentionally malicious, but they were always worthy of note.

The Bourbon initiative to introduce vaccination made temporary fugitives of subjects in regions beyond Puebla. A cluster of reports of fearful Indians fleeing into the mountains arrived from towns in the valleys around Celaya, in the fertile Bajío region that produced many of the comestibles for Mexico's mining centers. Celaya became a distribution hub for vaccine once the Balmis expedition passed through, with vaccinators and children from populations in the surrounding countryside arriving regularly to transport the material back home. In many cases this happened without a hitch, according to reports submitted to Guanajuato's intendant.[62] In a few, villagers made themselves scarce, disappearing within the region's volcanic mountain ranges or blending into other populations to wait out the disruption. In Salvatierra, twenty miles from Celaya due south, the royal order on vaccination had barely arrived, the administrator reported, "when parents of families, in their extreme ignorance, hid their children, taking them up to the mountains once news reached them of those [children] who were being collected in other parts." These parents were uncertain about the purpose and not easily persuaded that collections were for vaccination, "because they always presumed they were being sought out for other, diverse fates, while those who came to understand the purpose took the operations to be dangerous, and would not adopt them."[63] In nearby Chamácuaro the official reported thirty-three successful operations on children with lymph from Celaya. He had paid some of the children from his own pocket (*de mi faldriquera*) and would have continued doing so to entice the entire village, but this had not been possible "because the majority left for the mountains, some saying that their children were child martyrs [*mártires antes de tiempo*], and others that it was the intention of the magistrate and surgeon to take illegitimate possession of them. This is what the ignorant said."[64] In Yuriria (Yuririapúndaro), vaccine transported from Celaya by three children and a skilled practitioner (*perito*) sent to learn the procedure spoiled when other children "immediately left with their mothers for the hills and other places" and could not be vaccinated.[65]

As they departed, parents reportedly leveled some condemning and even shocking charges. Preparing to revive vaccinations in 1807, the new district governor of Nochixtlán, northwest of Oaxaca's capital, sought out the parish priest to learn why vaccine had expired. The priest informed him of Santiago Coda's commission and journey through the region in 1804, when vaccine had been left in the hands of a surgeon, Pedro Xijón, and *curandero* named Juan Abendaño. The surgeon explained that when treating various injuries in the district seat and surrounding pueblos he had requested that heads of families bring their children to him for vaccination. But "these parents, far from doing it, had fled with their little ones to other pueblos, saying that they would not allow *una brujería* to be done with them, and as a result lymph had run out, and the operation ceased."[66] The charge of witchcraft, which so effectively cast doubt on the legitimacy of their own healers and healing practices, had reportedly been leveled to condemn the surgeon and his vaccine as villagers voted on its adoption with their feet.

The same result obtained in Mexicaltzingo district in 1808, during a renewed campaign in central Mexico. The local authority wrote that while as many as possible had been vaccinated in the head town and San Mateo Churubusco, Indian tributaries in several other villages were objecting, apparently horrified by the operation. Some fathers and mothers had fled with their children to conceal them in the surrounding mountains, having persuaded themselves that the operation was a ruse to brand them with the mark of the king.[67] The figure of the king invoked there was far from the beloved, beneficent figurehead, so often exempted from charges of injustice or corruption that were leveled against local administrators. Nor was this the figure who appeared in messianic rumors reported after 1810, when some expectation apparently surfaced that the dethroned king, Ferdinand VII, would return triumphantly to reclaim his rightful place.[68] Instead, departing parents accused the sovereign of enslaving his subjects, equating vaccination with a royal brand, and an illegitimate abuse of power.[69]

The sources are mostly silent about differences of gender, class, or race. Reports operated at a middle level of generalization, in which the "dramatic structuring" of these performances of flight is most visible, to the detriment of the idiosyncratic.[70] In an exceptional case, Manuel López Sobreviñas, subdelegate of Acayucan, 150 miles south of the port of Veracruz, complained in 1817 that many in his district but primarily *pardos*—a label used for persons of mixed African, European, and Indian ancestry—"are stubbornly against this incomparable benefit to humankind. They resort to fleeing to the *montes* with their children so that a malady [*mal*] that God does not send is not put into them. This," he remarked incredulously, "is the language they use." The administrator added that *pardos* were further sowing discord among *indios*, who had been seen scratching and washing the arms of their children to impede the action of the vaccine, in effect reversing earlier progress.[71]

Acts of flight, sometimes prominently featured in reports, formed familiar patterns of negotiated rule. During Mexico's colonial period Indian subjects, along with enslaved and free communities of African descent, had at their disposal the option to flee into what Gonzalo Aguirre Beltrán called "regions of refuge," denoting the ecological backlands that might provide shelter against harsh political or economic circumstances. These were often sparsely settled places of rough terrain, where villagers might wait out forced labor drafts, tributary exactions, and ill treatment, among other stresses of Spanish sovereignty.[72] Facing acute food shortages in the summer of 1778, residents of Tixtla district left their villages in search of sustenance along the coast to the south, consuming along the way roots, gourds, wild herbs and fruits, and cactus hearts. The royal governor and parish priest sought exemption from two-thirds of the year's tribute levy for the stricken populations as a result of the disruption (and called on witnesses who deemed these foods "harmful to their health" and the cause of outbreaks of dysentery and *tabardillo*).[73] Migrations in times of disease, sterility, or starvation, or away from burdensome taxation or abusive labor drafts, catalyzed legal as well as extralegal practices of remediation. Flight bled into performances of negotiation, paving the way to some response from administrators, in the form of tribute reduction, a legal advocate in a larger town, or a safe harbor to wait out a political storm with friends or family.[74]

If flight was a plausible, conventional, and even anticipated form of social action, it also provided administrators responsible for vaccine with ready-made excuses for poor performance or inaction, who by condemning flight highlighted the obstacles they had to overcome. Reports perpetuated a distinction between *gente de razón* (literally people of reason—the common phrase designating persons of European descent, affiliation, or affinity) and those presumed less reasonable in judgment. Chamácuaro's official, when describing the response of "los ignorantes," insisted that most inhabitants "de razón" there and elsewhere in his jurisdiction were traveling with their children directly to the source of vaccine in Celaya. The distinction in turn reflected realities of medical care, where castes and classes had differential access to the procedure because administrators typically declined to ask indigenous agriculturalists to abandon their work to travel to district seats. But practitioners were rewarded according to the magnitude of difficulty they claimed to have encountered in their work. The physician commissioned to introduce vaccine in Texcoco during the disease outbreaks of 1806 and 1807 reported 1,295 vaccinations over forty days in the head town, three barrios, and four pueblos, "notwithstanding the great repugnance with which parents as well as children look on the operation: they believe that it will cause them great harm, and the regular experience that nothing happens to the vaccinated does nothing to dispel this judgment." In the margin of this document, submitted to the Protomedicato for a stipend, the president scribbled his recommendation, "four pesos daily." It was an implicit validation of the physician's conclusion that, if too few had been vaccinated, "it has not depended on me, but rather on the terrified panic with which the Indians conceive of the operation."[75] Scenes of flight, panic, and general disorder thus arrive through a glass darkly.

Still, some peasants did flee and in doing so participated in a distinguished tradition of colonial protest. Rumors alleging kidnapping or child martyrdom originated in the circumstances and social worlds of those who repeated them; although they often took on a life of their own, they were "rooted in at least some shallow soil of fact."[76] In Acapulco, where reports of kidnapping stalled the campaign, Balmis and his team arrived after painstakingly collecting twenty-four children from various cities in New Spain to take along to the Philippines as carriers. Though caretakers had been paid considerable sums of money—in some cases up to 150 pesos—and their children not forcibly taken, as rumor had it, such reports of compulsory enlistment, which highlighted certain aspects of vaccine's transmission, took the shape of compelling stories about force, duplicity, and vulnerability.

So did reports that vaccination was a variety of state-sponsored witchcraft germinate in the facts of medicine's practice. Plausibly or not, administrators, physicians, and aficionados in New Spain and abroad had been touting vaccine as a kind of panacea, the thing that would cure what ailed you. Experimentation was prescribed in regulations issued for major cities in hopes that other uses would be uncovered with time. Regulations for the Central Vaccination Junta in Mexico City called vaccine's other preservative virtues undeniable, particularly against cutaneous diseases: it protected against scrofula and rickets and might even be used as a kind of tonic to fortify the delicate and sickly constitutions of patients and protect against future illnesses. The junta was directed to perform tests on patients suffering from elephantiasis and ergotism, or gangrene (*fuego de San Antón*), and because prior observations in Constantinople had shown vaccine's usefulness as a preservative against plague (*peste*), "we hope that it can similarly protect against the illnesses commonly known as black vomit and yellow fever," which were similarly pestilential, putrid, and malignant. The controversial 1810 version added other diseases including dropsy and, among teething children, diarrhea and dysentery. Instructing physicians to continue experiments, Article 13 specified that vaccination "clears up cataracts [*las nubes de los ojos*] and, without other aid, restores vision loss caused by *gota serena* [amaurosis]," and reiterated expectations about protection against yellow fever.[77]

This spirit of discovery encouraged more than one intrepid vaccinator. In Valladolid the surgeon of the royal hospital vaccinated three girls from the Colegio de Niñas Educandas for intermittent fevers (*fríos* or *tercianas*, tertiary fever) after they were bled without effect. One resident, don Josef María Luna, reportedly experienced relief after vaccination for an eye ailment ("por enfermedad en los ojos"), perhaps cataracts. Others showed favorable outcomes following vaccination for various unspecified illnesses.[78] Remarking on these developments, Balmis proclaimed vaccination's protective benefits against smallpox "the least of its virtues in view of the miraculous and sudden healings we witness."[79]

Not all were convinced. Besides parents in Nochixtlán, who deemed vaccination *una brujería* as they took to the hills, Oaxaca's bishop, Antonio de Bergosa y Jordán, expressed skepticism years later in corresponding with the viceroy. For years an active supporter of vaccination's practice in his diocese, as he noted, he recounted how his opinion had soured after contracting an illness in the blazing heat of Oaxaca and Tehuantepec. This illness had led Bergosa to submit to vaccinations on three separate occasions—in Puebla, Mexico City, and Oaxaca—at the hands of "expert practitioners," as Balmis had advised, but without effect. Although Bergosa would continue to support vaccine's use against smallpox, his personal experience flatly contradicted the claims being made that it was a "remedio universal," citing a letter from Balmis of March 7, 1811. He wrote: "If only what the director had set down in writing and perhaps has been published in Spain were true, I would give him thanks for the invention, but I regret that this can be added to the many medical falsities with which the credulous are deceived."[80] His criticism reflected years of frustration with prevailing political and economic circumstances, but the central message, articulated in official correspondence, resembled that of some of Oaxaca's rural parishioners: the assurances being made about vaccine's powers were not realistically fulfilled.

In their skeptical affinities and wariness of duplicity, the universes of literate and illiterate might not have been so far apart. It was a time when educated doctors were no less guilty of rumormongering within an ongoing, politically charged, transcontinental polemic that drew on many secondhand reports in support of one position or another. Reports about immunization's underhanded appropriation as a weapon of biological warfare, for instance, serve as a reminder of the global scope of the debate, which took place in a multitude of media, in the most rarefied intellectual circles of Europe and in the agricultural countryside of New Spain.[81] Nevertheless, poor, indigenous inhabitants received the brunt of elite scorn. In the summer of 1804, members of San Luis Potosí's city council threw up their hands in a letter to the viceroy following successful preliminary propagation of vaccine. While they had sufficient fluid to transport to the entire province, there were in the city, its barrios, and surrounding villages people of good judgment and learning ("de juicio, e instrucción"), and some who timidly submitted to those who ministered to them, but also many lacking intelligence ("de muy escasas luces"), miserable, suspicious of everything, and scared or intimidated when presented with any novelty, even of proven benefits.[82] As another city official put it, Indians and the poor were *gentes torpes*, slow-witted folk who by and large could not manage vaccinations on their own.[83] This class of people was most often described as ignorant and childlike, fleeing to the hills in the face of arriving physicians in such numbers and dramatic fashion that one might conclude that few in the countryside participated in campaigns, if not for registers indicating otherwise.

If the wealthy urban classes construed peasants as timid, irrational, distrustful, or simply dim objects of imperial medicine, others acknowledged the need for special consideration, negotiation, or instruction, if only because such precautions ensured that anticipated obstacles not become threats to colonial rule. Not just riots but the threat of riots, the British historian E. P. Thompson wrote in his study of English crowds, might compel rulers to behave in conciliatory ways, bargaining over the price of bread, for example, when sensitivity toward crowd pressure derived in part from a socioeconomic reality in which the well-being of the upper classes depended on the service and contentment of the lower. In colonial Mexico, by threatening to relinquish any obligations to the common good, Indian subjects might "dramatize the gravity of their circumstances." Cautious threats of flight might "signal to ruling authorities, not least the viceroy, that a local situation was dangerously out of kilter."[84]

During public health campaigns the initiation of a process of reconciliation just as often began with words. Rumors and the possibility of flight pointed to a real or potential breakdown of a functioning colonial order.[85] Remediation became the responsibility of local administrators, priests, and others who might ease the worries of the pueblo. Put otherwise, mass exodus contained elements of a self-fulfilling prophecy, confirming as it did elite awareness of patterns of colonial protest. Indians behaving in ways that had become calcified as stereotypical meant that administrators had not taken the appropriate precautions to militate against undue burdens and unfavorable outcomes. The mere threat of flight, following this line of thought, would have shaped the provision of public health measures over time, so long as administrators remained attentive to the outcome and eager to avoid it.

In this view, gossiping laypeople ended up leveraging notions of fragility and irrationality in interesting ways. When parents in Acapulco fretted that their children would be taken with the expedition to the Philippines, the local official went from house to house to persuade families that their belief was unfounded. It was a tactic that, according to Balmis, who witnessed the intervention, yielded fruit: 337 children brought cheerfully by their parents to the administrator's home, with sessions attended by Acapulco's bleeder, at the insistence of the physician of the royal hospital, so that he might duplicate the method in surrounding pueblos. This achievement was even greater, Balmis thought, considering that besides the governor and hospital physician, Acapulco lacked *ayuntamiento* members, parish priest, or any other subjects ordinarily available to help appease ("despreocupar") the pueblo.[86]

Efforts by administrators, priests, and physicians to persuade in these campaigns had the effect of demonstrating that these were not forceful and even acknowledged that the costs and hardships of public health for the poor and marginalized were high. In the renewed campaign in 1820, Mexicaltzingo's district governor pledged compliance but explained that in the past there had been much opposition, "and principally among the Indians, who utter the falsity that what is administered to their children to liberate them from smallpox is uncertain, pronouncing instead that it is an iron, or brand that marks them, leaving them signaled as slaves." He added optimistically that it would help if the archbishop was apprised of the situation, and parish priests instructed to "combine forces with me in their respective parishes" to persuade parishioners to present their children, "removing from their minds the error that they are marked as slaves."[87] On the cusp of Independence, when religion would again be invoked to provide stability in the new political order, the proposed solution echoed decades of wisdom on immunization, perhaps reinforced by perceptions of clerical involvement in the insurgency: put rural priests at the front of battle lines to temper a suspicion, uncertainty, and fragility everywhere seen and remarked. In consideration of the observation that medical campaigns were far from perfect; that physicians and administrators struggled continuously with shortages of funds and personnel; that vaccinations were often attempted as an afterthought, rather than primary interest, with funding assembled in an ad hoc fashion, such gestures could telegraph a kind of care and carefulness that masked these aspects of practice.

On the other hand, the possibility of reconciliation was considerably diminished without trusted mediators. The *cura* from Puebla's Sierra Norte, who suffered a crisis of authority among his impatient parishioners, eventually conceded his own lack of moral influence. Junguera noted that the rebellious residents of Santiago barrio, recently elevated to the status of pueblo, were worrying residents of Hueyapam about vaccination, and he suspected that both in turn had been influenced by residents of nearby Teteles, a pueblo of *gente de razón* and "seductive adviser of both." Seeking to explain his lack of authority in these pueblos (which he now studiously avoided, "fearful of an uprising"), he deduced a reason from an incident three years earlier, when he had reprimanded residents of Santiago for a special assessment (*derrama*) its governor had made, likely for a festival or ongoing legal dispute. For this its residents had spewed many *groserías* at their pastor and further abuses at the Catholic Church. The priest recalled another incident, in which he had reprimanded a previous governor who entered the sacristy with head covered. Apparently not inclined to hold the priest or the church building in high regard, when ordered to remove his hat the official was adamant that he did not want to. Now tasked with overseeing vaccinations, Junguera had to rely on a justice who lacked the means to implement measures and a local governor whose admonitions, issued after a contingent of residents had traveled to the district seat to request an exemption, had been ignored. As a result, he confessed, "I find myself without satisfactory resources to achieve the desired goal."[88] And there things would stand. The introduction of vaccine collided with an already tense political situation, in which a battle of wills between parishioners and their priest, exacerbated by the growing pains of a barrio asserting its independence, a pastor's inexpert handling of conflict, and intervillage alliances structured by race, all plausibly contributed to reception, and fueled something resembling an autochthonous imperial ideology, in which vaccine became a tool of forced enlistment and royal abuse.

If village politics cannot be reconstructed in every case, local power struggles are a reminder not to take questions of belief, or commitment to the literal content of rumors, too far. Like the charge that vaccine was a priest's nefarious ploy to augment his fees from burials, rumors of enlistment, enslavement, kidnapping, and martyrdom were useful political weapons. While some probably uttered and heard things in a literal sense, a reading along these lines sends one in pursuit of questions of rationality and sobriety of belief, which privileges a logic external to the charged context of the speech act and echoes the elite sources that reported them, too often only to condemn them. As an analogy (a comparative reflection on distinct realities) reports vividly located a feature or effect shared across multiple practices, namely the buboes and lesions that vaccination left on the body. Complications, though infrequent, were painful and frightful and only exacerbated this physical reality. In Miahuatlán district a single complication (of 6,753 vaccinations) in Santa María Osolotepec involved sixteen-year-old Juan Pérez, who was soaked while traveling back to his ranch following his vaccination and fell ill. Juan's father returned him to the vaccinator-phlebotomist, who observed that eruptions of pox on the boy's body had formed horrific blisters that made it appear as if he had been badly burned.[89]

This was the empirical soil, to evoke Thompson again, in which opinion took root and blossomed. Transformed into a reasonable, if not simply true or false, pastiche and elaboration on circumstances and appearances, the marks comprised a nontrivial reality, pregnant with meaning that transcended the question of immunization's effectiveness against smallpox, to say nothing of the many other diseases for which it was being advertised. Calling to mind the stigmata of a martyr, villagers transformed the Christian trope into commentary on the underlying premise of colonial public health initiatives, in which a child was scarred and "sacrificed" for the good of Spain, industry, and economic growth. Well-placed rumors amounted to linguistic surprises, tricks, or tactical ruses that produced their effects in particular situations.[90] Rumormongering thereby effected a dissection, laying bare the inner mechanisms of the technique for others to see and rendering the practice exposed by means of a striking economy of words and images.

Just a few years earlier, the viceregal government had considered the effects of speech when it ultimately declined to prohibit opinions contrary to inoculation. The incident suggests the epistemic value placed on accumulated experience as a component of enlightened public health policy, as well as the importance of public opinion and notoriety, or *voz pública*, as its articulation. Speech had a deep history and broad significance in this time and place. Testimony admitted in secular and ecclesiastical courts, like testimonials circulating beyond, amounted to verbal expression of publicly held opinion; oral testimony acquired institutional force and epistemic weight in these settings, the equivalent of certified knowledge in the status it was accorded.[91] Similarly, to discuss immunization was to enter an arena in which a few words or gestures could magnify the significance of an untimely death and shape the outcome of a campaign. Public denunciations and judgments, like so many judicial cases, did not always reconcile with the "facts." But charges to the effect that a village's children were being taken by the magistrate, priest, or surgeon for other schemes had consequences in addition to disarmed vaccinators and aborted campaigns. It might mean, for instance, lost revenue as administrators worked to resettle fleeing populations. Rumors were more than spun webs of significance for those who repeated them, in cultural anthropologist Clifford Geertz's classic formulation; they were webs that entangled administrators and practitioners and occasionally threatened to wreck the vaccinating machine.[92]

Medical, political, religious, and legal institutional cultures intersected in these campaigns, when expressions of what laypeople observed and insisted became social fact. Informal performances of remediation indelibly marked immunization's introduction and reinforced paternalistic structures of rule. Against reforms that sought purposefully to undo Mexico's juridical and social divides, efforts to mitigate abrupt change and facilitate more acceptable interventions fulfilled a tacit colonial pact, reconceived at the end of Bourbon rule, in which the ruled in New Spain placed limits on the latitude afforded the ruler. The foundations of a colonial project—in which *indios*, castes, and the poor were seen as *miserables*, childlike and fragile, to be instructed and protected for God and king—were reinforced in these years, perhaps nowhere more than in the provision of modern medicine.

CONCLUSION

Scholars of nineteenth-century attempts to introduce "Western" medical practices to Native American communities show that when modernizers did not hail new therapies and medications as replacements, or hunt the old practices or systems into extinction, they were likelier to be incorporated into familiar repertoires.[93] A uniformly derogatory and suspicious stance toward local healing practices would have had severe negative implications in colonial Mexico; if assaults were rarely successful, they were also exceptional. Agents of reform did not have at their back an all-powerful, unified state entity, willing or able to impose its will on populations. The medical profession encompassed a range of attitudes and interests, with physicians in pursuit of fees or recognition, in some cases closely monitored by bureaucrats and regulating institutions, but also in possession of their own opinions, dispositions, ideas of propriety, and preconceptions of the peasants they confronted—a far cry from unthinking pawns of institutions able to carry out their agendas through them.[94]

As with parish priests, these archetypal personalities must be extracted from stereotypical representations. When they did not recognize their limited abilities and authority, they were compelled to, as the figure in which medical dogma and the expectations of communities came into tension. Elite commentaries on the countryside as a place of deficiencies and superstitions faced villagers willing to leverage their positions as members of corporate republics to compel outsiders to respect local customs, social conventions, and healing preferences. Anyone who unwaveringly pursued intellectually faddish philosophies would have been in gross neglect of their patients' needs and thus unworthy of their trust. At the end of the day more than a few remained what Bartolache termed *recetadores*, or enthusiastic prescribers of medication.[95] Indulgence was the price paid for cooperation.

In the end the universalist aspirations of the age would have to wait for a more opportune moment. Still, many residents came to terms with global processes in these years, and as they did public health campaigns witnessed a great deal of viable political action, in the form of flight or in the signaling of discomfort or dissatisfaction through familiar idioms. Laypeople passed judgment about the serious matter of health by subjecting administrators, healers, and priests to criteria that assessed their medical, spiritual, or personal worth. Rumors were a sophisticated means by which to articulate an experience of losing autonomy, of relinquishing control over one's body or children, and of explaining the actions of authority figures and outsiders. Analogical connections addressed some salient reality, and in the process creatively unmasked the reasons of state and the pretensions of Enlightenment medicine, in such a way as to preserve the dignity of speakers against the uncertainties of change. The tendency of elite reporters to impute primarily a stubborn irrationality to their untutored charges has dulled our perception of their sharp critical faculties. Expressions of analogical thought—the foundation of creativity and theory—might provide a way out of this interpretive impasse. They remind us how peasants become theorists and producers of knowledge about immunization alongside doctors, scientists, and historians. Their skepticism—as well as hope, anxiety, and faith—was no less part of the world of the literate, and they should be integral to the stories we tell about the dilemmas of public health and technological change.

Conclusion

During the presidency of Porfirio Díaz (1876–1911), a period of relative social and political stability known as the Pax Porfiriana, Mexico's authoritarian government pursued international investment with help from scientists, technocrats, and medical professionals, who projected an image of national progress at home and abroad. Created in 1841 to assume the duties of sclerotic medical and hospital institutions, the Consejo Superior de Salubridad (Superior Council of Health) contributed by advertising advances in science and medicine.[1] The national narrative was reinforced by a special issue of the council's *Boletín* published to commemorate the centennial of Edward Jenner's discovery. A short article on immunization in Mexico, a history of Jenner's experiments by the city vaccinator, a paean in verse by the council's resident chemist, and documents reproduced from the Royal Vaccination Expedition underscored the authority of the city's medical and scientific authorities as well as the few expert hands responsible for preserving vaccine in Mexico, including Francisco Xavier de Balmis, Antonio Serrano, José Miguel Muñoz, and Luis Muñoz, the son.[2] On display was the confidence and urbanity typical of science in this period, in which men with technical learning circulate durable and fixed ideas, techniques, matter, and meanings from one trained hand to the next, with few trials, disputes, or failures.

Below this flawless veneer, renewed vaccination campaigns after 1882 in Mexico continued to respond to disease outbreaks, coordinated by an array of municipal, state, and federal bodies, councils, and private and public practitioners.[3] In the summer of 1889 the two men commissioned to vaccinate in Santa Veracruz parish, in downtown Mexico City, pressed its *cura*, Daniel Escobar, to use the sacristy or the baptistery of the church for operations. As they informed him, they had used these spaces elsewhere and considered them to be most suited (*a propósito*) to the procedure. Escobar parried the request by citing vaccination's profane nature, and "the circumstances of the people brought to vaccinate, who are from the *pueblo bajo* and leave the spaces they occupy befouled with all kinds of filth." These persons could not be trusted to behave decently if unsupervised. Weighing in on the matter, the ecclesiastical government determined that the sacred spaces of the church should not be used for the procedure.[4] That the vaccinators had done so previously—and thought they would again—reveals cracks in the official version of modern science, and confusion over the proper boundaries of medicine first evident in Mexico's early experiences with immunization.

Historians now regularly approach the era of Bourbon reform and modernization as a complicated partnership between state and society, which engendered contradictions, false starts, and modifications as enlightened clerics, patriotic district governors, nuns in convents, and Indian villagers renegotiated the boundaries of overlapping colonial authority.[5] Reforms in preventive medicine similarly looked to private initiative, generated confusion over jurisdictional boundaries, and reflected imperfectly the agendas and philosophies of Bourbon ministers. The patriotic dimensions and nationalist significance of the global public health initiative have perpetuated debates over origins as well. Who contributed more, Spaniards or creoles? Did the program begin in Spain, with the king's councils and advisers? Or was vaccination an American enterprise, in the sense that it drew on the know-how of Amerindians, creoles, municipal bodies, and local sources of cowpox fluid? There is little doubt that physicians, municipal bodies, governors, private residents, prelates, and priests were actively searching for cows with signs of pox throughout Spanish America, or acquiring it from other sources, months before the European inception of a global expedition.[6] Would these initiatives have yielded a coordinated program of prevention approaching the scale eventually witnessed? The stakes of the question are high, as evident in the blunt assertion that "the Expedition begins with the Royal Order of September 1, 1803, in which the wishes of the king are communicated to all overseas authorities.... It is after this moment, and not before, that certain viceroys and captains general begin to concern themselves with obtaining vaccine as soon as possible."[7]

Without denying the impact of royal orders, the program underwent numerous modifications and elaborations in crossing from the realm of theory to practice. It is a straightforward matter to show how a figure no less central than Balmis, the director, definitively modified the Bourbon plan as he puzzled over problems of administration, population, and regional variation. In vaccination regulations for New Spain's provincial capitals, issued in consultation with local administrators, vaccination juntas and buildings for public vaccinations (*casas de vacunación*) already reflected adjustments.[8] Considering how distance from metropolitan authority introduced challenges to following royal orders, Balmis endeavored to place vaccine under the care of committees rather than the local governors (corregidores) who oversaw it in Spain. He favored municipal buildings (*casas consistoriales*) for vaccinations, moreover, because the hospitals that were designated for use in a royal *cédula* of April 21, 1805, instead of reassuring parents of the care of a medical professional, planted unnecessary fears. "The idea of congregating in hospitals," Balmis observed, "is for many shameful and revolting, and for others risky." The best route was to eliminate "any notion of sickness, pain, or danger, [and nothing is more] advisable than to see the vaccinated continuing their ordinary life out in the open air, without preparation or diet, as if the operation had not been performed on them." By providing a *casa decente*, people would be vaccinated "without the horror and repugnance with which hospitals, hospices, and other houses of mercy are held."[9] The notion that directors, subdirectors, physicians, and the clergy mainly instantiated the royal vision, finalized with the expedition's departure from Spain, ignores adjustments made along the way, not least of which were those encouraged and endorsed by the director himself.[10]

More to the point, these modifications and accommodations were foretold in numerous late colonial episodes of disease and remediation. The story begins in streets and shrines, with people and saints in prayer and procession, rather than in hospitals or with statutes and legal codes, because the earliest designs for programs of disease prevention began there, in procession. Well before the inception of plans to acquire and propagate Jennerian vaccine, residents of colonial Mexico were contributing the common sense, logistical aptitude, and ritual meanings that would shape the technology at the center. Literate and illiterate, professionals and laypeople confirmed, over decades of coping with disease, that hospitals were frightful places of last resort that were unsuitable for treatment owing to their associations with disease and death. Spain's ministers thought that vaccine should arrive "beneath a canopy," but colonial projects of evangelization and conquest, viceregal ceremony, and the visual and embodied cultures of parish and devotional life suggested the eyes and ears as suitable routes to true understanding. In literary projects of vernacular translation and public instruction, creole *letrados* encouraged laypeople to wield instruments of measurement to regulate their health, to examine visual reproductions of plants and machines, and to experiment with useful medicinal plants, endeavoring to enlist a greater segment of society in shielding the population against disease.

Government initiatives and institutions occasionally converged with these homegrown efforts to enlighten, educate, and remedy. In 1813 the acting Spanish government, looking to advance medical education and other measures to combat disease, solicited information on the status of the medical sciences in New Spain. The inquiry noted that the Crown had established anatomical theaters, chairs of medicine, and botanical gardens for this purpose. Had the Protomedicato been licensing additional practitioners, and if so were Indians among those studying medicine, surgery, and botany? If not, what might be done "to provide this instruction, which would be of great usefulness in their pueblos, where generally this assistance is lacking"? This forward-looking vision of medical training and practice sought to incorporate rural populations into official institutions, where competent healing was imagined to originate.[11] In New Spain this acculturating impulse existed alongside a countervailing interpretation that construed the countryside as more than just a place of healing deficiencies. At least some public figures, pursuing other ways to improve health, recognized the wealth of medical knowledge and experience held by untrained and unlicensed rural communities.

The public rituals, conventions of communication, and implicit understandings that informed patterns of response to disease suggest that the most assertive personalities are best understood within the culture into which they were born, to which they were sensitized, or in which they were compelled, if only briefly, to labor. When Balmis acknowledged viceregal conventions, by encouraging the gift of a coin to the poor, for instance, he advanced his cause. When he sought to restrict vaccine's administration to elite practitioners specially trained and certified by vaccination boards (a restriction implied in royal decrees), he failed. Although "the practice of vaccination may be so simple and easy that mothers will eventually execute it by themselves," he insisted that distinguished professors of medicine and surgery must be selected for this important mission.[12] This position, justified by the complex interaction of vaccine matter with the human body and the need to recognize successful operations, was in constant tension with Mexico's social, medical, and political realities. Spanish American prelates and district officials noted that the ideal was untenable in most places, where dearth and deprivation prevailed and the perceived safety, accessibility, and cost-effectiveness were decisive in the procedure's general acceptance and use.

More sustained focus on these conditions over decades brings to view other judgments and models of public health. The obvious point of contrast is with the plantations of the Caribbean, where thousands of inoculations took place under the supervision of Esteban Morel, as recounted in the opening pages of this book. If not effortless, Morel presumably never took the trouble to compose a treatise in defense and support of inoculation, because promotional efforts were superfluous. The violent logics of plantation slavery and profit decided in favor of immunization, granting only a tiny fraction of the population the liberty to choose.[13] In New Spain, by contrast, where residents battled epidemics through elaborate rituals of penitence and supplication, a smattering of healing manuals, and therapeutics such as bleeding, purging, and sweat baths, enthusiasts of measurement and experimentation sought other ways to induct the populace into enlightened modes of disease management and self-care. Public health and disease prevention were envisioned vertically, above all, through an idiom that linked subjects to patrons and benefactors—and ultimately to God and king—and not horizontally, as a sacrifice made on behalf of a community of equals.

In this society, petitions requesting special consideration for Indian tributaries under duress embedded ancien régime expectations that the royal figure would execute his paternal duties and moral obligations during crisis.[14] The Spanish state buttressed the social order by consenting to such petitions for tributary relief, provisioning supplies of food and water, and redirecting communal funds toward urgent needs. Priests, hacienda owners, governors, physicians, viceroys, and other patrons earned the right to exercise authority through generous and conspicuous displays of benevolence, and agents of state-sponsored public health programs found themselves compelled to respect these traditions. Processions and celebrations marking the entrances of vaccinators bespoke a gift economy that is uniquely revealing of this universe of obligations, within which members of Indian republics were positioned to set the terms of the exchange.

In the end, adaptations were germane to the mechanics and claims to legitimacy of this highly mediated absolutist state. When village elders in Oaxaca protested isolation measures on the understanding that their children would be subjected to afflictions worse than smallpox; when in Puebla, absent a royal vaccinator, estate workers took it upon themselves to vaccinate one another; when parents stalled campaigns by decrying vaccine as an instrument of their enslavement or enlistment; when a regalist bishop prematurely made allowance for lay and clerical vaccinations, they acted through paternalistic routines that were inflected by ideas about cultural capacity, the imprint of centuries of colonial rule. Where infrequent violence and relative tranquility in the Mexican case might be explained by the alignment of colonial interests with the state project, and the latter's imposition on a subdued society, the reality appears to have been otherwise: medical reform facilitated by a class of self-interested representatives and power brokers who drew on timeworn strategies from multiple discursive and symbolic domains to tailor overly ambitious projects. More often than not, vaccine arrived accompanied by trumpets rather than truncheons, in missives from the pulpit, in chords of music, hymns of praise, and light displays, with coins and cookies to entice the impoverished sectors, and in the hands of barbers, aficionados, and parish priests. If coercive measures of quarantine, social control, and vaccination were rare, the upheavals of insurgency made them even more so.[15]

Beyond the epidemiological impact, the effects of this period of disease prevention and control were profound. Just as the expedition was launched, Francisco Lizana y Beaumont, Mexico's new archbishop, was writing the Spanish metropolis about the waning influence of the Catholic Church in all aspects of life in New Spain: attacks on ecclesiastical immunity and privileges would further weaken the authority of priests, he warned, who were the cornerstone of Spain's presence in the Americas.[16] A global campaign to vaccinate reaffirmed their role, along with a concurrent royal *cédula* mandating the extraction of fetuses in postmortem caesarean operations on pregnant women.[17] But these medical initiatives reiterated what matters of disease and health regularly demanded—namely, the participation of ecclesiastics in public life.

The involvement of priests in the bodies and ailments of their parishioners is vividly illustrated in the résumé of Julio Antonio Monroy, the fifty-six-year-old pastor of Santa María Amealco. His recollection of thirty years of nearly uninterrupted pastoral work begins in February 1810 in the parish of Tlalnepantla, north of Mexico City. A time of upheaval, Monroy overcame his own infirmities and fears of infection to confess and assist parishioners during the *peste* of 1812, "whose ravages are remembered even today with bitterness." In Tepetitlan parish after 1821 he crossed a flooding river to heal and confess the sick, and once performed a caesarean section, "by means of which he successfully extracted a child, who survived some minutes after having been administered the healing waters of baptism." Monroy listed postmortem caesarean operations to baptize the unborn again as acting *cura* of Chapa de Mota parish, citing a lack of medical practitioner, along with instruction of his Otomí-speaking parishioners in the mysteries of the Catholic faith. Finally, banished from his parish by the governor of Querétaro during the political crisis of 1833, Monroy ministered elsewhere to victims of Mexico's first cholera epidemic. All of this, in addition to repairing or restoring liturgical ornaments, vestments, altarpieces, chapels, bells, and musical instruments, he counted among "the duties [*deberes*] of a priest." And he was in good company among Mexico's rural clergy in emphasizing the provision of medicine, care, and food in periods of epidemic disease.[18]

The heroic self-presentations offered in these résumés require a skeptical reading. But by indicating encounters with priests and medical procedures that endured after Independence, they also invite us to revisit familiar teleologies about religion and medicine. As historians have corrected outdated Black Legend notions about Spanish America (and the deficit of scientific activity and medical expertise once thought to characterize the region), they continue to contemplate the relation of religious practice, rhetoric, people, and experience to narratives of modernity.[19] Historian Pamela Voekel's study of funerary practices and the communal dimensions of death and salvation in late colonial Mexico has done much to reassess the shift in authority from religion to medical empiricism during the Enlightenment. In the wills of a sector of upwardly-mobile merchants, physicians, clerics, and government bureaucrats in Mexico City and Veracruz, Voekel found evidence of enlightened piety in the form of flagging interest in saints and the elaborate mortuary rituals of baroque Mexico. The sensibilities of these *sensatos* facilitated an alliance with public health officials over reforms of cemeteries and the use of public spaces. It was a precarious marriage that supposedly ended in the nineteenth century, when the enlightened clerics who pronounced in favor of empiricist approaches to medicine and health found their theological justifications for cemetery reform undermined by the new professional and evidence-based epistemology. When assessing the rise of modernity, in other words, "medical empiricism" can seemingly only be consummated through a vigorous negation of religious precursors and participants.[20]

This urban story cannot be the only one if we hope to account for the experience of the majority of the population who lived elsewhere. Given that Bourbon rulers and viceregal institutions never managed to increase the numbers of certified medical personnel available to civilian populations (in contrast to the military), there is good reason to be suspicious of the hegemony of "medical empiricism." Infected states, pursuing the Enlightenment emphasis on health and immunity as a means of population growth, had a way of pulling into the breach a coterie of other healers and caretakers, who espoused multiple frameworks of healing and whose work was not always officially sanctioned. Civil authorities leaned on the moral influence and technical expertise of pastors who, along with saints and other Catholic mediators, performed indispensable duties in disease outbreaks. In the process the Catholic Church—its personnel, liturgical spaces, genres, prayers, and sacraments—acquired or maintained practical relevance through years of burgeoning medical practice, helping to underwrite the persistence of religious epistemologies and rituals into the Republic.[21]

After Independence, civil authorities continued to harness religion to the needs of society and the new nation, while the clergy warned of the dangerous legacies of Enlightenment rule, in the form of mitigated influence, impiety, and even secularization.[22] The diminished influence of the church was real, but this had as much to do with the temporary power vacuum atop the ecclesiastical hierarchy and confused jurisdictional boundaries as with a permanent shift in religious sensibilities. Despite the institutional predicament, in sermons the high clergy still viewed themselves as essential mediators between a reforming liberal state and its populace, while popular expressions of Catholic pride elsewhere in society suggest a continued investment of legitimacy in religious agents.[23] The terms in which rural priests fashioned their pastoral careers in post-Independence Mexico likewise pointed in calculated ways to their relevance and utility. They even acquired new significance, if language touting disease eradication and human health worked as a form of patriotism in the ideology of the new republican order.

Taken too far, the prevailing focus on cities as centers of collection, enlightened administration, regulation, and intellectual life—with their institutions of higher learning, hospitals and anatomical theaters, libraries, artistic academies, and printing presses—can obscure the local processes of remediation and deliberation that made technology applicable and gave abstract learning concrete place. The recovery of these settings continues to encourage a rethinking of the locus of scientific fashioning in the Enlightenment, when nonliterate ways of knowing and rural trajectories and institutions facilitated assessment, review, and revision.[24] Physicians, magistrates, ecclesiastics, and informally trained healers, some in the service of the Bourbon monarchy, worked in tandem and in tension with the designs of colonial and republican states. They drew on the flexible, locally situated, practical knowledge that the anthropologist James Scott has reserved for peasants and other targets of reform; schemes for human improvement became reality because of the range of intermediary perspectives that constituted them.[25]

In the end, the varieties of practical knowledge brought to bear are not easily classified as peasant, indigenous, viceregal, creole, American, Spanish, or Atlantic. In 1818, Cuautitlán's district governor, after nearly two hundred vaccinations performed during a smallpox outbreak, marveled that "this antidote is not only a preservative against smallpox infection, but also extends to the extermination of chronic ulcers and sores, as many children who suffered from this sickness have recuperated in full." Drawing on a viceregal culture of experimentation, one encouraged in regulations for vaccine issued throughout the Americas, he repeatedly sought announcement of his findings in *periódicos* or *gazetas* for public consumption and emulation elsewhere.[26] A climate of discovery and change produced uncertainty but also faith and expectation among healers, officials, and laypeople, who together certified (and occasionally recorded) what they saw and heard. In December 1819 the vaccinator-phlebotomist in Zacatecas agreed with the parents of three-year-old Euntaquio Martínez, believed to be mute, who attributed his miraculous recovery—in the form of a fully uttered sentence—to vaccination. Months later the same practitioner recorded the case of nineteen-month-old Luisa Velasco, who was cured of a congenital skin condition, for which her father acknowledged vaccine's marvelous role.[27] The creativity with which people read the body's signs gave vaccine the fructifying meaning that nourished it, in a dense ritual ecosystem that generated more than a little epistemic confusion about the technology's meaning and place. The confusion was hardly resolved in Mexico City's parishes at the end of the century.

Public health was again prioritized in the relative peace following the Mexican Revolution. Efforts to educate the public about immunity included a Day of Vaccine in Mexico City, on September 27, 1923, with more extensive campaigns in the wake of obligatory vaccination laws in 1925. In December 1931 public health officials, wary of the thousands of pilgrims who converged annually on Mexico City for Guadalupe's feast, organized a fifteen-day vaccination campaign. In the countryside, post-revolutionary vaccinating brigades composed of medical students, nurses, and other practitioners (some were entirely female) arrived to vaccinate and train locals. In June 1949, Francisco Chavarria Velasco, the physician in charge of a brigade in Michoacán, suspended the campaign in San Antonio pueblo after failing to coax its "rebellious" population. Only the parish priest, exhorting from the pulpit, prevailed upon parishioners to submit to ministrations, according to Velasco's report. Three years later, on June 16, 1952, Miguel Alemán declared smallpox eradicated from Mexico.[28]

If a story of success, it is hardly a triumphal one. Infectious disease and its attendant scapegoating remain omnipresent. During the H1N1 outbreak in the spring of 2009, for example, with Mexico City at a standstill and fears of a global pandemic rising, dozens of the faithful, wearing masks to protect against infection, appeared in procession with a statue of the Cristo de la Salud—an intercessor not seen since an 1850 outbreak of cholera.[29] National and international media outlets, seeking to place blame as reports of outbreaks multiplied, noted that Mexicans are prone to delay visits to licensed healthcare professionals.[30] Such characterizations, revealed as overblown in the aftermath, harbor an irony in light of what we know about early modern medicine, when techniques of prevention and treatment were embraced in the most remote regions despite or because of the ritual life of the population.

As medical experts and healthcare workers struggle to inform wary parents of the risks and advantages of a shot in the arm, a question at the core of public health and nation-building efforts resounds. Can biomedical technologies and health measures be established in concord with religion, folk practice, and freedom of choice? In pursuing matters of trust, expertise, and science in translation, this history of early experiments with preventive practice suggests the simplicity of this opposition.

In light of ongoing debates about the safety of vaccines, the role of experts in society, the erosion of scientific authority, and the role of the media in shaping belief and public opinion, it seems we are living through the same transition as before, with matters of culture and communication at the fore. And the end of this transition is nowhere yet on the horizon.

Notes

INTRODUCTION

1. Biographical details are from Esteban Enrique Morel, "Disertación sobre la utilidad de la inoculación, escrita de encargo de la nob[ma] Ciudad de Mexico," AHDF 3678 exp. 2; and Schifter Aceves, *Medicina, minería e inquisición*, 37. Unless otherwise noted, all translations into English are the author's.

2. Morel, "Disertación," 59v.

3. Ibid., 1r. On Morel's struggles with Mexico City's *ayuntamiento*, see Schifter Aceves, *Medicina, minería e inquisición*, 18–19.

4. For a recent volume in this direction, see Paquette, *Enlightened Reform in Southern Europe and Its Atlantic Colonies.*

5. Baltasar Ladrón de Guevara, "Discurso sobre la policia de Mexico: Reflexiones, y Apuntes sobre varios objetos que interesan la salud pública y la Policia particular de esta Ciudad de Mexico, si se adaptasen las providencias o remedios correspondientes," AHDF 3627 exp. 43, items I, II, VII, VIII, X, XVIII, XIX, quotation from para. 154. The archival copy is a *borrador*, with corrections. For a transcription with introduction, see González-Polo, *Reflexiones y apuntes sobre la Ciudad de México*. Guevara cited his role in the establishment of *comisarios de barrio*, which he had proposed in September 1778 and executed in the following years. A decade later, however, he considered them a failure owing to the lowly status of the people who had been commissioned to oversee *policía* in the new *cuarteles*.

6. Beezley, Martin, and French, *Rituals of Rule, Rituals of Resistance*; Viqueira Albán, *Propriety and Permissiveness*; and Bailey Glasco, *Constructing Mexico City*.

7. Owensby, *Empire of Law and Indian Justice in Colonial Mexico*, 58–77. The lawyer Hipólito Villaroel's treatise on the "political illnesses" of Mexico City (1785) is sometimes cited as evidence of elite disciplining efforts, but his disapproving gaze was also turned on the vices and excessive liberty of the upper classes, who were no less threatening to good order. Villaroel would have known: he was accused before the Juzgado General de Indios of abuses committed during his time as district governor (*alcalde mayor*), including distributions of merchandise to villagers in the practice known as *repartimiento de comercio*. See Borah, "Alguna luz sobre el autor de las *Enfermedades políticas*," 62–66.

8. Núñez de Haro y Peralta, *Nos el Dr. D. Alonso Nuñez de Haro y Peralta, por la gracia de Dios*, 1779.

9. Tissot, *Aviso al pueblo acerca de su salud*, 10–11 (the Spanish edition of

Avis au peuple sur sa santé). Though fears of depopulation were overdrawn, the size and health of the population "was considered an essential component of the wealth of nations" (Rusnock, *Vital Accounts*, 39).

10. Campomanes y Sorriba, *Discurso sobre el fomento de la industria popular*, 52.

11. Torre Villar, *Instrucciones y memorias de los virreyes novohispanos*, 1070 (item 237).

12. Warren, *Medicine and Politics in Colonial Peru*, especially the introduction.

13. On free trade *reglamentos* and the strategic importance of New Spain, see Stein and Stein, *Apogee of Empire*, 69–80 and 143–175.

14. Brading, *Miners and Merchants*, 47–51.

15. Scholars debate the degree to which this effort was imposed by the secular state or endorsed by the ecclesiastical hierarchy. For the view that stresses the role of a heterogeneous ecclesiastical hierarchy, see Connaughton, "Transiciones en la cultura político-religiosa mexicana," 447–466. In support of this regional perspective is the varied timing of secularization: in Puebla, for instance, the process began as early as the seventeenth century due largely to the efforts of Bishop Palafox y Mendoza.

16. The principal blueprint for "defensive modernization" undertaken under Charles III appeared as early as 1743 in José del Campillo y Cosío's *Nuevo sistema de gobierno económico para la América*, which was incorporated wholesale into Bernardo Ward's influential *Proyecto económico* in 1762, discussed in Brading, *Miners and Merchants*, 25–54, 63–65, and 74–92. See also Phelan, *People and the King*, chapters 1 and 2.

17. Taylor, *Magistrates of the Sacred*, 13–14.

18. Gálvez, *Informe sobre las rebeliones populares de 1767*, 63–64. Kuethe and Blaisdell, "French Influence and the Origins of Bourbon Colonial Reorganization," 595–596, downplay the Francophile Gálvez's role in favor of other ministers and prior efforts internal to Spain. For a recent view that stresses emulation and international influence (especially English and French), see Paquette, *Enlightenment, Governance, and Reform in Spain and Its Empire*. On obstacles to the abolition of *repartimiento* in Oaxaca, see Guardino, *Time of Liberty*, 91–101 and 116–121.

19. On regional variation, see Mazín Gómez, "Reorganización del clero secular novohispano."

20. Joseph de Gálvez to Señor Virrey de Nueva España, Aranjuez, April 15, 1785, AGN Epidemias 7 exp. 1, 4–5. Reasons for suspending publication of the *bando* in New Spain were given by the man who served as his secretary: the Conde de Gálvez apparently preferred to pass royal orders to justices and parish priests, for immediate communication of the measures to their subordinates and parishioners. Fernandez de Cordova to Viceroy, Mexico City, September 17, 1797, ibid., 29.

21. *Extracto de la obra publicada en Madrid el año pasado de 1784 con el título de Disertación Físico-Médica*, AGN Epidemias 7 exp. 1, 9–14. After an original printing of four thousand copies, a revised edition printed in New Spain in 1786 included anecdotal evidence of success by the prescribed method to convince readers of the benefits of its adoption.

22. In the port of Veracruz, fear of contagion propagated by goods and persons arriving on ships from Havana in the spring and summer of 1790 moved municipal officials, in consultation with Viceroy Revillagigedo and the Protomedicato in Mexico City, to subject ships to quarantine in harbor and individual pieces of mail to fumigation when they could not be so detained. When the frigate *Nuestra Señora de la Piedad* arrived from Campeche with three enslaved women purchased in Havana, who were apparently recovering from smallpox, the governor prevented the women from disembarking in port, and the captain was fined 1,000 pesos for contravening orders not to carry sick passengers. Whether or not he paid, officials were deadly serious about the propagation of infection. Correspondence on the reputed outbreak of smallpox in Havana (more common than exceptional there) and emergency measures in Veracruz is in AGN Epidemias 7 exp. 2. (The final documents on the enslaved women are by the captain, Diego de Mérida, requesting permission to sell them and claiming that they did not show signs of *viruelas* in two and a half months in his home after traveling from Havana; and the viceroy's legal assessor, who advises that the *esclavas* be examined to see whether they are free of contagion and can be sold; see Mérida to Viceroy, Veracruz, June 23, 1790, ibid., 95–96 and following.)

23. The new philosophy of governance correlated the health and productivity of populations to increased tax revenue, trade, and military strength; problems of disease became urgent globally, as evidenced by the way absolutist states employed quantitative studies of populations, achieved by counting births and deaths and tracking life expectancy, health, and average age, as measures for more efficient and enlightened statecraft. Porter, *Health, Civilization, and the State*; Rosen, *History of Public Health*; Rusnock, "Biopolitics," 49–68; and Foucault, "Politics of Health in the Eighteenth Century," 166–182.

24. Guevara, "Discurso sobre la policia de Mexico," item XX (titled "Concurrencia eficaz y necesaria de la jurisdicción arzobispal o eclesiástica para la policía de México").

25. Fray Joseph Mariano to Pedro Fessar, San Juan, January 22, 1796, AGN Historia 531 exp. 3, 39–41.

26. On the *higienista* "foot soldiers" and their regulation of sexual practices, see Bliss, "Science of Redemption." On the "scientific" groundwork for many urban renewal and public health campaigns, see Stepan, *"Hour of Eugenics."* McCrea, *Diseased Relations*, 83–94, notes that in Yucatán physicians prescribed expensive beverages like brandy and opiates for outbreaks of cholera in the 1850s, which were inaccessible or impractical for the region's poor residents.

27. See Espinosa, *Epidemic Invasions*, chapter 3 and 63–66. Mariola Espinosa notes a cruel irony in the fact that the disease targeted with such zeal was not one that had much prevalence in the local population. Chalhoub, "Politics of Disease Control," makes a similar observation for Brazil.

28. The *revolta contra vacina* brought poor and working-class residents from crowded tenements and favelas of the capital's most marginal districts into the streets for days in November 1904, where longstanding grievances and resentment over the government's invasive hygienic policies found violent expression. On the centrality of the medical issue, see Chalhoub, *Cidade febril*, 101–102 and 121–162, which places the moment within a longer history of vaccination. Others

have deemphasized the importance of vaccination, including Needell, "*Revolta Contra Vacina* of 1904"; Nachman, "Positivism and Revolution in Brazil's First Republic"; and Meade, *"Civilizing" Rio*, 90 and 75–120.

29. Scott, *Seeing Like a State*, 51–52.

30. Few, *For All of Humanity*, 150–152 and 248n39. In Guatemala, inoculation campaigns were entangled in a growing interest in caesarean operations to save and baptize the unborn fetus in the event of its mother's death. Few portrays this process both in terms of biomedicalization (the colonization of bodies through medical discourse and practice) and as a more compassionate expression of "medical humanitarianism" that gives way to coercion and surveillance owing to the scale on which Jennerian vaccine was enacted (163–164). That the Guatemalan case shows a characteristically modern state apparatus—one capable of making bodies legible through public health measures, accurate censuses, and the experience or threat of violence (199–200)—is not entirely borne out by evidence in the chapter on the expedition. The Mexican case seems to indicate greater variability across space and time.

31. Grandin, *Blood of Guatemala*, 74–76. For Peru, coercion in Lima and along the South American path of the vaccination expedition appears minimal. Historian Adam Warren has found orders for priests to persuade their parishioners and the occasional posting of a soldier outside a vaccination site, but few instances of opposition, induced by uncertainties and inconsistencies in the official program, lack of funds, and the reasonable fears and apathy of parents. Warren, "Piety and Danger," 145–160, 174, and for San Miguel de Piura, where villagers "actively took part in the destruction of the vaccine project," 165–166.

32. Joseph Antonio Rincón, San Martin Tileagete, February 20, 1780, AGN IV 5724 exp. 12, 42r-v. This newly classified section was paginated in somewhat haphazard fashion; other identifiers, such as dates, authors, and places, should be followed in the likely event that the pages are rearranged.

33. On rumor as a substitute for public discourse in this setting, see Lomnitz, *Deep Mexico, Silent Mexico*, chapter 7.

34. The phrase is from the late French historian François-Xavier Guerra, who institutionalized the study of Spanish American independence movements at the Sorbonne. On Guerra's influence on studies of revolutionary liberalism, see Ávila, "De las independencias a la modernidad," 76–112. For the position sketched here, see Guerra, *Modernidad e independencias*, 11–15, 46–47, 85–113, and 275–318; and Guerra, "Spanish-American Tradition of Representation and Its European Roots."

35. The Royal College of Surgery in the Indian Hospital (established in 1770), the Royal Botanical Garden (established in 1788), and to a lesser extent the Royal College of Mining (established in 1792) contributed to reforms in epidemic management in Mexico. All were located in Mexico City, although each institution had important rural connections and dimensions. Continuing in this vein, there is a growing literature on the Enlightenment that connects the history of early modern Mexico to Spain and the rest of Europe by examining the writings of elite creoles within an Atlantic world framework, highlighting processes of identity formation and patriotism in and through the great debates of the period. See, for example, Paquette, *Enlightenment, Governance, and Reform in Spain and*

Its Empire; Paquette, *Enlightened Reform in Southern Europe and Its Atlantic Colonies*; and Cañizares-Esguerra, *How To Write the History of the New World.*

36. Guerra and his colleagues contributed to this revision, as in the edited volume by Guerra and Annick Lempérière, *Los espacios públicos en Iberoamerica*, especially the introduction, 9–10. The concept of a bourgeois sphere, these critics pointed out, was a European paradigm that did not apply to Latin American reality at the time of Independence. The individual case studies nevertheless affirm the centrality of political revolution as the key crisis transforming thought and action in what became the Republic of Mexico: of thirteen chapters, ten focus on the Independence wars in Latin America and their aftermath; of four that devote significant portions to the colonial period, two (one by Guerra) emphasize old forms of sociability in corporatist ancien régime society, in contrast to modern forms of political practice. The exceptions on "public spaces" prior to Independence are provocative analyses of critical publics in late colonial Spanish America, by Annick Lempérière and Renán Silva.

37. On the more radical modernity of the Spanish American Baroque, see Cañizares-Esguerra, *How To Write the History of the New World*, 344. He observes that the history of science in the colonial Spanish world, "by and large, does not belong in the 'non-Western world.' The scientific practices and ideas that became dominant were those brought by Europeans as they strove to create stable, viable colonial societies." See Cañizares-Esguerra, *Nature, Empire, and Nation*, 46–47. The absence of indigenous science is explained by the flattening of social hierarchy experienced by formerly complex Aztec, Inca, and Maya civilizations, with an accompanying decline of the priests, scribes, and intellectuals who produced scientific knowledge and asked the important theological and cosmological questions prior to the arrival of the Spanish. What remained was a hybrid "folk Catholicism," Cañizares-Esguerra argues, largely popular knowledge relegated to the margins of colonial society.

38. In Greek and European medical practice, "crisis" designated a turning point in an illness, the moment in which it culminated, after which the patient's condition either improved (often by expelling some corrupted humor from the body) or declined. The words "crisis" and "critique," as in "critical days" of an illness, are etymologically related, the one implying the other.

39. Epidemics also compelled these friars to become healers, and to the extent that they were received as effective in their art, they made inroads among communities of neophytes. On the Jesuits in New Spain, see Reff, *Disease, Depopulation, and Culture Change*; for the Guaraní of South America, see Chaves de Resende, "Entre a cura e a cruz," and Prieto, *Missionary Scientists.*

40. See Florescano and Malvino, *Ensayos sobre la historia de las epidemias en México*; Austin Alchon, *Native Society and Disease in Colonial Ecuador*; Newson, *Life and Death in Early Colonial Ecuador*; Cook, *Born To Die*; Cook and Lovell, *"Secret Judgments of God"*; and Hernández Palomo, *Enfermedad y muerte en América y Andalucía.*

41. See Márquez Morfín, *La desigualdad ante la muerte en la Ciudad de México*, on the typhus and cholera epidemics of 1813 and 1833; Cuenya Mateos, *Puebla de los Ángeles*, on the city of Puebla during the epidemic of 1737; and Molina del Villar, *La Nueva España y el matlazahuatl*, on the 1737 epidemic in

Mexico City and the Valley of Mexico, the relation of epidemics to famine crises, and their effects on migration and land tenure.

42. Father Jácobo Sedelmayr to Juan Antonio Balthasar, 1749, quoted in Radding, *Wandering Peoples*, 123.

43. In other words, "the official obsession with the pathological generates an almost surreal record of the normal." Starn, foreword to Calvi, *Histories of a Plague Year*, xiv.

44. "Breve exposicion de la Epidemia que está reinando en Mexico y sus alrededores," signed Juan de Balenchana, Francisco Montes de Oca, and Joaquin Piña, Mexico City, April 30, 1824, AHDF 3674 exp. 21.

45. Intermediaries in the mature colony were readily available in the resources of the Catholic Church. Devotional images came to acquire such roles in much the same way as magistrates, priests, and village elders, all crucial figures linking rural populations to urban centers and global processes. See Taylor, "Between Global Process and Local Knowledge."

46. In part this has been achieved by widening the geographic focus of the Enlightenment (*ilustración* in Spanish) to consider the production and reception of new knowledge, values, or theories among a wider range of people and across national borders. See Darnton, "High Enlightenment and the Low-Life of Literature"; Golinski, *Science as Public Culture*; Stewart, *Rise of Public Science*; Bolufer Peruga, "De la historia de las ideas a la de las prácticas culturales," 21–52; and the essays in Manning and Cogliano, *Atlantic Enlightenment*. Art historian Daniela Bleichmar approaches the natural history expeditions that traversed Spanish America in the final decades of the eighteenth century in search of plants, minerals, and other useful goods through a visual sensibility, or "visual epistemology," evident in the importance scientists placed on the thousands of illustrations they produced. See Bleichmar, "Visible and Useful Empire," 290–310, and *Visible Empire*, especially 38–39. On religion as an analytical category in Enlightenment studies, see Sheehan, "Enlightenment, Religion, and the Enigma of Secularization," noting that religion can be usefully understood in its anthropological, social, ideological, and institutional aspects, along with the emphasis on "belief" of eighteenth-century societies.

47. Farge, *Subversive Words*. Studies of the press in Latin America's insurgency period stress that the true political import of the written word can only be understood in relation to the spoken word, even after Independence, when nation-builders were far more likely to associate writing with civilization. See the contributions to Jaksic, *Political Power of the Word*, especially Earle, "Role of Print," and Serrano and Jaksic, "Church and Liberal State Strategies on the Dissemination of Print." We would do better to speak of *hearing* and *speaking* publics as well as reading publics.

48. Corbin, *Village Bells*, x.

49. Corbin, *Foul and the Fragrant*, 15, 44–45, and 49.

50. Historian Mary Ryan has described women's grievances in the 1863 draft riots of New York as "both just and reasoned, if tragically misdirected." She warns that boundaries "must be permeable to even distorted voices" of such excluded people. See Ryan, "Gender and Public Access," 286. Critical theorist Nancy Fraser proposes avoiding a priori definitions of the common good by fo-

cusing on "subaltern counterpublics": groups with distinct issues and styles of reasoning and conversing whose concerns (e.g. women's rights) have import for the broader society and cannot be set apart. See Fraser, "Rethinking the Public Sphere," 129, 116–118, and 122–132. These contributions emphasize multiple publics in conflictive interaction, resurrecting Gramsci's notion of hegemony and hegemonic processes whereby groups struggle over contested meanings; see Eley, "Nations, Publics, and Political Cultures," 319–325.

51. Sahlins, *Islands of History*, 7–8.

52. Carreón Nieto, *Epidemias y desastres en el Obispado de Michoacán*, 50–55.

53. Historians and demographers disagree about the epidemiological impact of inoculation and vaccination in Mexico. Some aver that death rates declined even with inoculation, others that the nature of the available data makes it difficult to disentangle those factors that might have contributed to improve human health, including nutrition and care. For the former position, see publications by Cramaussel, especially "Epidemias y endemias"; for the latter, see McCaa, "Inoculation." These debates and methodological challenges aside, it is equally certain, whatever the biomedical efficacy, that residents were far more familiar with the practice after 1804, long before legislation making immunization against smallpox obligatory proliferated at the federal, state, and municipal levels in the 1880s and 1890s. For an overview of this legislation and struggles to enact it, see Carrillo, "Por voluntad o por fuerza."

54. New interpretations are facilitated by access to more of the record, including the recent classification in Mexico's national archive of a cache of unbound documents spanning roughly 1805 to 1821. Such virgin source material considerably enriches the picture by filling out some of the gaps for the years of the Mexican insurgency.

55. While this thematic approach to the early decades of immunization in Mexico offers analytical and interpretive advantages, it leaves out much of the narrative of the Royal Philanthropic Vaccination Expedition. For detailed accounts, see the studies cited in the Bibliography by Francisco Fernández del Castillo (*Los viajes de don Francisco Xavier de Balmis*), Michael Smith ("Balmis en la Nueva España" and *"Real Expedición Marítima de la Vacuna" in New Spain and Guatemala*), and Susana María Ramírez Martín ("Fuentes bibliográficas para el estudio," *La mayor hazaña médica de la colonia*, and *La salud del Imperio*).

56. *Gazeta de Madrid*, no. 84 (October 14, 1806), "Suplemento": "managing in both places to introduce the fluid, fresh and fully active...a task that the English have not been able to achieve on the various occasions that they tried, by transporting on ships of their East India Company samples of pus, which arrived inert."

57. *Gazeta de México* 12, no. 12 (May 26, 1804), "Suplemento," 93–96.

58. The politics of this rivalry in Peru is fully examined in Warren, *Medicine and Politics in Colonial Peru*, chapter 3, especially 104–112.

59. The political charge of literature on the expedition is briefly revisited in the Conclusion. For a full account of efforts to vaccinate in advance of the expedition, see Smith, *"Real Expedición Marítima de la Vacuna" in New Spain and Guatemala*.

60. Available in nineteen states, as of 2012, according to Marcuse, "Prudent Personal Belief Exemption Policies."

61. For observations about the affinities between rising vaccination skepticism in the United States and certain strands of environmentalism, see Conis, *Vaccine Nation*, chapter 6.

CHAPTER 1

Devotions of Affliction

Epigraph: Exodus 5:3 (King James).

1. At the twenty-fifth session, councilors reaffirmed the intercession of saints, veneration of relics, and the cult of images.

2. For the Valley of Toluca, see Pizzigoni, *Life Within*, especially chapters 1 and 6.

3. Braudel, *Structures of Everyday Life*, vol. 1, 90–92; even the wealthiest regions of Europe witnessed periodic epidemics that subverted or reversed long-term growth in population.

4. Some historians of medicine have found a common, invariant structure in the social reception of crisis and its resolution in disease episodes across place and time. See, for instance, Charles Rosenberg's treatment of an epidemic's dramaturgic forms and aspects in *Explaining Epidemics*, 278–292, first published as Rosenberg, "What Is an Epidemic?" Reflecting on the AIDS epidemic in 1989, Rosenberg saw in its progression a typical historical structure, including an initial perception and revelation; attempts to manage "randomness" by placing the revelation into moral, physiological, and environmental terms; negotiation of public response, including acts of solidarity and reassurance; and the subsidence and retrospective evaluation of the event. This model of social response helpfully draws attention to the ways in which communities endow crises with meaning, through culturally specific patterns of response. (See also Slack, introduction to *Epidemics and Ideas*, 3, wondering whether a "common dramaturgy" existed in all epidemics.)

5. The devastating Lisbon earthquake of 1755, for example, whose aftershocks were literally and figuratively felt across Europe, was seen as a major turning point, although recent scholarship indicates a less sudden or complete change in mentality. Braun and Radner, *Lisbon Earthquake of 1755*.

6. Most recently, see Carreón Nieto, *Epidemias y desastres en el Obispado de Michoacán*.

7. Fields, *Pestilence and Headcolds*, holds out the possibility of fresh insights from letters to Spain, ex-voto images in public and private collections, and sections on health in the sixteenth-century *relaciones geográficas*. Fields has argued that laypersons and professionals shared many ideas about healing, as evident in prescriptive texts directed at the elite of New Spain.

8. The source has provided historians with a wealth of information about the development of Marian devotions in colonial Mexico. For instance, see Taylor, "Virgin of Guadalupe in New Spain"; and Brading, *Mexican Phoenix*, 120–132, who has been especially critical of its tedious baroque style. Cabrera composed

his chronicle in accordance with the conventions of sacred history, which elevated *exornación* (adornment) into a stylistic principle of historical truth; as Cabrera put it, certain flourishes were required by the historian's time. See Cabrera, *Escudo de armas*, xxxiv–xxxv.

9. The viceregal government ordered all copies removed from circulation, perhaps because of complaints about the book's criticisms of the city's physicians. See Molina del Villar, *La Nueva España y el matlazahuatl*, 167–168.

10. These aspects were documented in other sources, making it possible to corroborate some of Cabrera's descriptions. See items for May 24, 25, and 26, 1737, in Sahagún de Arévalo, *Gacetas de México*, vol. 2. The understanding of *baroque* employed here is commensurate but not identical with the one put forth by Maravall, *Culture of the Baroque*, in which a propensity for ornamentation and exaggeration in art and architecture has the effect of engaging viewers as coparticipants in the resolution of their puzzles.

11. Voekel, *Alone before God*.

12. Cabrera, *Escudo de armas*, 158.

13. Sahagún de Arévalo, *Gacetas de México*, vol. 2, 78. On typhus, see Porter, *Greatest Benefit to Mankind*, 26; Molina del Villar, *La Nueva España y el matlazahuatl*, 65–66; and Cabrera, *Escudo de armas*, 59–60. The Greek etymology of "typhus" denotes smoke or vapor, perhaps deriving from the perceived ambient source of infection.

14. Cope, *Limits of Racial Domination*, 89–91.

15. For instance, in 1719 the parish priest of Santiago Tlatelolco complained that he could not isolate the "sheep" of his flock because Indians were becoming indistinct from Spaniards, among whom they lived in the rest of the city. Parishioners refused to dress in traditional clothing, self-identified as mestizo, and intermarried at high rates with Spaniards, *negros*, *mulatos*, and mestizos. "Dictamen de Conciencia por Fr. Miguel Camacho Villavisencio," 1719, Bancroft Library, M-M 135, fol. 18.

16. From summaries of the original *actas* for January 24 and January 25, 1737, in Riva Fernández, *Guía de las actas de Cabildo*, vol. 5.

17. January 28, 1737, in Sahagún de Arévalo, *Gacetas de México*, vol. 2.

18. Molina del Villar, *Por voluntad divina*, 64–68.

19. Cabrera, *Escudo de armas*, 252.

20. Ibid., 67–68.

21. Molina del Villar, *Por voluntad divina*, 62.

22. Bando, February 16, 1736, in *Ordenes de la Corona*, 1529–1812, vol. 1, Bancroft Library, M-M 170.

23. Juan Antonio Arzobispo to Crown, Mexico City, July 10, 1738, AGI Audiencia de México leg. 506.

24. Bando, June 6, 1737, in *Ordenes de la Corona*, 1529–1812, vol. 1, Bancroft Library, M-M 170.

25. A royal *cédula* of 1755 stated that furtive production of cane brandy, harmful to the health of natives, also harmed the royal treasury and weakened commerce by reducing the demand for legitimate *vinos*. Real Cédula, August 22, 1755, in *Ordenes de la Corona*, 1529–1812, vol. 1, Bancroft Library, M-M 170.

26. Cited in Gruzinski, *Conquest of Mexico*, 83 and 85. See also Pardo-Tomás, "'Antiguamente vivían más sanos que ahora.'"

27. Taylor, *Drinking, Homicide, and Rebellion*, 40–41.

28. On these reforms, see O'Gorman, "Reflexiones sobre la distribución urbana colonial de la ciudad de México," 38–40. On the aftermath of the riot, see Cope, *Limits of Racial Domination*.

29. The earlier decree made distinctions when assigning punishment for transgression: Spaniards risked the loss of properties and expulsion, those *de color quebrado* (the darker strata) two hundred lashes and six years in the galley.

30. December synopsis, in Sahagún de Arévalo, *Gacetas de México*, vol. 2, 77.

31. Juan Antonio Arzobispo to Crown, Mexico City, April 16, 1737, AGI Audiencia de México leg. 504, 3r-v, cited in Molina del Villar, *La Nueva España y el matlazahuatl*, 152.

32. Christian, *Apparitions in Late Medieval and Renaissance Spain*, 14–15 and 83.

33. López de Hinojosos, *Summa, y recopilacion de Chirugia*, 190v–196.

34. Ibid., 193r–194 and 198r-v. The chronicler Diego Muñoz Camargo, another eyewitness, considered this the third major *pestilencia* in severity, after 1519 and 1545. He attributed the decline to population losses and the vigilance of Viceroy Martín Enríquez and the Spaniards he dispatched throughout New Spain to look after the health of the indigenous populations. "And so there was great care in healing them temporally and spiritually, with fasting, assistance, processions, and *disciplinas*, until it pleased God that such great pestilence unleashed on the world for our sins should cease." See Muñoz Camargo, *Relaciones geográficas de Tlaxcala*, 76.

35. Florencia and Oviedo, *Zodíaco mariano*, 58–63.

36. Ibid., 347.

37. Ibid., 292.

38. On Zapopan, see Taylor, *Theater of a Thousand Wonders*, 190–193.

39. Molina del Villar, *La Nueva España y el matlazahuatl*, 153. The paralysis of urban institutions in disease crisis was not uncommon in early modern Europe. In 1630 the administrative organization of Turin, with a population of roughly thirty thousand, collapsed as doctors, councilors, and mayors fled the city. See Cavallo, *Charity and Power in Early Modern Italy*, 52. On the effects of the flight of wealthier citizens to healthy cities in Italy, see Carmichael, *Plague and the Poor in Renaissance Florence*, 100–101. Mexico City's *ayuntamiento* functioned continuously for reasons that might have included the poor travel conditions of Mexico's central valley and news of the epidemic's greater devastation elsewhere.

40. Cabrera, *Escudo de armas*, 101. For the reminder from the *ayuntamiento*, see December 13, 1736, in Riva Fernández, *Guía de las actas de Cabildo*, vol. 5.

41. December 17, 1736, in ibid..

42. Cabrera, *Escudo de armas*, 102.

43. Ibid., 103.

44. Ibid., 103–104.

45. Ibid., 126. On the near-completion of the sumptuous Altar de los Reyes inside the cathedral, a baroque that "has found its wings," see Weismann, *Art and Time in Mexico*, 49.

46. Cabrera, *Escudo de armas*, 103.

47. Entry for January 20, 1737, in Sahagún de Arévalo, *Gacetas de México*, vol. 2.

48. What remained of wax, as well as the income generated, was handed over to the Jesuit College upon Loreto's return. Cabrera, *Escudo de armas*, 104–105.

49. Ibid., 106.

50. Ibid., 133. The goal was that Guadalupe be "moved by prayers, to do what hands were not permitted." The frontispiece of Cabrera's chronicle, of Guadalupe hovering among suffering victims and patrons in city streets, was meant to illustrate its fulfillment (see figure 1.1).

51. Cabrera, *Escudo de armas*, 135. A sense of the crowds comes from Manuel de Arellano's painting of Guadalupe's transfer to her new sanctuary on April 30, 1709, in which the space around the sanctuary bursts with people and saints, including Santiago on his white horse; see Pierce, Ruiz, and Bargellini, *Painting a New World*, 190–193. In 1754, Mariano Fernández Echeverría described Indian congregations arriving on Saturdays throughout the year in various costumes to perform for Guadalupe; see *Baluartes de México*, 61.

52. Gurevich, *Medieval Popular Culture*, 42–45.

53. AHDF Ayuntamiento 437a, "Compendio de los libros Capitulares," 351v. María del Carmen Carreón Nieto's work on the 1759 volcanic eruption in the *tierra caliente* of Michoacán shows something similar: the numerous church patriarchs, saints, and Christ images in the region that were beseeched seem to betray local preferences rather than universal patronage, despite the popularity of Guadalupe in the diocese and the special role of Saint Joseph as patron of lighting and earthquakes. Carreón Nieto, *Epidemias y desastres en el Obispado de Michoacán*, 92–103.

54. Osores y Sotomayor, *Colegios de la ciudad de México*, 45–46. On the measles outbreak of 1727, when Jesuits confessed the sick, disposed of corpses, and distributed alms of food, medicine, and clothing through private donations and funds from Jesuit colleges, see Decorme, *La obra de los jesuitas mexicanos*, 341. For the royal order on fraudulent reporting of harvests on Jesuit estates, see *Real Cédula sobre diezmos en el pleyto contra las jesuitas*, 12, whose conciliatory tone and ambivalent placement of blame suggests the influential role of the Jesuits in colonial society.

55. Good Death Societies became especially popular in Spain in the sixteenth century, where *Ars Moriendi* (Art of dying) literature proliferated widely. The genre addressed a long-standing concern with the provision of correct ritual measures for passage into heaven or purgatory during the *agonía*. In Europe, Jesuit authors dominated the production of such literature, often simple pamphlets with correct procedures for last rites: a final, thorough confession; the viaticum, nourishment to accompany the deceased; and extreme unction, for the final hours preceding death. Authors sometimes recommended the presence of family or members of confraternities to pray for the soul of the dying; increasingly, as Alejo de Venegas emphasized, they advised a "good, constant preparation for death." Cited in Eire, *From Madrid to Purgatory*, 28–32.

56. Following Susan Schroeder's study, "Jesuits, Nahuas, and the Good Death Society," 64.

57. Ibid., 63–74.

58. According to the gazette, San Sebastián was at the center of a procession on February 28, several weeks later. The suggestion here is that a significant alignment of religious figures and days—of personality and time—increased the efficacy of the procession for some of the faithful.

59. Desjarlais, "Presence," 159.

60. Brading (in *Mexican Phoenix*, 120–123) notes Cabrera's eagerness to evoke "a powerful image of a Christian commonwealth, a Catholic city, where both priests and laymen exposed themselves to the danger of infection in order to minister to the needs, both physical and spiritual, of the sick and poor."

61. Cabrera, *Escudo de armas*, 248. Members of this parish engaged in a lively struggle with those of Santiago Tlatelolco, who were reportedly hesitant to relinquish their Christ of the Column for the former's procession due to the scarcity of miraculous sculptures in the city. Ibid., 243–244.

62. Ibid., 251. Compare this proximity to bodily effluvia with the laboring monks of Saint Mary's in Barcelona during the plague year of 1651, who when confessing reportedly held a torch between themselves and the sick and extended the communion wafer at the end of a silver rod "because it is said that the plague is carried by one's breath." Parets, *Journal of the Plague Year*, 48. Perhaps more priests in Mexico City took this approach than Cabrera allows.

63. Cabrera, *Escudo de armas*, 252.

64. Ibid., 242.

65. Ibid., 262.

66. Urban planner Kevin Lynch has theorized that in experiencing their cities, residents construct mental maps with landmarks or nodes that take shape by junctions of movement or concentrations of particular activities, where awareness of surroundings is especially acute. These might encompass a street corner, larger districts, or, "when conceiving the environment at a national level, the whole city itself may become a node." See Lynch, *Image of the City*, 72.

67. Molina del Villar, *Por voluntad divina*, 68.

68. León García, "Espacio, olor y salubridad en Toluca," 166–169.

69. This episode, along with others involving saints and devotional objects, has been interpreted as an expression, in Christian terms, of communal cohesion; see Gibson, *Aztecs under Spanish Rule*, 134.

70. Cabrera, *Escudo de armas*, 253.

71. Ibid., 150–151.

72. In Spain most flagellant processions took place during Holy Week, when they emulated the suffering and crucifixion of Christ. Verdi Webster, *Art and Ritual in Golden-Age Spain*, 29. In New Spain scourging and processions of flagellants were recorded as early as the sixteenth century and prompted contemporary observers to speculate that the practice sublimated pre-Conquest pagan rituals. Ricard, *Spiritual Conquest of Mexico*, 121. The Jesuits, among the most accomplished healers of colonial Mexico, were famous for their great scourging processions in the missions of northwestern Mexico. In one seventeenth-century case these entailed switches of maguey fiber, at the end of which were balls of wax embedded with cactus thorns to draw blood and atone for the community. Reff, *Disease, Depopulation, and Culture Change*, 262–263.

73. Verdi Webster, *Art and Ritual in Golden-Age Spain*, 6–13.

74. Anthropologists in the Andean highlands have observed that familiar social types often provide a model by which to conceptualize human-divine relationships; see Harris, "Coming of the White People." On typical social relations in the dress of saints and deities, see also Trexler, *Religion in Social Context*, 382 and 392.

75. On November 7, 1786, the *Gazeta de México* reported an atypical procession for the miraculous image of Saint Francis during an outbreak of fevers in Valladolid that included crowns of thorns on the faithful and penitential cords around their necks.

76. Cabrera, *Escudo de armas*, 91.

77. López de Hinojosos (*Summa, y recopilacion de Chirugia*, 17r) defined phlebotomy as a cut or incision in the veins, "by which to evacuate the abundance of the four humors, which are blood, cholera, phlegm, and melancholy." In the humoral conception one or another of these humors dominated depending on the time of day, which determined where and how much to bleed.

78. Cabrera, *Escudo de armas*, 254.

79. Christian, *Local Religion in Sixteenth Century Spain*, 22.

80. On passionate emotions "inscribed on things that are durable," see Durkheim, *Elementary Forms*, 232.

81. A fifth edition of a devotional pamphlet on the self-renovation of the Cristo Renovado appeared eight years earlier. Early, *Colonial Architecture of Mexico*, 70. On the popularity of this crucifix and other Christocentric devotions in the eighteenth century, see Taylor, "Two Shrines of the Cristo Renovado."

82. Cabrera, *Escudo de armas*, 454–456. On the procession of the Cristo Renovado and Archbishop Vizarrón's offer of plenary indulgence, see the entry for May 3, 1737, in Sahagún y Arévalo, *Gacetas de México*, vol. 2.

83. Torre Villar, *Instrucciones y memorias de los virreyes novohispanos*, 1066–1073 (item 247 quoted).

84. Rodríguez, *Contaminación e insalubridad en la ciudad de México*, takes a top-down view, stressing the small numbers who looked after problems of sickness and public health, including members of the *junta de policía* in Mexico City, viceroys, royal judges, architects, and men of medicine and science, such as José Antonio Alzate y Ramírez and José Ignacio Bartolache (both discussed in Chapter 2 of this volume). In her work on funerals and burial reform, Voekel, *Alone before God*, has moved away from this focus on administrators in favor of a social or class movement in Mexico City and Veracruz.

85. Rodríguez, *Contaminación e insalubridad en la ciudad de México*, 110, passim. See also Viqueira Albán, *Propriety and Permissiveness*; and Voekel, "Peeing on the Palace."

86. Carlos Tristan del Poso, Mexico City, September 17, 1696, AHDF 3668 exp. 1, 1–3; Real Protomedicato, Mexico City, September 17, 1696, ibid., 7–8. Members of the Audiencia and the viceroy, reviewing these reports, moved to have streets and irrigation canals cleaned and *indios forasteros* removed from the city that year. Gaps in knowledge about *policía* and public health for earlier periods stem from the destruction of documentation in the 1692 riot. On sanitation and health, see also Dávalos, *De basuras, inmundicias y movimiento*.

87. Cooper, *Epidemic Disease in Mexico City*, 20. See Cope, *Limits of Racial Domination*, 28–29, on perennial funding shortfalls for infrastructural upkeep and repair.

88. Cabrera, *Escudo de armas*, 265.

89. For Italy, historian Brian Pullan describes a dark consequence. Rather than lead to systematic, preemptive transformations in social policies by governments, sixteenth-century plagues produced a degree of elation or relief resulting from the connection drawn between disease and the elimination of poverty, commonly achieved through the elimination of the poor. Pullan, "Plague and Perceptions of the Poor," 121.

90. Ayuntamiento to Viceroy, Mexico City, October 22, 1779, AGN IV 2796 exp. 5, 3–6.

91. Ayuntamiento to Viceroy, Mexico City, November 15, 1779, ibid., 88r-v; Alonso Arzobispo de México to Viceroy, Mexico City, November 19, 1779, ibid., 89–90; and Ayuntamiento to Viceroy, Mexico City, November 29, 1779, ibid., 12–13. On the prolonged struggle over burial reform in Mexico City, see Voekel, *Alone before God*. Burial close to the altar and its saints facilitated the protection of the soul of the deceased and also indexed the social status of his or her family.

92. Ayuntamiento to Branciforte, Sala Capitular de Puebla, November 6, 1797, AGN Epidemias 16 exp. 4, 130–132. In 1797 Puebla's *ayuntamiento* was reviewing documentation from the previous smallpox epidemic, an illustration of the way that emergencies contributed to the formation of institutional memory.

93. See Viqueira Albán, *Propriety and Permissiveness*; and Voekel, "Peeing on the Palace," and *Alone before God*, stressing changing sensibilities among upwardly mobile middling sectors. For a demographic view, see Bailey Glasco, *Constructing Mexico City*, 26 and 100, arguing that reform was a consequence of population growth, a sense that the city was being overwhelmed by people, without sufficient services to accommodate them.

94. Pérez Toledo, *Trabajadores, espacio urbano y sociabilidad*, chapter 1, draws on a 1794 survey of more than four thousand establishments and their workers, collected by individuals from the *ayuntamiento* assigned to each sector.

95. Bailey Glasco, *Constructing Mexico City*, 137–138 and 143–144; and Rodríguez, *Contaminación e insalubridad en la ciudad de México*, 141–180.

96. For Toluca, see León García, "Espacio, olor y salubridad en Toluca."

97. "Noticia de las providencias tomadas por esta N.C.," Sala Capitular de México, October 31, 1779, AGN Epidemias 16 exp. 8, 291–297.

98. AGN Epidemias 1 exp. 5, especially "Noticias de lo que se observó en la Epidemia de Viruelas del año de 1797," 480–482; and AGN BN 1024 exp. 1, 243–244. See also the meeting minutes from the Junta Principal's sessions in the archbishopric palace, "Libro en que se asientan los Acuerdos de la Junta principal de caridad para la Epidemia de Viruelas," AGN BN 754 exp. 1, 11–13 and 24v–29v. In Puebla the Junta de Caridad similarly assigned the city's twenty-two physicians and surgeons to sixteen *cuarteles*, distributed printed forms to collect data, and solicited alms from private persons and corporations. See AGN Epidemias 6 exps. 3 and 4.

99. García Jove to Francisco José Urrutia, Real Protomedicato, January 17, 1787, AHDF 3674 exp. 5; Juan Francisco de Velasco, Mexico City, January 19,

1787, ibid.; and Juan Antonio de Yermo, Joseph Uribe, and Antonio de Vivanco, Mexico City, January 8, 1787, ibid.

100. This tally omits ceremonies of statecraft (for instance, thanksgivings for the birth of a royal heir, *entradas* of royal officials, issuing of decrees and papal bulls) as well as regular functions for the Christian liturgical year (for instance, Corpus Christi or a saint's feast day) unless specified in response to crisis.

101. *Gazeta de México*, September 26, 1786.

102. Ibid., June 13, 1786.

103. Ibid., May 6, 1786.

104. Ibid., April 5, 1785.

105. Ibid., May 16, 1786.

106. Ibid., July 29, 1794. Drought simultaneously afflicted residents of Durango, who in retrospect attributed several weeks of rainfall in the summer of 1795 to a *novenario* performed for the Virgin of Loreto, "its avowed Patron of timely rain." Ibid., September 18, 1795.

107. Ibid., April 5, 1785.

108. Ibid., November 6, 1787.

109. The cry of the exiled to God in Psalm 130—that is, "De Profundis clamamus ad te, Domine."

110. AGMP Expedientes 210 leg. 2536, 117r-v.

111. *Gazeta de México*, March 22, 1786.

112. Ibid., October 10, 1786.

113. Ibid., August 21, 1787.

114. Ibid., September 26, 1786.

115. Sala Capitular de México, October 26, 1797, AGN Epidemias 1 exp. 4. According to parish and hospital registers, weekly mortality rates escalated in October and peaked in November, with more than a thousand burials in a single week. See AGN Epidemias 1 exp. 1.

116. Cosme de Mier, José Mariano de Fagoaga, etc., to Viceroy, Sala Capitular de Mexico, November 6, 1797, AGN Epidemias 6 exp. 1, 3r-v; and Alonso Arzobispo de Mexico to Viceroy, Mexico City, November 6, 1797, ibid., 4r-v.

117. Viceroy to Ayuntamiento, n.p., October 30, 1797, AGN Epidemias 1 exp. 4, 395r-v; and Viceroy to Pedro Marin, Orizaba, October 11, 1797, AGN Epidemias 5 exp. 1, 15.

118. Viceroy to Archbishop, n.p., November 9, 1797, AGN Epidemias 6 exp. 1, 5r-v; and Viceroy to Real Audiencia, n.p., November 20, 1797, ibid., 9r-v.

119. Baltasar Ladrón de Guevara to Viceroy, Mexico City, November 20, 1797, AGN Epidemias 6 exp. 1, 11r-v.

120. *Gazeta de México*, November 29, 1797.

121. Guevara, "Discurso sobre la policía de México," AHDF 3627 exp. 43, paras. 250 and 262.

122. When the Cristo de la Penitencia was brought to Guadalajara for a *novenario* during the *peste* and food shortages of 1785, the *ayuntamiento* paid the majority of the cost (75.5 pesos) of 346 pounds of wax. "Expediente formado sobre los costos que tubo la traslacion del Smo. Christo de la Penitencia," Guadalajara, April 26, 1785, AMG AE 1/1785 paq. 7 leg. 25.

123. In the 1736 epidemic, Puebla's city council sponsored processions, made

donations to the prior of the convent hospital of San Juan de Dios and Nuestra Señora de Bethlehem for their sick poor, and secured permission from the viceroy to redirect funds destined for aqueduct construction and other public works to the many other hospitals whose *mayordomos* requested aid. "Noticia. Que prolixamente se ha sacado de los libros de cabildo de los novenarios y demás demostraciones espirituales, que catolicamente se han celebrado en las epidemias, y retiros de lluvias en los años de 1737, 1748, 1762 y 1771," AGMP Expedientes 210 leg. 2536.

124. Scholars studying this emergency have benefited from the copious documentation compiled in Florescano, *Fuentes para la historia de la crisis agrícola de 1785 y 1786*.

125. *Gazeta de México*, July 12, 1785.

126. Ibid., April 18, 1786.

127. Ibid., July 26, 1785.

128. Fernando Perez Marañon to Viceroy, Guanajuato, October 5, 1813, AGN Epidemias 13 exp. 6, 268–269.

129. Guadalajara's city council was fined in 1799 for missing public functions, then reprimanded in 1803, when the single representative who attended ceremonies for Saint Rose was rendered ridiculous carrying the ceremonial maces alone. The Audiencia's *fiscal* reminded councilmen that these public functions were to be decorous. Fiscal de lo Civil, Guadalajara, September 2, 1803, AMG AE 1/1803 paq. 19 leg. 96.

130. Religious corporations moving to sponsor public acts often framed their requests in terms of the petitions of residents. In the summer of 1808 the curate of Guadalupe's sanctuary, writing to Guadalajara's city council to request members' presence at the planned *triduo* (three-day prayer devotion), insisted that disease had moved the city's faithful to request her intercession, while the prioress of the convent of Dominicanas de Jesús María reported that residents had been compelled to solicit God's mercy with a *triduo* for San Sebastián, "universal patron of pests." Joseph Francisco Arroyo to Cabildo, Santuario de Nuestra Señora de Gaudalupe, June 8, 1808, AMG AY 1808 "Libro de Cabildo" leg. 2; and Sor Maria Francisca de la Concepción Priora to Cabildo, Convento de Dominicanas de Jesus Maria, June 20, 1808, ibid., 26–31.

131. Burdette, "Miraculous Crucifixes and Colonial Mexican Society," 192–199, and "*Caritas* and the Christ of the Seven Veils."

132. During devastating rainstorms in the summer of 1817, the Franciscans planned a nine-day "sacrificio de gracias" to implore the aid of Our Lady of Zapopan (declared in 1734 by the city its official protector against lightning and epidemics) in the convent church. Francisco José de Aparicio to Ayuntamiento, Guadalajara, August 15, 1817, AMG AE 11/1817 paq. 32 leg. 191.

133. Viceroy to Ayuntamiento, Mexico City, October 23, 1779, AGN IV 2796 exp. 5, 19–20; Viceroy to Ayuntamiento, Mexico City, October 23, 1779, ibid., 21r-v: "que los dueños de tienda de Pulperia y demás vecinos pongan luminarias de leña y ocote con mixtos u olores que indica por ser mui benéficas a la salud"; and Viceroy to Ayuntamiento, Mexico City, October 25, 1779, ibid., 22r-v: "que se use de algunos tiros de cañón por ser la pólvora conducente a purificar el ayre."

134. Guevara's treatise on *policía* is discussed in the introduction. In May

1810, months before Father Miguel Hidalgo uttered the cry that originated Mexico's insurgency, Remedios was brought from the church of Santa Veracruz to the Cathedral for a *novenario*, for which the city council issued a ban on carriages, fireworks, and sales of liquor along the path of the procession to maintain decorum. Mexico City, May 10, 1810, AHDF Ayuntamiento 3902 exp. 66.

135. *Gazeta de México*, no. 52 (December 6, 1785), 456.

136. For statistics showing a peak in the production of religious publications in Mexico City in the second half of the century, see Taylor, *Theater of a Thousand Wonders*, 97. On print in publicizing shrine devotions, see ibid., 401–407; and Donahue-Wallace, "Picturing Prints in Early Modern New Spain," 340–342.

137. Anderson, *Imagined Communities*. This chapter proposes a rather different kind of identity gelling through print, crisis, and communal rituals.

138. On the letter to Voltaire, the religious icon in Russia, and Catherine's own considerable devotional practice, see Levitt, *Visual Dominant in Eighteenth-Century Russia*, chapter 7 (quotation from 196). "Given the central place of the icon in Russian Orthodoxy theology and everyday practice," Levitt concludes, "suspicion of [miraculous] icons could probably never have been more than mild, a wariness of extremes and abuse" (216). On the September 1771 riot, see Alexander, *Bubonic Plague in Early Modern Russia*, chapter 7.

139. For the latter, see Carreón Nieto, *Epidemias y desastres en el Obispado de Michoacán*.

140. Alexander, *Bubonic Plague in Early Modern Russia*, 297. William Christian has argued that the elite/popular dichotomy is best discarded in an age in which illness was largely immune to medical solutions, highlighting the overlaps in practice of kings and commoners in sixteenth-century Spain: "In Toledo women who wished to be cured of *çiçiones* (probably malaria) would sweep the church of Santiago on Saturdays. When Charles V had malaria, he too swept the church" (Christian, *Local Religion in Sixteenth Century Spain*, 157).

141. For the British case, see Guerrini, "Newtonianism, Medicine and Religion."

142. On earthquakes, which moved residents across the social spectrum to flee to shrines, see Ramírez and Taylor, "Out of Tlatelolco's Ruins." A diarist in Orizaba with royalist sympathies and reverence for religious images and holy men, who mainly recorded troop movements and other developments related to the insurgency, reported processions with San Antonio following lightning strikes in the summer of 1813, along with prayers, hymns, masses, and processions with Christ of the Calvary and the town's patron saint for the "earthquakes, *peste*, drought, and hunger" delivered by God in 1819, "irritated with the inhabitants of this Villa because of their many sins." "Libro noticioso que contiene algunos apuntes particulares, acaesidos en esta villa de Orizava y otras noticias que an yegado aqui de sujetos fidedignos, 1812–1821," Bancroft Library, M-M 178, 21–23 and 143–145. Our Lady of Remedios periodically sat on her illuminated throne in Mexico City's cathedral for "lack of rain, *enfermedades* [illnesses], and other needs," in 1822, 1825, and 1826, AHDF 3902 exp. 66. For a tabulation of appeals to Remedios through 1810, see Granados Saladinas, "Mexico City's Symbolic Geography," 170–172.

143. Prieto, *Memoria de mis tiempos*, vol. 1, 88–91.

144. Cañeque, *King's Living Image*, isolates the political culture and rituals of rule surrounding the viceregal court as a proxy for viceregal power. See Osowski, *Indigenous Miracles*, on the importance of miraculous images within this colonial hierarchy.

CHAPTER 2

Periodically Healthy

Epigraph: *Gazeta de México* 2, no. 9 (1786).

1. Doctor y Maestro Pedro Puglia to Conde de Revillagigedo, Guanajuato, October 27, 1790, AGN Historia 460 exp. 10; and Revillagigedo to Puglia, Mexico City, November 3, 1790, ibid., 79–80. For Puglia's background, see Brading, "Power and Justice in Catorce," 377–379.

2. On the politics of collection, see Schiebinger, *Plants and Empire*; Findlen, *Possessing Nature*; Parrish, *American Curiosity*; Murphy, "Translating the Vernacular"; and Barrera, "Local Herbs, Global Medicines."

3. The garden drew the opposition of some influential colonial institutions and actors, notably members of the Protomedicato and the Royal and Pontifical University, who correctly perceived their autonomy and authority under threat. On these rifts and the slow and laborious process of domestication (*domiciliación*) of modern chemical and botanical practice, theory, and nomenclature there and in the Royal College of Mining in the 1780s and 1790s, see Aceves Pastrana, *Química, botánica y farmacia en la Nueva España*, 75–112. On the expeditions and their human and scientific dimensions, see Lafuente and López-Ocón, "Tradiciones científicas y expediciones ilustradas en la América hispana del siglo XVIII"; Lafuente and Valverde, "Linnaean Botany and Spanish Imperial Biopolitics"; and Pino Díaz, *Ciencia y contexto histórico nacional en las expediciones ilustradas a América*.

4. In Spain, reformers looked to research hospitals, botanical gardens, and observatories in Barcelona, Cádiz, Madrid, and Seville for the institutionalization of Enlightenment learning, as well as the military. On the role of these institutions in the modernization of Bourbon Spain, see Puerto Sarmiento, *La ilusión quebrada*; Burke, *Royal College of San Carlos*; Lafuente, "Institucionalización metropolitana de la ciencia española," 91–118; and Granjel, *Anatomía española de la ilustración*, on dissections and anatomical instruction in hospitals and royal academies.

5. The Société Royal de Médecine gathered correspondence from a network of physicians, defined and solicited the necessary data, facilitated its assembly, and provided support to local governments and medical practitioners. See Rusnock, *Vital Accounts*, 108–119.

6. Lanning, *Royal Protomedicato*, 11–12, notes this restricted sphere but argues that understandings of public health were limited to education, examination, and licensing, an excessively narrow view of the concept as contemporaries employed it at the time.

7. Saldaña, "Ciencia y felicidad pública en la Ilustración americana," 151–207, especially 167–168.

8. Saladino García, *Ciencia y prensa durante la ilustración latinoamericana*, 63–81, quote on 324–325.

9. Moravia, "Enlightenment and the Sciences of Man," 247–268; and Riskin, *Science in the Age of Sensibility*, on the "sensibility" of the empirical sciences that emerged as empiricists trained themselves to be open to the world and to questions of an aesthetic and moral nature. See also Porter, "Medical Sciences and Human Science in the Enlightenment," 53–87.

10. Valdez Garza, *Libros y lectores en la* Gazeta de literatura de México, 36–50, outlines European antecedents, alongside the occasional reports or *relaciones* of notable happenings from Mexico's colonial past, as a source of emulation, beginning with the earliest gazettes (1722 and 1728). Citing European fashion, she suggests, was calculated to help publishers to justify their efforts.

11. On periodicals as a source of proto-national identity, see Cruz Soto, "El nacionalismo de José Antonio de Alzate." Valdez Garza, *Libros y lectores en la* Gazeta de literatura de México, argues that periodicals manifest the desire of creole journalists to integrate into the Republic of Letters, as this legitimized, validated, or authorized their work, following Clark, "The *Gazeta de Literatura de México* (1788–1795)."

12. Porter, introduction to *Popularization of Medicine*, 1. This process is often seen as the effect of the expansion of the printing industry, a developed consumer marketplace, more consolidated medical authority, and rising literacy rates. For instance, see Porter and Porter, *Patient's Progress*, on a new marketplace and expanding consumer society in England's eighteenth-century industrialization. For an alternative model of diffusion in France, see Ramsey, *Professional and Popular Medicine in France*. Furdell, *Publishing and Medicine in Early Modern England*, 35 and 130–134, describes a more subversive experience in Tudor and Stuart England, with a shift in responsibility and authority away from professional physicians and toward family members and friends. For critiques of the concepts "popularization" and "popular," see Porter, introduction to *Popularization of Medicine*; Slack, "Mirrors of Health and Treasures of Poor Men," 237–273; Wear, "Popularization of Medicine in Early Modern England," 17–41; and Fissell, "Readers, Texts, and Contexts," 72–96, for a cohesive argument in favor of "vernacular" as an alternative.

13. On the printed page as a substitute for other arenas of debate and scientific performance, see Achim, *Lagartijas medicinales*, 167–169. For scientific demonstrations as a site of convergence for establishment and amateur, professional and lay, see the contributions to Bensaude-Vincent and Blondel, *Science and Spectacle in the European Enlightenment*.

14. The questionnaire and reports are collected in Acuña, *Relaciones geográficas del siglo XVI*, vol. 3. Tlacolula, item 17: "beber yerbas medicinales"; Miquitla, item 17: "yerbas del monte que van a buscar indios médicos"; Talistaca, item 17: "el nombre de las cuales no saben, más de conocerlas de vista." See also Ucila, item 26: "no saben cómo se llaman los nombres de las d[ic]has yerbas [ni] en lengua *mexicana* ni castellana."

15. Ibid., Teozacualco, item 26; Peñoles, item 17; and Papaloticpac, item 17.

16. Ibid., Tepeucila (with Papaloticpac), item 26, as well as *yolosuchil*, "heart-shaped flower." Teticpac, item 26, reports the names for a "hot" and "cold" herb,

along with the "bitter herb," *chichicmotl*. Tetiquipa, items 17 and 26, lists the purgatives *raíz de Michoacán*, *chichicpatli*, and *cacalosuchil*, the last flower described as violent and rapid in its effects. Tilantongo, item 17, lists the Mixtec and Nahua names for a "cold" medicine.

17. Ibid., Tecuicuilco, item 26.

18. Ibid., Peñoles, item 17: "curan a tino, sin saber dar razón de lo que hacen ni aplican." See also Teozapotlan, item 26: "today we understand that they know little about herbs, and the reason is that the *doctrina* priests saw that they practiced and mixed many superstitions into their cures and medicines; and removing the superstitions, the rest was lost."

19. In the appearance of *raíz de Michoacán* one senses how new nomenclature for botanicals was already penetrating at the local level to facilitate commerce in these plants, as they were extracted from these contexts for new destinations. On trade in this and in the purgative *cañafístula* (*Cassia fistula* L.), and a measured assessment of evidence that these New World plants were partially assimilated into European medical practices in this period, see Huguet-Termes, "New World Materia Medica in Spanish Renaissance Medicine."

20. Bell, *How To Do It*, 5. The eclectic nature of this genre is illustrated by Aristotle's *Masterpiece*, or *Master-Piece*, a compilation of roughly half-dozen sources on conception, childbearing, and women's illnesses that dominated the Anglophone market in the eighteenth century. See the essays in Rosenberg, *Right Living*, especially Fissell, "Making a Masterpiece."

21. Cárdenas, *Problemas, y secretos maravillosos de las Indias*: "Prólogo al lector"; Part I, chapter 2; Part II, especially chapters 7, 11, and 18; Part III, chapters 1 and 15. Quote from 236v: "*Medicinam de terra creavit altissiumus*, que es como dezir que puso Dios virtud en las yervas y cosas de la tierra para conservarse el hombre y librarse de las enfermedades."

22. This figure excludes editions of popular manuals in Spanish translation printed in Europe, only some of which circulated in New Spain. Data are from catalog searches and Perdiguero, "Popularizando la ciencia," 163–164.

23. Fields, *Pestilence and Headcolds*, chapter 4.

24. Cárdenas, *Problemas, y secretos maravillosos de las Indias*, 194v. Elsewhere Cárdenas remarked on the blindness that resulted from smallpox when *indios miserables* lacked the means to protect their eyes (223r–v). It is fair to say that he was generally more interested than his peers in saying what it was that was happening, and why, than in prescribing what to do practically, which may be why Cárdenas has drawn so much attention from historians.

25. López de Hinojosos, *Summa, y recopilacion de Chirugia*, "Al benigno lector."

26. Farfán, *Tractado brebe de medicina*, 143r–144v; and Acuña, *Relaciones geográficas del siglo XVI*, vol. 3, Tecuicuilco, item 26.

27. Esteynèffer, *Florilegio medicinal*, "Dedicatoria."

28. López, *Tesoro de medicinas*, "Prólogo."

29. Francisco Losa, *La vida que hizo el siervo de Dios Gregorio López en algunos lugares de esta Nueva España* (Mexico City, 1613), cited in Guerra, introduction to *El tesoro de medicinas de Gregorio López*, 16.

30. Ibid., 20–21, cites Luis Muñoz, official of the royal treasury in Madrid, re-

porting that a copy of the manuscript was highly esteemed in the Royal Convent of the Incarnation in Madrid. Apparently the treasury of divinely inspired medical knowledge was gifted by Luis de Velasco, viceroy of New Spain (1590–1595, 1600–1611), and was thus considered sufficient demonstration of honor for the convent and its regal patrons.

31. Tissot, *Aviso al pueblo acerca de su salud*, 20. Tissot remained a humoralist, judging by his manual, where he defined good health as a state of equilibrium. According to Emch-Dériaz, *Tissot*, 73, "he rejected bleeding, purging, vomiting, and heroic drugs as the primary agents of recovery" and promoted instead the powerful salutary benefits of nature.

32. Tissot, *Aviso al pueblo acerca de su salud*, 21–22.

33. On the Spanish editions of Tissot's manual, see Perdiguero, "Popularizando la ciencia," 165–167, and Perdiguero, "Popularization of Medicine during the Spanish Enlightenment," 109–113.

34. On Buchan, see Rosenberg, "Medical Text and Social Context," 26.

35. Perdiguero, "Popularizando la ciencia," 167–168.

36. *Gazeta de México* 2, no. 30 (March 13, 1787), "Aviso que comunican los Doctores D. Miguel Fernandez, D. Joaquin Pio Eguia Muro, y el Br. D. Joseph Vasquez."

37. *Gazeta de México*, no. 44 (August 9, 1785), 370.

38. *Gazeta de México* 2, no. 44 (November 6, 1787), 444; and *Gazeta de México* 3, no. 16 (September 16, 1788).

39. Venegas, *Compendio de la medicina*, "A el que leyere este Libro."

40. Whereas Hinojosos's *Summa, y recopilacion de Chirugia* advised the reader that by "dragma" was meant the weight of a silver *real* ("dragma, es peso de un real senzillo de plata"), Venegas went further: "The medical pound is 12 ounces. / An ounce is 8 *dragmas*. / A *dragma* is 3 *escrúpulos*. / An *escrúpulo* is 24 grains. / A grain weighs as much as an *alberjón* seed. / By handful we mean whatever fits in the hand. / By *tomado*, what the tips of three fingers hold. / By glass, half a flask [*cuartillo*]. / And by spoonful, half an ounce."

41. Venegas, *Compendio de la medicina*, 68–69.

42. Ibid., 359.

43. Tissot, *Aviso al pueblo acerca de su salud*, 26.

44. Venegas, *Compendio de la medicina*, "A el que leyere este Libro."

45. Earle, *Body of the Conquistador*; Cañizares-Esguerra, *Nature, Empire, and Nation*, chapter 4; and Norton, *Sacred Gifts, Profane Pleasures*, 132–140.

46. *Asuntos varios sobre ciencias, y artes*, no. 12 (December 28, 1772). Alzate's journals are available in two modern editions: Alzate, *Obras I. Periódicos*, and Alzate, *Gacetas de literatura de México*.

47. On European reading practices, see Melton, *Rise of the Public in Enlightenment Europe*, chapter 3. For the historiography of printing in Spanish America, see Calvo, "Politics of Print"; and for comparison, see Warner, *Letters of the Republic*. On shifts in organizing information, including newspapers, encyclopedias, maps, and statistical charts and graphs, see Headrick, *When Information Came of Age*; and on the impact of the printing press, see Eisenstein, *Printing Press as an Agent of Change*.

48. Uribe-Uran, "Birth of a Public Sphere in Latin America."

49. Saladino García, *Dos científicos de la Ilustración hispanoamericana*, 222–223.

50. There is a vast literature on this major figure of the Mexican enlightenment, whose patriotism made him suspicious of European system builders and the Linnaean system and moved him to defend creole Americans, their climate, and their intellect against disparaging commentaries, in print and in correspondence. It has been suggested that, feeling isolated after the departure of the Jesuits in 1767, Alzate sought company in the virtual world of his publications, even reaching out beyond the literate, who formed his primary audience. For his life and work and discussions of his eclectic reading habits, see Peset, "Símbolos e ideas en torno al concepto de naturaleza," 68–69; Saladino García, "José Antonio de Alzate y Ramírez," 37–55; Saladino García, *Dos científicos de la Ilustración hispanoamericana*, chapter 3; and Cañizares-Esguerra, *How To Write the History of the New World*, 281–286.

51. Alzate used his own resources to offset printing costs and keep his papers afloat; see his remarks in *Gazeta de literatura* 2, no. 23 (July 12, 1791).

52. *Diario literario de México*, no. 1 (March 18, 1768).

53. *Asuntos varios sobre ciencias, y artes*, no. 1 (November 2, 1772), "Prólogo del autor."

54. Clark, "*Gazeta de Literatura de México* (1788–1795)," 13–14. A streamlined style and lack of clear breaks on the page confound more precise identification of authors of particular sections. The resulting blurring of authorship was typical of a genre that borrowed learning from multiple sources.

55. *Gazeta de literatura*, no. 1 (January 15, 1788), "Prólogo del autor."

56. For Alzate's reactions to what he viewed as Mexico's outdated and unthinking pedagogical practices, see Saladino García, *Dos científicos de la Ilustración hispanoamericana*, 97–101.

57. Moreno, *Ensayos de historia de la ciencia y la tecnología*, 49–91.

58. *Mercurio volante, con noticias importantes y curiosas sobre varios asuntos de física y medicina*, no. 1 (October 17, 1772) and no. 2 (October 28, 1772), reprinted in Bartolache, *Mercurio Volante*, 3–14. All references to Bartolache's publications are to the Moreno edition.

59. *Mercurio volante*, no. 1 (October 17, 1772).

60. *Mercurio volante*, no. 2 (October 28, 1772), 13–14.

61. *Mercurio volante*, no. 5 (November 18, 1772), 45–54.

62. Bynum, Lock, and Porter, introduction to *Medical Journals and Medical Knowledge*, 2. This collection represents a broader effort by medical historians to take seriously the format of periodical publications, their mechanisms, and their special influence on the world of early modern medical practice.

63. Alzate, "Un indio de la Nueva España, Qué especie de hombre es, cuáles sus carácteres morales y físicos?" in *Memorias y ensayos*, 155.

64. Not unique to Alzate, these ideas were explicitly delineated in the *Gazeta de literatura*, nos. 14 and 15 (March 22 and April 12, 1790), "Observaciones sobre la práctica de la Medicina." Cañizares-Esguerra, "Nation and Nature," extrapolates from this interest in homegrown remedies the invention of a homogenous proto-national space based on the natural world; naturalist discourse, in this interpretation, supported New World affiliations.

65. *Asuntos varios sobre ciencia, y artes*, no. 3 (November 16 and 23, 1772).

66. *Gazeta de literatura* 2, no. 6 (November 16, 1790).

67. *Gazeta de literatura* 3, no. 1 (October 27, 1792), no. 5 (January 8, 1793), no. 10 (April 9, 1793), and no. 12 (May 11, 1793), 90; and Esteyneffer, *Florilegio medicinal*, 343, 357, 404, and 411, prescribing a dusting of its powder on the hair to treat head lice.

68. *Gazeta de México*, no. 35 (April 15, 1785), 286–287.

69. On the importance of association to the editors of the *Encyclopédie* and their debt to Francis Bacon, see Goodman, *Republic of Letters*, 24–28.

70. Alzate's borrowing and special admiration for French learning are discussed in Clark, "'Read All About It.'"

71. Furdell, *Publishing and Medicine in Early Modern England*, 101, and chapter 5. Without easy access to classical learning, historian Elizabeth Lane Furdell has argued, women worked as empiricists, experimentalists, patrons, and publishers of science and medicine, much of it aimed at popularizing medical practice among women, and thereby contributed to a process of encroachment on the professional domain of men.

72. Discourses of racial difference were similarly anchored to skeletal studies, which ascribed to the physiognomy of European men the "standard of excellence" to which others were held. Schiebinger, *Mind Has No Sex?*, chapters 7 and 8, and Schiebinger, "Anatomy of Difference," 387–405. On sexual difference helping to justify the exclusion of women from a public sphere coded as male, see Landes, *Women and the Public Sphere*, chapter 2. Tomaselli, "Reflections on the History of the Science of Women," stresses that nonmedical experiences and disciplines offered other views and that the medical sciences were not always privileged sites of discourse. On the exclusion of women healers in New Spain, see Hernández Sáenz, *Learning To Heal*, 269–270.

73. *Diario literario de México*, no. 1 (March 18, 1768). Another potential effect of rejecting barriers of gender, class, and education was to found their authority in a public forum in which they themselves would serve as privileged mediators, as Achim, "From Rustics to Savants," 283, has argued.

74. Viesca Treviño and Sanfilippo, "La medicina en las *Gacetas de Literatura*," 253–264.

75. *Asuntos varios sobre ciencia, y artes*, no. 1 (November 2, 1772), "Prólogo del autor."

76. *Mercurio volante*, no. 15 (February 3, 1773) and no. 16 (February 10, 1773), 171.

77. Eudiometry evolved simultaneously in Britain and Italy, where it was applied in epidemics by enlightened states convinced of the benefits of healthful air. Schaffer, "Measuring Virtue," 281–318.

78. Etlin, *Architecture of Death*, 17–34; and Voekel, *Alone before God*.

79. *Asuntos varios sobre ciencias, y artes*, no. 13 (January 4, 1773). Alzate also looked to the best European discoveries, such as the bellows pump, which might remove corrupted air from hospitals for the benefit of patients in New Spain and thereby improve their reputation among patients and physicians alike. *Asuntos varios sobre ciencias, y artes*, no. 6 (November 30, 1772). Mexico City's hospitals

were publicly known as especially insalubrious places; see *Gazeta de México*, no. 7 (April 7, 1784).

80. Saladino García, *Dos científicos de la Ilustración hispanoamericana*, 9 and 138–141.

81. *Mercurio volante*, no. 3 (November 4, 1772) and no. 4, (November 11, 1772).

82. Transcriptions from Silva Prada, "El uso de los baños temascales," citation on 37. The issue of the utility of the *temascal* to the Spanish population was complicated, according to Dr. Oliver, with water baths preferred owing to the ways dry heat exacerbated their drier and more choleric constitution (49).

83. For studies of *temascales* as spaces of diversion, sociability, suppression, and vice, see Gruzinski, "Las cenizas del deseo," 255–283; and Tortorici, "'Heran todos putos.'"

84. Guevara, "Discurso sobre la policía de México," AHDF 3627 exp. 43, paras. 199 and 258.

85. Rodríguez, *Contaminación e insalubridad en la ciudad de México*, 169–173.

86. Cody, "Index to the Periodicals," 444–445: "Practical problems in the field of medicine most engaged Alzate's attention as an editor."

87. *Gazeta de literatura* 2, no. 21 (June 14, 1791), 164–168. On the history of engraved images, see Donahue-Wallace, "Picturing Prints in Early Modern New Spain," which examines prints as a source of clerical identity and as works of art consumed by the upper classes. Alzate's focus on cost suggests that he intended something more like the hundreds of thousands of devotional prints circulating in colonial Mexico at the time, which were portable, accessible, and much more common.

88. *Mercurio volante*, nos. 11–14 (January 6, 1773 to January 26, 1773), 109–152, quotation from 121–22. The manual was widely consumed in French, English, and Spanish translations, appearing in London, Madrid, and Paris in the eighteenth century and in North American cities in the nineteenth and twentieth, but apparently less familiar in the Spanish world when Bartolache reprinted it.

89. *Mercurio volante*, no. 12 (January 13, 1773), 124.

90. Tribunal del Protomedicato, Mexico City, January 8, 1773, Bancroft Library, M-M 135, 13. Compare a 1786 medical report to municipal and viceregal authorities, in which abuse of food and alcoholic beverages and nudity of the poor, who are described as "por lo común desordenada," are adduced for this sector's greater ruin and vulnerability to noxious atmospheric effects, alongside general dirt, decomposition, and infected air. Tribunal del Protomedicato, Mexico City, May 19, 1786, AHDF 3674 exp. 4, 21–22.

91. These ideas were well represented in the healing guides surveyed above. Agustín Farfán asserted that women who menstruate irregularly suffer because their blood has thickened excessively, the result of overeating, much idleness (*ocio*), and little exercise; the women of New Spain in particular were seen as particularly "desreglada [*sic*]" in their eating habits. See Farfán, *Tractado brebe de medicina*, 33v–34r, and Tissot, *Aviso al pueblo acerca de su salud*, 14, which cites "vida desarreglada" as a factor in the dissolution of good health.

92. *Mercurio volante*, no. 6 (November 25, 1772), 55–64. Minor causes stem-

ming from atmospheric conditions were identified but not stressed in the same way as those relating to lifestyle.

93. Jaffary, *False Mystics*, 139–144 and 159, has observed that the symptoms of this newly classified medical disease overlapped with observed behaviors of female mystics, and that the medical literature resembled older church directives and discourses surrounding women's virtue, vice, and morality. An outbreak of *saltos* among nuns in the convent of La Purísima in San Miguel el Grande (Allende) might have been an expression of protest against the imposition of common life (*vida común*) in the 1760s. See Chowning, *Rebellious Nuns*, 105–118.

94. On the ideology of objectivity, see Daston and Galison, "Image of Objectivity" and *Objectivity*.

95. Nicolás José de Torres and Juan Gregorio de Campo to Viceroy, Mexico City, March 26, 1762, AGN Hospitales 144, reproduced in Velasco Ceballos, *La cirugía Mexicana*, 411–413.

96. Crucial in this was the establishment of the College of Surgery at the Royal Indian Hospital in 1770, after which patients of the city's hospitals were occasionally used as anatomical subjects until the college's transfer to the building of the defunct Mexican Inquisition in 1833. See Howard, *Royal Indian Hospital of Mexico City*, chapter 4, on the college's founding.

97. For discussion of fermented beverages, see Chapter 1 in this volume. On stereotypes about plebeian drinking and criminal activities in Mexico City, see Cope, *Limits of Racial Domination*, 37–38. For similar medical "discoveries" in Nueva Granada, see the 1783 report on the previous year's epidemic from the viceroy, Caballero y Góngora, and physician José Celestino Mútis, cited in Frías Núñez, *Enfermedad y sociedad en la crisis colonial*, 73–74.

98. Goodman, *Republic of Letters*, 164–165, traces the emergence of the Republic of Letters to older genres of literary and epistolary correspondence and argues that it was fundamentally defined by its epistolary format.

99. *Asuntos varios sobre ciencias, y artes*, no. 11 (December 14, 1772).

100. *Asuntos varios sobre ciencias, y artes*, no. 12 (December 28, 1772). The French "vinegar of the four thieves" was prescribed by Moscow's medical community in the same moment; see Alexander, *Bubonic Plague in Early Modern Russia*, 183. In the June 12, 1788, issue of his *Gazeta de literatura*, Alzate again solicited an "instructive report" addressing the reasons for the city's exceptional cases of tertiary fever, stipulating that it be based on facts, not theory; a response appeared in the April 25 and May 12, 1789, issues.

101. *Gazeta de México* 2, "Prólogo."

102. *Gazeta de México*, no. 6 (March 24, 1784).

103. *Gazeta de México*, no. 7 (April 7, 1784).

104. *Gazeta de México*, no. 33 (March 22, 1785), 266.

105. *Gazeta de México*, no. 37 (May 10, 1785), 297–300.

106. *Gazeta de México* 2, no. 15 (August 8, 1786). Venegas cited the January 18, 1785, issue announcing that there were only three physicians available to minister to Guanajuato's sizable populace, to support his claim that medical personnel in the viceroyalty were severely lacking. Venegas, *Compendio de la medicina*, "A el que leyere este Libro."

107. *Gazeta de México*, no. 48 (October 4, 1785), 400–401. The entry was

corrected with the addition of a negating particle in a subsequent issue, to clarify that it was *laypeople* in Oaxaca who esteemed its virtues; see 409.

108. *Gazeta de México*, no. 36 (May 3, 1785), 289–290. For Caballero's observations on hot-air balloons and remarks on his literary references, see *Gazeta de México*, no. 44 (August 9, 1785), 364–366.

109. On social inequalities and other obstacles to exchange that characterized these sometimes intimate, often fleeting relationships, see Achim, "From Rustics to Savants"; on the accumulation of healing knowledge in the Jesuit missions of Paraguay in the seventeenth century, see Prieto, *Missionary Scientists*, chapter 3. Londa Schiebinger, in *Plants and Empire*, 82–89, has discussed "noise" or barriers to exchange between naturalists in the "biocontact zones" of the West Indies.

110. *Gazeta de México*, no. 51 (November 22, 1785), 441.

111. Tarantola, "Four Thousand Years of Concepts Relating to Rabies" 6, observes that not all who are bit by a rabid animal subsequently contract the germ, which would have encouraged belief in the effectiveness of these various treatments. I am indebted to Roger Gathman for bringing this variety to my attention.

112. *Gazeta de México*, no. 20 (October 6, 1784); no. 30 (February 8, 1785); no. 31 (February 22, 1785).

113. *Gazeta de México*, no. 39 (June 7, 1785), 315.

114. *Gazeta de México*, no. 41 (July 5, 1785), 330–331.

115. Aceves Pastrana, *Química, botánica y farmacia en la Nueva España*, 55–74, and "Átomos y luces en los periódicos de Alzate y Ramírez," 221–250. For Buffon's objections, see Headrick, *When Information Came of Age*, 27–29.

116. *Gazeta de México* 2, no. 9 (May 16, 1786), 109–111: "meter la hoz en mies agena."

117. For a time in the 1730s the gazette offered readers news of local remedies and antidotes against rabies, venereal infection, and other contagious diseases. As Guedea, "La medicina en las gacetas de México," argues, these reports reflected casual interest in collecting any newsworthy items, rather than a deliberate, programmatic project.

118. *Gazeta de México* 2, no. 24 (December 19, 1786).

119. *Gazeta de México* 2, no. 11 (June 13, 1786), 129.

120. *Gazeta de México* 2, no. 36 (June 5, 1787). The descriptions and applications suggest that correspondents were describing the same yellow-flowered plant, which went by a variety of regional names: *guachichile*, *espinosilla*, *hierba del tabardillo*, *mirto cimarrón*, *hierba de la Virgin*, and so on.

121. For the price of approximately 1 *real* an issue, over a subscription period of twenty-four to twenty-eight issues (3 or 4 pesos) residents could read accounts of these debates and discoveries in real time. New Spain's gazette had no more than four hundred subscribers, while its first daily, the *Diario de México*, peaked at its 1805 premiere with seven hundred. These figures can be misleading: the latter also sold, for a half *real*, at a dozen locations around Mexico City, and reading practices dictated that copies would have been shared and read aloud. On the *Gazeta de México*, see Saladino García, *Ciencia y prensa durante la ilustración Latinoamericana*, 72; and Delgado Carranco, "Un acercamiento a la segunda época del *Diario de México*," 83–94.

122. The phrase is from Tilley, *Africa as a Living Laboratory*, 26, referring

to "scientists and technical officers" in a subsequent period of colonization who provided the categories "that helped make vernacular knowledge visible and communicated it beyond the locality within which it arose."

123. On the process by which Valdés secured permissions to publish, see Ruiz Castañeda, *La tercera gaceta de la Nueva España.*

124. Viceroy to Real Tribunal, Mexico City, March 11, 1786, AGN Historia 460, no exp., 53–54. In 1797, Viceroy Branciforte moved to end the practice of publishing "secret remedies" by ordering Valdés to submit these to the Protomedicato for ratification first. Its power to censor was soon challenged, and in 1807, Viceroy Iturrigaray exempted the editors of Mexico City's publications from any compulsory review by the medical body prior to advertising new drugs. See Lanning, *Royal Protomedicato*, 364–365.

125. *Gazeta de México* 8, no. 46 (November 29, 1797), 379.

126. An instructional pamphlet on inoculation, authored by Mexico's Protomedicato, was propagated in the gazette; notices from its pages were reprinted and dispatched during epidemics to facilitate the work of caretakers and institutions; and eventually the efforts of officials and patriots on behalf of vaccine campaigns were publicized in its pages. In Orizaba during the 1797 smallpox epidemic, for instance, the viceroy distributed a dozen copies of Bartolache's 1779 instruction and of gazette issue number 42 for use by residents commissioned to assist in each of the villa's *cuarteles*. Viceroy to Ayuntamiento, Orizaba, October 11, 1797, AGN Epidemias 5 exp. 1, 18–19; and Regidor Suarez to Pedro Andres Marin, Orizaba, September 14, 1797, AGN Epidemias 5 exp. 2, 95r. This print culture indirectly encroached on the Protomedicato's functions, as when the tribunal discounted the idea of producing another simplified instructional pamphlet, citing the variability of outbreaks and circumstances and the availability of the manuals of Tissot, López, and the *Florilegio medicinal*. Tribunal del Protomedicato, Mexico City, May 19, 1786, AHDF 3674 exp. 4, 27r.

127. Recent studies of early modern scientific practice have attempted to appreciate the roles, often poorly delineated, of practitioners "from all social strata, but often occupying a middle ground between university-trained scholars, immersed in texts, and workshop-trained artisans, immersed in a world of technique." On these "relative newcomers to the historiography of science," see Smith and Findlen, introduction to *Merchants and Marvels*, 16–17.

128. *Mercurio volante*, no. 7 (December 2, 1772), 65–75.

129. Too little is known about reading practices in these years. There were reading societies, such as the one composed of lawyers, clergymen, university students, and others that the proprietor Antonio Nariño periodically assembled in his home in Santa Fe de Bogotá, in the 1780s and 1790s, to purchase, circulate, and discuss copies of books and journals. See Renán Silva's summary in "Prácticas de lectura, ámbitos privados y formación de un espacio público moderno," 90–93.

130. Voekel, *Alone before God*, especially 174–175. The influence of these creoles no doubt justifies scholarly focus on them. Alzate was a corresponding member of the Basque Royal Economic Society of "Amigos del País," a voluntary civic association that solicited ideas and funded projects for improvements in agriculture, industry, and manufactures. See Bleichmar, *Visible Empire*, 28–29. His journals were an extension of this activity, and of his correspondence with

Viceroy Revillagigedo on urban sanitation and renewal, the mines of New Spain, and population. On these epistolary sources, see Rodríguez, *Contaminación e insalubridad en la ciudad de México.*

131. Perdiguero, "Popularizando la ciencia," 170.

132. Achim, "Making Lizards into Drugs," 183.

133. *Gazeta de México* 7, no. 34 (May 30, 1795), "Continuación del Suplemento," 292.

134. Shapin, *Social History of Truth*, 338.

135. After the November 8, 1785, issue of the gazette identified two residents of the city of Querétaro who declined to contribute to relief efforts to supply food to the poor, a subsequent notice issued a retraction; in fact, they had contributed by offering loans. "El público" was asked "to discard the notion that it has perhaps formed against the good conduct, charity, and patriotic zeal of those two subjects." *Gazeta de México* 2, no. 8 (May 2, 1786), 107.

136. At the conclusion of the *Mercurio volante*'s run, Bartolache sold the remainders and turned his attention to promoting a proprietary pill of pure iron, for persons without access to a physician, to prevent and treat lack of appetite, stomach pains, heartburn, hysteria and "obstructions," and scurvy, for a peso an ounce, and less for "poor *indios*." See Bartolache, *Instrucción para el buen uso de las pastillas marciales, o fierro sutil* (August 19, 1774), in *Mercurio volante*, 183–189. A promise that an instruction would appear in Nahuatl (*idioma mexicano*) for non-ladino Indians was apparently never fulfilled. See Bartolache, *Noticia plausible para sanos y enfermos* (July 15, 1774), in *Mercurio volante*, 179.

137. Guevara, "Discurso sobre la policía de México," para. 276.

CHAPTER 3

"Massacre of the Innocents"

Epigraph: Conejares to Intendant, Villa Alta, February 10, 1797, AGN Epidemias 10 exp. 5.

1. July 13, 1796, AGN Epidemias 3 exp. 1, 1–5.

2. See Slack, *Impact of Plague in Tudor and Stuart England*, 44–50 and 199–226; Cipolla, *Public Health and the Medical Profession in the Renaissance*; and Cipolla, *Faith, Reason, and the Plague*, describing the clash of a clerical mentality that insisted on public rogations with one espoused by civil authorities and "rationalists" who sought to enforce cordons and other prohibitions on travel. Many of the countermeasures examined in this chapter were also enacted in Enlightenment Russia during a 1771 plague outbreak; see Alexander, *Bubonic Plague in Early Modern Russia*, chapter 7.

3. The *acusas* are in AGN IV 2796 exp. 5. See also Miguel Chacon y Diaz, Ramon Ximenez, and Francisco de Leon to Viceroy Flores, Querétaro, April 12, 1788, AGN Historia 460 exp. 2, 4–5, expressing concern that if *curanderos* and other *intrusos* in medicine were not subject to the same orders for reporting and separation, the measures would have no effect.

4. Real Tribunal to Manuel Antonio Flores, Mexico City, February 14, 1788, AGN Historia 460 exp. 2, 6–7.

5. *Extracto de la obra publicada en Madrid el año pasado de 1784 con el título de Disertación Físico-Médica*, articles VII, VIII, XII, XIII, XIV, XV, XVII, XVIII, XX. Its program resembles John Haygarth's rules for containing smallpox in Chester, published in 1784, which evolved in the context of inoculation and paid less attention to cleansing agents than the Spanish version. Booth, *John Haygarth*, 49–59.

6. Most administrators pledged obedience and sometimes reported measures taken. Taxco's official proposed the use of a hospital recently constructed at considerable cost in the district seat, adding that a method of prevention (*método preservativo*) composed by a medical practitioner had been sent to parish priests for translation into the "language of the Indians" and for implementation in parishes, to "prepare and purge the humors" in the event of infection. Fernando de Mendoza to Viceroy, Taxco, August 20, 1796, AGN Epidemias 3 exp. 1, 45v.

7. Felipe de Ortuño to Viceroy, Pachuca, September 3, 1796, AGN Epidemias 3 exp. 1, 55.

8. See Voekel, *Alone before God*, on public health reforms in Mexico City and Veracruz; Cooper, *Epidemic Disease in Mexico City*; Price, "State, Church, Charity, and Smallpox"; Villaseñor Cabral, "La Epidemia de viruela en Nueva España"; Thompson, "To Save the Children"; Espinosa Cortés and Miranda Ocampo, "La epidemia de viruela de 1796–1798"; Cramaussel, *El impacto demográfico de la viruela en México*, vol. 1, for regional studies; and Magaña Mancillas, *Epidemias y rutas de propagación*, which compiles the work of members of the Red de Historia Demográfica in Mexico, whose quantitative methods have reconstructed routes of propagation, demographic impact, and regional integration. Rolf Widmer Sennhauser's analysis of Tehuantepec, "Política sanitaria y lucha social en tiempos de viruelas," attributes the eventual reversal of policy and the "modern" turn to inoculation to the persistence of dominant classes, above all Spaniard and creole merchants in Chiapas, Oaxaca, and Tehuantepec, who sought to limit the impact of cordons and protect their financial interests at the expense of the indigenous communities of the region. This chapter adopts Sennhauser's fine-grained approach but adduces additional explanations for change.

9. In the words of Teotitlán del Valle's administrator: "Public health is of great concern, and I believe that God would look with displeasure on any devotions that could occasion the misfortune of many of His creatures." Esteban Melgar to Intendant, Teotitlán, October 6, 1796, AGN Epidemias 12 exp. 7, 345r-v (and correspondence on the festival's logistics in the same file).

10. In his 1775 review of the convent hospitals of San Juan de Dios in Mexico City, Pachuca, Texcoco, and Toluca, the archbishop of Mexico noted that the only patients were *pobres infelices* who had no other recourse. He observed that Indians feared hospitals and would rather die in their villages "without any care [*socorro*]" than enter them, citing inconsistent treatment that varied depending on the prior in charge. Velasco Ceballos, *Visita y reforma de los hospitales*, vol. 2, 139–146. The bishop of Puebla noted that though physicians preferred them, hospitals were an impossible solution for nursing infants and a category of shamefaced patients, among them girls beginning puberty, "who would prefer the horrors of death inside their own homes to assured health elsewhere." Obispo to Branciforte, Puebla, February 2, 1798, AGN Epidemias 6 exp. 4, 195.

11. Nicolas de Lafora to Viceroy, Oaxaca, March 7, 1780, AGN IV 5724 exp. 12, 60r-v.

12. These schoolteachers continued to be supported financially by the parents of their charges, who might drag their feet or refuse outright to make payments. Tanck de Estrada, *Pueblos de indios y educación en el México colonial*, 168–214, 334–394, and 426–447.

13. Guardino, *Time of Liberty*, chapter 3. On the *repartimiento* system as vital to indigenous producers, see Baskes, *Indians, Merchants, and Markets.*

14. Especially Antonio de Mora y Peysal, Oaxaca, July 2, 1795, AGN Historia 531 exp. 1, 23–24.

15. Signed by Fessar, with rubrics of several officials, ibid., 69.

16. Machuca Gallegos, *Comercio de sal y redes de poder*, 211–217, derives data from *alcabala* records to argue for an interregional framework, whose analytical value is reinforced in disease emergencies.

17. Fessar to Mora y Peysal, Tehuantepeque, July 21, 1795, AGN Historia 531 exp. 1, 42–43; and Tehuantepeque, September 12, 1795, ibid., 110–111. When endorsing quarantine as preferable to absolute prohibition on trade, Antequera's physicians cited medical experts (William Cullen and Herman Booerhaave) in support, while the viceroy referred to success by means of this approach in 1790 with goods arriving from infested Havana. See Oaxaca, September 22, 1795, ibid., 115–117; and Mexico City, October 28, 1795, ibid., 126.

18. A village weaver contravened quarantine to travel with his son through precipitous mountain ranges to sell his goods, eventually arriving in the heart of the infected Chontales district. The boy contracted smallpox and passed it to other children in his home and neighborhood. For the full itinerary, see AGN Epidemias 15 exp. 9, 240r-v.

19. Chance, *Race and Class in Colonial Oaxaca*, 144–151.

20. Melgar to Mora y Peysal, Teotitlán, September 28, 1796, AGN Epidemias 12 exp. 5, 195.

21. For details of the arrangement, see Melgar to Intendant, Teotitlán, October 3, 1796, AGN Epidemias 12 exp. 7, 337–338. Expenses generated in Teotitlán amounted to 1,203 pesos for hospitals, beds, and medications; 660 pesos for troops to guard the cordon; and roughly 2,900 pesos for the purchase of these textiles from weavers, returned to coffers once the goods were sold (and the excess from sales given to villagers). See Bernardo José de Rioja to Real Tribunal y Audiencia de Cuentas del Reino, Oaxaca, July 24, 1801, AGN Epidemias 15 exp. 2, 74–75; Melgar to Intendant, Teotitlán, January 9, 1796 [1797], AGN Epidemias 10 exp. 6, 231; Melgar to Intendant, Teotitlán, January 12, 1797, ibid., 232–233; and Melgar to Intendant, Teotitlán, January 22, 1797, ibid., 236.

22. Melgar to Intendant, Teotitlán, October 1, 1796, AGN Epidemias 12 exp. 5, 204–205; Intendant to Melgar, Antequera, October 4, 1796, ibid., 206–207; and Melgar to Intendant, Teotitlán, October 7, 1796, AGN Epidemias 15 exp. 2, 23. Melgar represented his *indio* charges as poor and in need of protection, without which they would perish below the leaky roofs of their homes.

23. Taylor, *Landlord and Peasant in Colonial Oaxaca*; Chance, *Conquest of the Sierra*; Carmagnani, *El regreso de los dioses*; Terraciano, "Crime and Culture in Colonial Mexico"; and Chassen-López, *From Liberal to Revolutionary*

Oaxaca, 442, on the persistence of territorial disputes through the nineteenth and twentieth centuries.

24. Bando, Tehuantepec, December 13, 1795, AGN Historia 531 exp. 2, 34v–36.

25. Isidro Flores, Cárcel de San Pablo Ayutla, October 15, 1796, AHJO VA Criminal 21 exp. 19, 7v-8r; and Isidro Flores, *escribano*, Villa Alta, October 19, 1796, ibid., 16–17.

26. Juan Martin, Isidro Flores, and Juan de la Cruz, Villa Alta, October 19, 1796, ibid., 15–18.

27. Marcos Ximenes, Geronimo Nicolas, and Jacinto Nicolas, Villa Alta, October 20–21, 1796, ibid., 19–22. The alliance between district seat and subject towns on the basis of ethnicity suggests that the process of political fragmentation into autonomous *repúblicas* looked different for the Mixe communities, in a region less disrupted by the effects of commercial agriculture than the Mixteca. On the latter, see Pastor, *Campesinos y reformas*, 175–176 and 189–190.

28. "El comun de San Pablo Ayutla," AHJO VA Criminal 21 exp. 19, 11r–12v.

29. Marcos Ximenes and *regidores* Josef Gomez and Geronimo Nicolas, to José Milangos, San Pablo Ayutla, October 15, 1796, ibid., 6–7: "estos Zapotecos son muy alzados."

30. "Justicias y principales de Tlahuitoltepec," ibid., 10v: "por desovedientes y mal hablados"

31. Certified report, Villa Alta, October 20, 1796, ibid., 18–19.

32. Auto signed Ruiz de Conejares, Villa Alta, October 15, 1796, ibid., 3, and his counterpart's report, José Melgar to Conejares, Tlacolula, October 15, 1796, ibid., 5, subscribing to the villagers' self-presentation as simple agriculturalists defending their land.

33. Auto signed Ruiz de Conejares, Villa Alta, October 22, 1796, ibid., 22v–23v.

34. Ruiz de Conejares to Intendant, Villa Alta, February 10, 1797, AGN Epidemias 10 exp. 5, 222–225.

35. José González to Manuel de Flon, Tehuacán de las Granadas, June 11, 1797, AGN Epidemias 10 exp. 4, 198–200.

36. Alexandro de la Pasqua to Intendant, Mextitlan, November 15, 1797, AGN Epidemias 3 exp. 12, 174–175: "pues para ellos todo es camino."

37. "Los diputados del Comercio (y Mineria) de esta ciudad," n.p., n.d., AGN Epidemias 10 exp. 2, 88r-v, discussed at the February 21, 1797, meeting of the Junta Provincial with the intendant present.

38. Don Juan María García, n.p., n.d., ibid., 89–90v, also discussed at the February 21, 1797 meeting.

39. As proof, they observed that the senior judge (*oidor decano*) of the Audiencia of Guatemala had traveled to Mexico City with fourteen children in tow without passing quarantine. Don Joaquín Vasco had been detained in Tehuacán several weeks earlier and seemed to believe the quarantine was entirely too inconvenient. Joaquín Vasco to Viceroy, Tehuacán, March 4, 1797, ibid., 100; and "Los labradores, y vecinos de Tehuacán," March 21, 1797, ibid., 110–111, signed by eleven men in steady, elegant script.

40. Borbón to Viceroy, Mexico City, March 24, 1797, ibid.

41. Borbón to Viceroy, Mexico City, May 2, 1797, ibid., 141v.

42. Deciding that it was impossible to pay miners two-thirds the value of their silver in Antequera as they proposed, the royal treasury attorney recommended opening the passage between Oaxaca and Mexico City for *arrieros* transporting silver, provided the mine was not infested, the muleteer not sick, and that clothes, harnesses, saddles, and bags were fumigated. Fiscal de Real Hacienda, Mexico City, March 23, 1797, AGN Epidemias 10 exp. 4, 213–215.

43. Fessar to Mora y Peysal, Tehuantepeque, July 12, 1795, AGN Historia 531 exp. 1, 31–32; and Fessar to Mora y Peysal, Tehuantepeque, November 10, 1795, ibid., 165–166.

44. Certificación, Esteban Melgar, Teotitlán, December 30, 1796, AGN Epidemias 15 exp. 9, 244.

45. The literature on gender in colonial Mexico is vast. On strategies for splitting patriarchal authority, see Stern, *Secret History of Gender*, 98–103, and the related discussion in Franco, *Plotting Women*, 9–22. On gender and violence in Oaxaca, see Taylor, *Drinking, Homicide, and Rebellion*; and Sousa, "Women and Crime in Colonial Oaxaca." For a hemispheric overview of gender parallelism, honor, and shame, see Kellogg, *Weaving the Past*.

46. Melgar to Intendant, Teotitlán, October 1, 1796, AGN Epidemias 12 exp. 5, 204–205; and the priest's *certificación*, Manuel Antonio Martínez, Casa Parroquial de Teotitlán, November 16, 1796, AGN Epidemias 12 exp. 7, 381r-v.

47. José Flores, "Instrucción sobre el modo de practicar la inoculación de las viruelas y método para curar esta enfermedad acomodado a la naturaleza y modo de vivir de los Indios, y demás castas de Gente rústica de los Pueblos de el Reino de Guatemala," Nueva Guatemala, October 25, 1794, AHJO VA Civil 31 exp. 14; and Mora y Peysal to Melgar, Oaxaca, September 30, 1796, AGN Epidemias 12 exp. 5, 200r.

48. Melgar to Intendant, Teotitlán, October 8, 1796, AGN Epidemias 15 exp. 2, 24–25; and Melgar to Intendant, Teotitlán, September 27, 1796, AGN Epidemias 12 exp. 5, 193.

49. Certificación, Melgar, Teotitlán, December 30, 1796, AGN Epidemias 15 exp. 9, 245v–246r; and Melgar to Intendant, Teotitlán, October 1, 1796, AGN Epidemias 12 exp. 5, 204–205.

50. Josefa Ximénes, Teotitlán, October 17, 1796, AGN Epidemias 15 exp. 9, 208.

51. Petrona Chávez, Teotitlán, October 17, 1796, ibid., 207v–208r.

52. Antonio López, Teotitlán, October 12, 1796, ibid., 199–201.

53. José Bernardo Aragón, Teotitlán, October 21, 1796, ibid., 212r-v.

54. Where not otherwise cited, the foregoing account is from Melgar's official statement, Teotitlán, December 30, 1796, ibid., 246r–247v; Félix Confite to Melgar, Teotitlán, October 8, 1796, AGN Epidemias 15 exp. 2, 26; and Melgar to Intendant, Teotitlán, October 8, 1796, ibid., 26r. In colonial Mexico acts of humiliation often centered physically or verbally on the face and head; see Lipsett-Rivera, *Gender and the Negotiation of Daily Life in Mexico*.

55. Intendant to Viceroy, Oaxaca, October 28, 1796, AGN Epidemias 15 exp. 2, 33–34; and Melgar to Intendant, Teotitlán, November 17, 1796, ibid., 44. The intendant's orders were to apprehend the *cabecillas* (rebel leaders), close off the district seat from neighbors, and avoid harming any *indios* unless absolutely un-

avoidable. On the behavior of soldiers, see Intendant to Tomas Martínez Carrillo, Oaxaca, October 5, 1796, AGN Epidemias 12 exp. 7, 340r.

56. Melgar to Intendant, Teotitlán, October 20, 1796, ibid., 367r-v; and Melgar to Intendant, Teotitlán, November 17, 1796, AGN Epidemias 15 exp. 2, 44.

57. Certificación, Melgar, Teotitlán, December 30, 1796, AGN Epidemias 15 exp. 9, 225.

58. Pedro Alavés, Teotitlán, October 11, 1796, ibid., 194–195.

59. Josefa Ruiz, Teotitlán, October 25, 1796, ibid., 214–215r; Juana Lorenzo, Teotitlán, October 27, 1796, ibid., 215v–216r; and Pascuala de la Cruz, Teotitlán, October 19, 1796, ibid., 210.

60. On the Friday before the riot, don Joaquín Villasante read to Teotitlán's deputation in Antequera the brief he had written, which likened their village to a prison. He advised them to check back in two weeks for a final ruling and assured them that they would soon be able to leave to sell their textiles. When shown the *parecer*, Marcos de los Ángeles, a translator who first introduced the villagers to the attorney, recognized the writing as his own and swore he had composed the complaint himself, from notes brought from the village. The admission provides a rare glimpse of the work of another legal agent and reinforces the impression that many (if not all) of the forty-seven male *oficiales de mantero* whose names appear did not authorize the complaint. Joaquín de Villasante to Thomas Antonio Paradela, Oaxaca, October 7, 1796, AGN Epidemias 15 exp. 8, 166–167; Joaquín de Villasante, Antequera, October 13, 1796, ibid., 168v–171r; Gaspar García, Teotitlán, October 12, 1796, ibid., 197–199 (on assurances from Villasante that the measures were authored by Oaxaca's intendant); and Marcos de los Ángeles, Oaxaca, October 13, 1796, ibid., 174–176.

61. Melgar to Intendant, Teotitlán, October 12, 1796, AGN Epidemias 15 exp. 8, 162r-v.

62. "A nosotros la República y Comunes Naturales y principales del pueblo y cabecera de Teotitlán del Valle ante vuestra señoría nos presentamos rendidamente," Teotitlán, October 11, 1796, AGN Epidemias 15 exp. 9, 193r-v (signed on behalf of the *república* by scribes and interpreters).

63. Magdalena Hernández, Teotitlán, October 17, 1796, ibid., 209r.

64. Manuel Bazan, Teotitlán, October 11, 1796, ibid., 196–197. (Bazan cited Lorenzo's personal interest in the infirmary.)

65. Bolder politicking beyond *cabildos* might have been an outcome of Bourbon interventions in governance, insofar as reform rendered local representative bodies redundant or less capable of carrying out functions. See Taylor, *Drinking, Homicide, and Rebellion*, 141–142, on a "loss of vitality" of rulers. Pastor, *Campesinos y reformas*, 199, argues that Bourbon policy followed, rather than produced, a decline in the functioning of local governments.

66. Ruiz de Conejares to Intendant, Villa Alta, October 8, 1796, AHJO VA Civil 30 exp. 2, 1v-4v (also in AGN Epidemias 12 exp. 3, 153–156). Oaxaca's intendant reported these objections to the viceregal government, which placed the onus of resolution back on him.

67. After stating the need to beseech divine mercy by rogations and the intercession of the Virgin Mary and saints, he enumerated six goals: (1) a suitable pesthouse for the sick in each pueblo; (2) patients separated by sex and cared for by

capable nurses; (3) larger pueblos split into barrios under the care of distinguished residents; (4) guards to prohibit communication between healthy and sick; (5) smallpox victims safely buried in *camposantos*; and (6) prohibition of *temascales*. Villa Alta, May 15, 1797, AHJO VA Civil 32 exp. 4, 2–5.

68. On the critical harvest time, see Joseph Mariano de Velasco to Conejares, Yahuive, May 29, 1797, ibid., 27–28.

69. Ignacio José Ximenez to Conejares, Tavaa, May 17, 1797, ibid., 9–10.

70. Nicolás Pelayo to Ruiz de Conejares, Zoochila, May 17, 1797, ibid., 6–8.

71. Fray Joseph Mariano to Pedro Fessar, San Juan, January 22, 1796, AGN Historia 531 exp. 3, 39–41.

72. Puxmetecan, May 28, 1797, AHJO VA Civil 32 exp. 4, 24–25; and José Antonio Menezes to Conejares, Atitlán, May 27, 1797, AHJO VA Civil 31 exp. 15, 46r-v.

73. Ignacio José Ximenez to Conejares, Tavaa, May 17, 1797, AHJO VA Civil 32 exp. 4, 9–10; and "La República y Principales del Pueblo de Tavaa," Villa Alta, May 18, 1797, AHJO VA Civil 31 exp. 15, 38r.

74. Mariano Marlanzón to Conejares, Santa Cruz Yagavila, May 28, 1797, ibid., 49r; and Justicias to Conejares, Yaneri, May 28, 1797, ibid., 51r.

75. "El Governador, Alcaldes, Regidores, Ancianos, y demás común de Naturales del Pueblo, y Cavezera de Santa María de la Asunción de Tlacolula" [1796], AGN Epidemias 7 exp. 2, 349–350; and "El común y naturales de Santa María Asunción de Tlacolula...ante Vuestra Excelencia parecemos y decimos" [1796], AGN Epidemias 12 exp. 7, 373–734.

76. Antonio de Zúñiga to Conejares, Choapam, March 10 and March 13, 1797, AGN Epidemias 10 exp. 2, 121–124.

77. Thompson, "Moral Economy of the English Crowd," and *Customs in Common*, 8.

78. José González to Manuel de Flon, Tehuacán de las Granadas, June 11, 1797, AGN Epidemias 10 exp. 4, 198v–199.

79. Conspicuous shifts from first-person plural to third person, referring to the "supplicants," followed by an abrupt midsentence shift back to first-person plural to register an appeal ("reclamamos y ocurrimos") before the viceroy, suggest a collaborative effort, most likely assembled by a scribe from complaints and arguments dictated by prisoners and their lawyer.

80. Francisco Ruiz, Santiago Vásquez, Baltasar Ruiz, Pascual Hipólito, Pedro González, Domingo Matheo, and Lucas Sosa, Real Cárcel de Oaxaca, April 24, 1797, AGN Epidemias 15 exp. 2, 65v–66v. Only González signed; the other prisoners made six crosses in a small cluster.

81. Tanck de Estrada, "Indian Children in Early Mexico," 13–32. For the Mixteca of western Oaxaca, Pastor (*Campesinos y reformas*, 404–407) calculates that 35 percent of deaths occurred before the age of four and 51 percent by the age of twelve. Pastor speculates that this reality delayed the formation of strong emotional bonds with offspring, but the willingness of families to risk punishment for sick infants and children and the physical and discursive attempts to strengthen or protect this bond seem to run counter to the conclusion.

82. On the heart as the metaphoric locus of passions in the commentary of eighteenth-century priests, at once a person's essence and cause of instability, ir-

rationality, and mercurial temperament, see Taylor, "'. . . de corazón pequeño y ánimo apodaco,'" 28. On Nahua bodily conceptions of the heart as equivalent to the soul (*ánima*), center of thought and feeling, see López Austin, *Human Body and Ideology*, vol. 1, 174–175 and 229–231.

83. Descriptions of the cramped quarters of the lower classes abound. The physician sent to investigate reports of fevers in Azcapotzalco, northwest of Mexico City, uncovered more than seventy sick in one day, many afflicted with what he diagnosed as *matlazahuatl*. He described "an unhappy mother confined [*reducida*] to a home no bigger than six *varas* long, and four wide, with a child in her arms, two on a sad *petate*, and perhaps another stretched out, and all infected by a cruel *peste*, without having medications to give them, foods to sustain them, or anyone who aches for their unhappy situation." José Villarreal to Igacio Garcia Jove, Tacuba, September 5, 1797, AGN BN 754 exp. 3.

84. In advocating for the special attachment of children to their parents, villagers had learned counterparts in Europe: on the nature of children in Buffon's writings, for instance, see Benzaquén, "Childhood, Identity, and Human Science in the Enlightenment," 37–44. On the cultural dimensions of healing, see Sullivan, "Religious Foundations of Health and Medical Power in South America," 395–448; and Scheper-Hughes and Lock, "Mindful Body." For clinical studies demonstrating the role of strong social support networks in recovery, see Scott, *Miracle Cures*, 123–127.

85. Yannakakis, *Art of Being In-between*, 45–60 and 122–125, has highlighted the cultural commonalities, sustained regional alliances, and political solidarities that cut across deep ethnic divisions.

86. José Antonio Meneses to Conejares, Atitlán, May 7, 1797, AHJO VA Civil 31 exp. 15, 46r-v. In written complaints, leaders focused on the guards placed on the roads that caused them and *sujeto* pueblos harassments and delays, as when quarantine rules were applied to parishioners who had come to the town for baptisms. "Alcaldes, Principales, Común y Naturales" to Conejares, Atitlán, May 27, 1797, ibid., 47r.

87. Joseph Mariano de Velasco to Conejares, Yahuive, May 29, 1797, AHJO VA Civil 32 exp. 4, 27–28.

88. Francisco Ruiz et al., Real Cárcel de Oaxaca, April 24, 1797, AGN Epidemias 15 exp. 2, 66r-v.

89. Certificación, Melgar, Teotitlán, December 30, 1796, AGN Epidemias 15 exp. 9, 246r–247v.

90. For acknowledgment of these sentiments, see the communication to Oaxaca's intendant in November 1796, in which the viceroy conceded that "if the parents of the sick, and especially mothers, absolutely insist on attending" to their children in Teotitlán del Valle, Melgar might allow it, so long as they remained in the infirmary and subject to the same precautions. Notably, this concession followed the riot and departed from the recommendation of his legal adviser. AGN Epidemias 12 exp. 5, 214r-v.

91. Mora y Peysal, Oaxaca, September 26, 1796, AGN Epidemias 12 exp. 3, 162–164.

92. Mora y Peysal to Fiscal, Oaxaca, December 30 1796, AGN Epidemias 10 exp. 1, 3r-v.

93. Diego de Villasante to Intendant, Antequera, February 7, 1797, AGN Epidemias 10 exp. 2, 49–50.

94. Francisco Bernardo Galindo to Promotor Fiscal, Oaxaca, February 4, 1797, AGN Epidemias 10 exp. 3, 168–169.

95. Francisco de la Riba to Intendant, Antequera, February 7, 1797, AGN Epidemias 10 exp. 2, 53–54.

96. For a familiar narrative of human populations primed for surveillance through anticontagion measures in French plagues at the end of the seventeenth century, see Foucault, *Discipline and Punish*, 195–209, which follows neat prescriptions as a basis for an analysis of power.

97. On sacramental adjustments in service to the preservation of family structure, see Brown and Hall, "Family Strategies and Religious Practice," 41–68.

98. Manuel Antonio Moreno to Promotor Fiscal, Oaxaca, February 4, 1797, AGN Epidemias 10 exp. 3, 170r-v. Moreno directed the parents to their parish priest, who forwarded them on to the intendant, who (it was said) sent the cadaver to Teotitlán for burial and placed the father in jail.

99. Pedro José Gomez Priego to Protomor Fiscal, Oaxaca, n.d., ibid., 173r-v.

100. Fr. Pedro Joseph Frasqueri, Procurador General y Prior, to Promotor Fiscal, Antequera, February 4, 1797, ibid., 171–172.

101. In epidemics, parents without means were most likely to forego burials; the result was chronic underreporting of deaths from infectious disease in parish registers, a well-known setback for historical demographers. These abandoned children were occasionally listed as *huérfanos*, with no parents to identify or claim them. (For instance, see the parish registers in AGN Epidemias 13 exp. 2 for the 1762–1763 epidemics of smallpox and *matlazahuatl* in Mexico City.)

102. Written in the same uncertain hand, similar themes, phrasing, and orthographic peculiarities are repeated on both pages: "contar" (*contra*); "eho" (*hecho*); "lell" (*ley*); "rell" (*rey*). "Digo que dios es benigno y todo es eho por dios," AGN Epidemias 10 exp. 3, 183–184.

103. During the Paris uprisings of 1750, the trope circulated in public as part of a rumor that the city's children were being abducted by the libertine King Louis XV. See Farge and Revel, *Vanishing Children of Paris*, 108–113.

104. "Mujer preñada" (pregnant woman) also rhymes nicely with "a Teotitlán caminaba" (walked to Teotitlán).

105. José de Gálvez and his brother Matías (d. 1784), viceroy of New Spain, conceived the intendancy system. See the introduction to this volume for their role in public health initiatives.

106. Gregorio José de Omaña to Viceroy, Oaxaca, February 3, 1797, AGN Epidemias 10 exp. 3, 163–165.

107. Mantecon to Bishop, Antequera, February 7, 1797, ibid., 174–182. The *promotor fiscal* also reported that the Indians of San Felipe pueblo had been contracted to build the new edifice but were neither paid nor fed for their efforts.

108. See the documents in AGN Epidemias 7 exp. 8, especially Joseph de Bargas to Revillagigedo, Mérida de Yucatán, April 11, 1793, 343r-v: "It is experienced that those who are inoculated...emerge happily from said epidemic, because of which I have tried to revive the same method to protect these inhabitants from the danger in which smallpox puts them."

109. AGN Historia 531 exp. 3, 71–78, cited in Sennhauser, "Política sanitaria y lucha social en tiempos de viruelas," 62; and Fessar to Mora y Peysal, December 10, 1795, AGN Historia 531 exp. 2, 199–200.

110. "Resultas de la Epidemia de Viruelas, principiada en la Villa de Tehuantepeque en 10 de Noviembre de 1795 segun Padron formado de todo su vecindario," Tehuantepeque, February 10, 1796, AGN Historia 531 exp. 3, 55.

111. Fiscal de lo Civil, Mexico City, April 17, 1796, ibid., 87–89.

112. For instance, Mora y Peysal to Subdelegate of Nexapa, Oaxaca, July 29, 1796, ibid., 215–216.

113. Joseph Maria Rosales to Fessar, Guelabeñe, July 2, 1796, AGN Epidemias 12 exp. 3, 124–125.

114. "Ocurrencias del Pueblo de Tequisistlan, desde el dia 16 de Junio," Tequisistlan, July 7, 1796, ibid., 136–138.

115. "Comparecencia de la republica ante el subdelegado," Santa Maria Petapa, May 20, 1796, AGN Historia 530 exp. 3, 144r–145v.

116. Cura Palacios to Luis de Ribas, n.p., June 28, 1796, and Luis de Ribas to Cura Palacios, Tehuantepeque, July 2, 1796, AGN Epidemias 12 exp. 3, 133r-v. Upon receiving this news, the subdelegate sent another official in his name, first contacting the Indian governor to plead with villagers to cooperate, for otherwise the viceroy and intendant would be angered "and would say that the Indians of San Juan are very bad, and this goes against my credit, because I have always said they are very obedient." Fessar to Governador de Guichicobi, Tehuantepeque, July 2, 1796, ibid., 134–135.

117. Intendant to Viceroy, Oaxaca, November 11, 1796, AGN Epidemias 12 exp. 5, 219–220.

118. Intendant to Viceroy, Oaxaca, November 25, 1796, ibid., 215v–216r.

119. "Teniente Letrado de Oaxaca y demás capitulares comisionados," Oaxaca, February 7, 1797, AGN Epidemias 10 exp. 2, 42–47.

120. The intendant's calculation of 483 susceptible residents (those who had not contracted smallpox previously, primarily children) prior to the start of inoculations indicates that most eligible members underwent the procedure. Mora y Peysal to Viceroy, Oaxaca, November 1, 1796, AGN Epidemias 12 exp. 7, 375r-v; and Juan Antonio Figueroa, Mariano José Carranza, Joseph Valerio Fernández, and Josef Fernández Darela, Antequera, February 7, 1797, AGN Epidemias 10 exp. 2, 55–59.

121. Promotor Fiscal Manuel Fernández Pantaleón, Letrado Licenciado Manuel Mimiaga, Letrado Licenciado Mariano de Castillejos, Oaxaca, February 7, 1797, AGN Epidemias 10 exp. 2, 60v–62v.

122. Bando, Oaxaca, February 8, 1797, ibid., 66–67.

123. Edict, Antonio de Mora y Peysal, Oaxaca, February 22, 1797, ibid., 96.

124. Intendant to Viceroy, Oaxaca, April 14, 1797, ibid., 135–140.

125. Intendant to Asesor General, Antequera, February 17, 1797, ibid., 70–71; Intendant to Viceroy, Antequera, February 28, 1797, ibid., 85r-v; and Intendant to Viceroy, Antequera, March 10, 1797, ibid., 102–103.

126. Fiscal Borbón, Mexico City, February 12, 1797, AGN Epidemias 10 exp. 1, 16v.

127. Fiscal Borbón, Mexico City, February 11, 1797, ibid., 10–13. In fact, the

instructions circulated to administrators included a prescient passage on the need to preempt parental fear of transfer in the open air; see *Extracto de la obra publicada en Madrid el año pasado de 1784 con el título de Disertación Físico-Médica*, Article 3.

128. Fiscal Borbón to Viceroy, Mexico City, February 12, 1797, AGN Epidemias 10 exp. 1, 15–26; and Tribunal del Protomedicato, Mexico City, February 11, 1797, ibid., Mexico City, 13–14.

129. Fiscal Borbón to Viceroy, Mexico City, February 12, 1797, ibid., 15–26. For deliberation over the creation and coordination of one of these institutions in the city of Puebla, see AGN Epidemias 6 exp. 3, especially the edict issued by the bishop of Puebla in accordance with the prescriptions of Article 9 of the viceregal decree, Salvador Obispo de la Puebla, Palacio de la Puebla de los Angeles, November 10, 1797, 65–66; and Obispo to Branciforte, Puebla, February 2, 1798, AGN Epidemias 6 exp. 4, 194–199, declaring the experiment with juntas a success.

130. Mexico City, February 28, 1797 [printed], AGN Epidemias 16 exp. 2, 28–30 (also in AHDF 3678 exp. 6). Following the clause permitting voluntary inoculation was another that affirmed the power of propitiation and prayer.

131. *Gazeta de México* 8, no. 10 (May 10, 1796).

132. Protomedicato to Viceroy, Mexico City, February 14, 1797, AGN Epidemias 10 exp. 1, 28r-v.

133. Cosme de Mier to Viceroy, Mexico City, August 28, 1797, AGN Epidemias 16 exp. 5, 189–190.

134. Protomedicato to Viceroy, Mexico City, August 17, 1797, ibid., 159r-v; and José Maria Alcala to Alonso Núñez de Haro, Mexico City, August 27, 1797, ibid., 182.

135. Cosme de Mier to Viceroy, Mexico City, August 31, 1797, AGN Epidemias 1 exp. 1, 20r, citing reports of the practice from San Pablo parish. Correspondence on the distribution of cemeteries between the archbishop, viceroy, and various parishes and religious convents in Mexico City is in AGN BN 754 exp. 3.

136. Without permission Luis José Montaña, considered one of the more capable physicians of the day, inoculated his own daughter with the pus from an eight-year-old Indian boy (one of the first to take ill in the capital) and thereafter joined in the push for a widespread campaign. Montaña to Cosme de Mier, Mexico City, August 28, 1797, AGN Epidemias 16 exp. 5, 184–185.

137. Testimony of Teresa Bastida, with rubric, AGN Historia 44 exp. 14, 332r-v; and Fiscal Alva to Branciforte, Mexico City, September 29, 1797, ibid., 334–335r. The rumors seem to have mixed up the identities and relationships between children within the same extended elite family.

138. Antonio Boso, Mexico City, September 22, 1797, AGN Historia 44 exp. 14, 362r-v; and Cosme de Mier to Viceroy, Mexico City, September 28, 1797, ibid., 319r.

139. "Boleras," n.p., n.d., ibid., 313v–316r; and Fernández del Castillo, *Los viajes de don Francisco Xavier de Balmis*, 66–70.

140. See Farge, *Subversive Words*, 60–66, on the ways that irreverence might lend plausible meaning to opaque mechanisms of rule. Melton, *Rise of the Public in Enlightenment Europe*, observes that rumors thrived under regimes (including the French) that stressed secrecy.

141. Cosme de Mier to Viceroy, Mexico City, October 2, 1797, AGN Historia 44 exp. 14, 353–354.

142. Alva to Viceroy, Mexico City, September 29, 1797, ibid., 336r and 342–344. The Protomedicato similarly worried that papers discrediting inoculation would influence the masses but that those who possessed "scientific judgment and patriotic sentiment" would be immune. Real Tribunal to Cosme de Mier, Real Protomedicato, September 19, 1797, ibid., 323v–324r.

143. An announcement in the gazette called Viceroy Bernardo de Gálvez the "true Father of the Patria," in reference to his charitable beneficence toward the city's Indian and poor hospital patients. *Gazeta de México* 2, no. 4 (February 28, 1786), 51. On the rhetoric of "wretched" Indians and "the infantilization of the indigenous population" vis-a-vis viceregal authority, see Cañeque, *King's Living Image*, 214–222 and 230–236; quote on 220.

144. "El Governador y Cabildo de Naturales del pueblo y cavezera de Yxhuacan," December 16, 1797, AGN Epidemias 3 exp. 16, 215–216. Members of the *cabildo* argued that all other resources had been exhausted, which legally authorized the use of *cajas de comunidad.*

145. Melgar to Intendente, Teotitlán, October 12, 1796, AGN Epidemias 15 exp. 8, 162r-v.

146. Fiscal de Real Hacienda Alva, Mexico City, April 16, 1797, AGN Epidemias 15 exp. 2, 60–64.

147. Taylor, *Drinking, Homicide, and Rebellion*, 120.

148. Valenzuela to Viceroy, Orizaba, October 11, 1797, AGN Historia 44 exp. 14, 354v–356r; and Viceroy to Cosme de Mier, Orizaba, October 12, 1797, ibid., 357r-v.

149. Gunn, *Queen of the World*, 175–176. On the persistence of ancien régime traditions during the French Revolution limiting expression of speech deemed impious, self-interested, hateful, or vulgar, see Walton, *Policing Public Opinion in the French Revolution*, 73–93.

150. For instance, small-scale plots inspired by the French Revolution saw alleged sympathizers arrested and persecuted at an alarming rate. After *motines* erupted in major mining centers of the Bajío with the expulsion of the Jesuits in 1767, moreover, dozens were executed for insubordination and many more sent to labor in galleys and *obrajes*. José de Gálvez, who as visitor-general took charge, had little patience for disobedience and was particularly wary of verbal challenges to royal authority.

151. On the premium placed on "humane treatment" in eighteenth-century scientific expeditions and its extension to pacification and religious conversion along frontiers of the Spanish Empire, see Weber, *Bárbaros*, 47–50 and 99–102 (following the historian Stanley Payne's estimate that around 5 percent of the population were affected by such enlightened ideas, perhaps "a few hundred thousand people").

152. Philosopher Seyla Benhabib and others have stressed the importance of witnessing the emergence and redefinition of relevant issues like the "public good" through crisis and debate, as opposed to their delimitation from the outset. Insofar as the issues are personal, the nature of the questioning shifts: "At stake are the reflexive questioning of issues by all those affected by their foreseeable

consequences and the recognition of their right to do so" (Benhabib, "Models of Public Space," 81).

153. Asesor General Valenzuela to Viceroy, Mexico City, February 15, 1797, AGN Epidemias 10 exp. 6, 244v.

154. Viceroy to Intendant, Mexico City, February 19, 1797, AGN Epidemias 10 exp. 1, 33r-v; and Viceroy to Intendant, Mexico City, February 28, 1797, AGN Epidemias 10 exp. 2, 84r-v.

155. With donations from wealthier residents, some 5,000 pesos initially were placed in the hands of cathedral priests and convent heads, to distribute in alms to the poor and destitute in five districts; 120-day indulgences were offered to residents, physicians, nurses, and priests to care, heal, and confess. "Nos el Doctor Don Gregorio de Omaña," Palacio Episcopal de Antequera, February 11, 1797, AGN Epidemias 10 exp. 3, 187–190.

156. Intendant to Viceroy, Antequera, March 3, 1797, AGN Epidemias 10 exp. 2, 98r-v.

157. "Nota de todas las personas que han muerto de Viruelas en la presente epidemia...desde principios de 7bre. de 1797," AGN BN 873 exp. 180.

CHAPTER 4

The Gift of Immunity

Epigraph: Junta Central, Izucar, April 30, 1806, AGMP Expedientes 198 leg. 2278.

1. In Monterrey, 1,650 inoculations in a population of 4,000; in Guanajuato, 11,000 inoculations out of 14,000; in Valladolid, 6,800 inoculations (these numbers are approximations). See García Flores, "Morbilidad y vulnerabilidad en una epidemia de viruela"; and Thompson, "To Save the Children." Data from Alexander von Humboldt for Valladolid is cited in Camacho Alberto, "Guanajuato y Valladolid de Michoacán durante la epidemia de viruela." For Mexico City no reliable accounting of inoculations was carried out, as members of the Junta de Caridad lamented, "Noticias de lo que se observó en la Epidemia de Viruelas del año de 1797," n.p., n.d., AGN Epidemias 1 exp. 5, 480–482.

2. Esquivel Navarrete, *Sermón eucarístico por la felicidad que logró la ciudad de Durango.*

3. It appears in the works, for instance, of Charles Marie de la Condamine and Esteban Morel, discussed in this chapter.

4. Cotton Mather, *Sentiments on the Small Pox Inoculated*, reprinted in Increase Mather, *Several Reasons Proving*, 75 (emphasis in original).

5. Razzell, *Conquest of Smallpox*, 1–17; Susan and Stanley Plotkin, "Short History of Vaccination," 1–15; Hopkins, *Princes and Peasants*; Schifter Aceves, *Medicina, minería e inquisición*, 13–15; and Wain, *History of Preventive Medicine*, 173–195. Robert Sutton is credited with using a lancet instead of needle to make a shallower incision just under the surface of the skin, which inspired surgeons to follow his lead.

6. Chalhoub, *Cidade febril*, 104–105, remarks on the appropriation and ap-

plication, on a global scale, of local medical knowledge and health practices for professional, imperial, and national ends.

7. Golinski, *British Weather and the Climate of Enlightenment*, 109–110. See also Saldaña, "Ciencia y felicidad pública en la Ilustración americana," 151–207, on the adaptation of mining and industrial techniques in Spanish America. A related argument about precision instruments is that they are typically less precise than is apparent in retrospect because their effects are first conditioned by a complex set of formalized and informal practices. See Shapin and Schaffer, *Leviathan and the Air Pump*.

8. Norman, *Design of Everyday Things*, 9. Borrowing from the conceptual psychologist J. J. Gibson, Norman calls these uses "affordances," as in the uses to which an object *affords* or lends itself.

9. Rigau-Pérez, "Introduction of Smallpox Vaccine in 1803," 400.

10. Mark and Rigau-Pérez, "World's First Immunization Campaign."

11. Major botanical expeditions to Chile and Peru (1777–1788), Nueva Granada (1783–1816), and New Spain (1787–1803), and a naval expedition to America and Asia led by Alejandro Malaspina (1789–1794), collected and catalogued flora and fauna, described the porous edges of Spain's American empire, and sent crates of plant species, drawings, and texts across the Atlantic for commercial, medicinal, and industrial purposes. See Bleichmar, *Visible Empire*, chapter 4, and 137–138 on the collecting and classifying objectives as distinct from the financial motives of these endeavors.

12. Saladino García, *Ciencia y prensa durante la ilustración latinoamericana*, 323.

13. Jacobs and Stewart, *Practical Matter*, suggest that Newtonian science might simultaneously appeal to industrialists, philosophers, and social reformers and alienate popular audiences and thus exacerbate a divide between high and low culture.

14. For instance, James Jurin's published works on smallpox and inoculation as secretary of the Royal Society relied on a network of informants that supplied him raw data, while his arguments and calculations appeared in French publications, including the *Encyclopédie* and the writings of Charles Marie de la Condamine. See Rusnock, *Vital Accounts*, 49–63 and 75–81.

15. Geographers and mathematicians demonstrated later in the century on the basis of parish baptismal registers that the French population had in fact grown. See Headrick, *When Information Came of Age*, 60–61 and 65–68.

16. On the contents of Campomanes's archive, his patronage of inoculation apologists, and the council's greater openness to reforms in preventive medicine under his leadership, see Riera and Granda-Juesas, *La inoculación de la viruela en la España ilustrada*, 21–27.

17. Rodríguez Campomanes y Sorriba, *Discurso sobre el fomento de la industria popular*, 52.

18. León Sanz and Barettino Coloma, *Vicente Ferrer Gorraiz Beaumont y Montesa*, 236.

19. Ferrer Gorraiz Beaumont, *Juicio, o dictamen, sobre el proceso de la inoculación*, 199–213. He was also concerned with the risk of physical deformity and death from inoculation as well as exposure of cities and towns to infection.

20. On this opposition, see Riera and Granda-Juesas, *La inoculación de la viruela en la España ilustrada*, 9–13.

21. Amar, *Instrucción curativa de las viruelas*, especially 144–145. The demographer Robert McCaa, referring to the cautious stance of Madrid's Protomedicato, stresses that aversion was based on research into the risk of exposure to contagion: "Strangely, medical historians, particularly of Spain and Spanish America, ignore the vigilance of Spanish authorities and instead celebrate each manifestation of the inoculationist's art as a victory for medical progress." See McCaa, "Inoculation," 5.

22. Menós de Llena, *Memoria contra la inoculación*, especially 42–53; and León Sanz and Barettino Coloma, *Vicente Ferrer Gorraiz Beaumont y Montesa*, 229 and 233–234.

23. Gil, *Disertación físico-médica*, 40–41.

24. O'Scanlan, *Ensayo apologético de la inoculación*, xxxiv–xxxvi (where he confronted the "calumnies" of Ferrer's major work).

25. Ibid., xxxiii–xxxiv.

26. Francisco Salvá y Campillo, perhaps the most prominent doctor in Barcelona and one of the first peninsular physicians to embrace the operation, wrote simply that inoculation ultimately conserved more human life than the alternative, and thus it could not be reasonably said that it contradicted the law of God. León Sanz and Barettino Coloma, *Vicente Ferrer Gorraiz Beaumont y Montesa*, 229–232.

27. *Gazeta de México* 2, no. 24 (December 19, 1786) and 3, no. 32 (May 26, 1789). O'Scanlan's works were subsequently advertised for sale in Veracruz and Mexico City, in the September 2 and 23, 1797, issues.

28. The entries provide a sense of inoculation's physical risk and moral ambiguity. Alzate's usual editorializing indicated that he endorsed its use and further study, but that he too was concerned about the possibility of contagion. In one footnote he stressed New Spain's role in this history by describing Morel's 1779 experiments with inoculation, discussed elsewhere in this chapter. A translated 1776 letter to a French journal, from one "Mr. Maupetit, prior of Casan," on the treatment of natural versus inoculated smallpox, concludes with the author's justification of his efforts: "You may be surprised to see how an ecclesiastic, not being a professor of medicine, dares to expound a method for curing smallpox: the great mortality it causes in Languedoc has driven me to observe it attentively and to seek the most efficacious means, if not to prevent, then at least to propose the simplest cure. Reason belongs to all *estados* [estates, professions], to all the sciences." *Gazeta de literatura*, no. 19 (June 8, 1790). See also *Gazeta de literatura* 3, no. 15 (July 3, 1793).

29. Venegas, *Compendio de la medicina* [1788], 360 (emphasis in original), and the editions in 1841 and 1853.

30. Schifter Aceves, *Medicina, minería e inquisición*, 37; and Morel, "Disertación sobre la utilidad de la inoculación," AHDF 3678 exp. 2, 15v, 24r. On the community of French expatriates in Mexico City at the time, see Houdaille, "Frenchmen and Francophiles in New Spain," 4–7.

31. For Bartolache's publishing activities, see Chapter 2.

32. Morel, "Disertación sobre la utilidad de la inoculación," 4–9.

33. Ibid., 11r-v and 21v.
34. Condamine, *Mémoire sur l'inoculation de la petite vérole*, 31–59.
35. Morel, "Disertación sobre la utilidad de la inoculación," 26r–27r.
36. Ibid., 30r.
37. Ibid., 37v.
38. Ibid., 32v–33r. The pseudo-pox was called *fatuas, espurias,* or *volantes* in France, and *locas* in Mexico.
39. Ibid., 40r-v, 41v.
40. Ibid., 13r.
41. Ibid., 52v–53v. Cotton Mather similarly observed that God had taught man to make himself sick, with artificial purges, "in a way that will save his Life." *Sentiments on the Small Pox Inoculated*, reprinted in Mather, *Several Reasons Proving*, 76–77.
42. Morel, "Disertación sobre la utilidad de la inoculación," 41v–42v.
43. Ibid., 57v.
44. Ibid., 58–61r. The identities of these children indicate the networks of sociability that bound men of enlightened science and medicine. Two were the son and daughter of Pedro Lafargue (LaFarge), "my esteemed fellow countryman," aged seven and eight, while a three-year-old girl from the Puente de la Merced had been delivered to Morel for inoculation by José Antonio Alzate y Ramírez.
45. Houdaille, "Frenchmen and Francophiles in New Spain," 14–15.
46. For transcriptions of the Inquisition testimonies, see Schifter Aceves, *Medicina, minería e inquisición*, 51–54.
47. These included the *Disertación fisico-medica* by Juan Spallarossa, physician in the Royal Hospital of Cádiz; the Spanish philosopher Benito Feijóo's *Teatro crítico universal* (book five, which presented inoculation as one of several preventives against smallpox); and the lectures of Antonio Genovesi, *catedrático* in Naples, who refuted the theological argument that inoculation was illicit *en conciencia* and deemed inoculation as worthy of royal support. See Alva to Branciforte, Mexico City, September 29, 1797, AGN Historia 44 exp. 14, 337r–339v.
48. The instruction appeared weeks later in *Gazeta de México* 8, no. 43 (October 28, 1797).
49. Alva to Branciforte, Mexico City, September 29, 1797, AGN Historia 44 exp. 14, 340r–342r.
50. On the government's overturning of its position on August 31, 1797, see Cooper, *Epidemic Disease in Mexico City*, 100–117.
51. Esquivel Navarrete, *Sermón eucarístico por la felicidad que logró la ciudad de Durango.*
52. Herrejón Peredo, *Del sermón al discurso cívico*, 367 (quotation), 374–375.
53. Nos el Doctor don Antonio Bergosa, Villa de Etla, December 7, 1804, AGI Indiferente 1558a, 818–821.
54. Following Mariana Valverde's study of the sociology of legal knowledge about vices, *Law's Dream of a Common Knowledge*, 20–21.
55. Ramírez Martín, "Fuentes bibliográficas para el estudio." These tabulations are suggestive rather than conclusive: the author includes two publications by José Ignacio Bartolache that were only marginally about inoculation, an unpublished letter from Archbishop Núñez de Haro, and omits many more unpub-

lished works, including those discussed here. Nevertheless, the contrast is striking: "ecclesiastical" publications accounted for only 2 percent of the total in Spain, and 5 percent in other Spanish American territories.

56. Examining official Maya documents from early colonial Yucatán, linguistic anthropologist William Hanks writes variously of "ambivalent genres," "boundary works," "blended genres," and "colonial genres" to describe historical change as witnessed in emergent Yucatec discourse. See Hanks, "Discourse Genres in a Theory of Practice"; and Hanks, "Language and Discourse in Colonial Yucatán [1996]," in *Intertexts*, 271–311.

57. For the Nueva Granada background, see Frías Núñez, *Enfermedad y sociedad en la crisis colonial*, 129–190.

58. Flores described epidemic routes, his rush to Guatemala's capital to inoculate when smallpox arrived from Oaxaca in 1780, and his implementation of inoculation in 1794 as president of Guatemala's Protomedicato after other measures failed (and reported fourteen thousand inoculations, forty-six deaths). Proposal submitted by Doctor Joseph Flores, Madrid, February 28, 1803, AGI Indiferente 1558a, 327r and 329r–330r.

59. Ibid., 325r–326r and 330–333. Guatemalan physicians subscribed a special *correo* to Mexico, where cowpox was supposed to exist, but it arrived inert from New Orleans via Veracruz.

60. Paquette, *Enlightenment, Governance, and Reform in Spain and Its Empire*, 74.

61. Proposal, Madrid, February 28, 1803, AGI Indiferente 1558a, 331.

62. On the combative leader of the expedition, see Smith, *"Real Expedición Marítima de la Vacuna" in New Spain and Guatemala*, 16–17; Ramírez Martín, *La salud del Imperio*, 90–91 and 94–96; and Fernández del Castillo, *Los viajes de don Francisco Xavier de Balmis*, 32–35, 89–96, and 134–135. As Fernández del Castillo noted, while Balmis might have adopted a more conciliatory stance in New Spain, it is also true that another person lacking his nonconformist nature might never have completed an expedition of that scale.

63. "El Ministro que hace de Fiscal," Madrid, March 17, 1803, AGI Indiferente 1558a, 321–323. An early version of Flores's dual-ship plan, which had the physician Lorenzo Vergés accompany the new viceroy to Nueva Granada to deliver cowpox lymph, appears to have been scrapped when the physician died. On this variation of the plan, see Frías Núñez, *Enfermedad y sociedad en la crisis colonial*, 189.

64. Palacio Real, July 31, 1803, AGI Indiferente 1558a, 399–400.

65. San Ildefonso, September 3, 1803, ibid., 465–466.

66. Balmis to Flon, Mexico City, August 29, 1804, AGMP Expedientes 198 leg. 2278; and Flon to Balmis, Puebla, September 4, 1804, ibid., 182–185.

67. *Recopilación de leyes de los reinos de las Indias*, vol. 1, book I, title I, law IV.

68. Dutcher Mann, "Opus Dei, 'The Work of God'," 266–278. Countervailing forces among the religious orders sought to stem the tide of what they considered the excessive enthusiasm of their indigenous converts, particularly in matters of music, dance, and image worship. See Ricard, *Spiritual Conquest of Mexico*, 176–193; and Taylor, *Magistrates of the Sacred*, 252–258.

69. Viqueira Albán, *Propriety and Permissiveness*; and for theater publics in eighteenth-century Europe, see Melton, *Rise of the Public in Enlightenment Europe*, chapter 5.

70. *Demostración* was more common. *Ceremonia* referred to the formal overtures that precede or accompany an intended action, which only partially overlaps with the English "ceremony" to mean an act of celebration.

71. On this case, see Brading, *First America*, 494–495.

72. Manuel Ignacio Obispo de Puebla to José Antonio Caballero, Puebla, September 28, 1804, AGI Indiferente 1558a, 695–696; and Conde de la Cadena to José Antonio Caballero, Puebla, October 27, 1804, ibid., 712–714. Public acts in Puebla served as a model elsewhere.

73. Estatutos, Puebla, October 29, 1804, AGN Epidemias 4 exp. 3, 94–99, Article 11. Article 12, missing from Mexico City's statutes, refers to the frequent appearance of putrid fevers among the "casta de Indios" and recommends that the juntas make careful observations of the frequency of such fevers, but secretly, because otherwise unsatisfactory results might discredit the procedure among this sector. In these ways the Indian population was singled out as exceptional, both culturally and physiologically.

74. Respuesta del Sindico Procurador, Guadalajara, November 22, 1804, AGN Epidemias 4 exp. 8, 256v–259r; Ayuntamiento to Audiencia, Guadalajara, November 27, 1804, AGI Indiferente 1558a, 866–867; Pedro Catani to Bishop Cabañas, Guadalajara, November 20, 1804, ibid., 864–866; signed testimony of Fernando Cambre (escribano mayor), Guadalajara, December 7, 1804, ibid., 876r-v; and certification of Fernando Cambre, Guadalajara, December 9, 1804, ibid., 878–879.

75. Ayuntamiento to José Antonio Caballero, Sala Capitular de Celaya, November 29, 1804, ibid., 748–751.

76. Junta Central General Filantrópica de Vacunación Pública, Izucar, April 30, 1806, AGMP Expedientes 198 leg. 2278, 344–354.

77. Balmis to Iturrigaray, Mexico City, September 5, 1804, AGN Epidemias 10 exp. 7, 320r-v; the copy in AHDF 3678 exp. 17, 18–26, is reproduced in Fernández del Castillo, *Los viajes de Don Francisco Xavier de Balmis*, 229–241.

78. Cf. Andrés Pérez de Velasco's manual for curates (Puebla, 1766), quoted in Taylor, *Magistrates of the Sacred*, 265: "What will this [devout] Indian think...if he sees the priest elevate and lower the consecrated Host quickly, without special feeling or reverence?...[W]ill he learn from this Mass the respect and reverence that is owed to Christ Our Lord in the Eucharist?"

79. Francisco Arzobispo to Mariano Dionisio Alarcon, Mexico City, January 10, 1806, AGN IV 3885 exp. 4, 6–8. The prelate quoted the Latin Vulgate: "Honor the physician out of necessity / for God created him....Give a sweet sacrifice and an offering of fine flour, anoint it / and give the physician his place." Eccl. 38: 1–2, 11–12.

80. Juan Cruz Obispo to José Antonio Cavallero, Guadalajara, January 17, 1805, AGI Indiferente 1558a, 799–800.

81. Cited in Taylor, *Shrines and Miraculous Images*, 38: "las cosas santas han de ser tratadas santamente."

82. "Cuenta de los gastos hechos," Guanajuato, December 1, 1804, AGN Epi-

demias 4 exp. 15, 474r-v; and "Gastos causados en obsequio de la Real Dirección de la Bacuna," Sombrerete, December 17, 1804, ibid., 460r.

83. The head town of San Juan del Rio, with roughly fifteen thousand inhabitants, set its annual expenses for the feast of Corpus Christi at 56 pesos, for masses, processions, musicians, wax, *sacristanes*, and fireworks (the other major expense for the year was a *maestro de escuela*, at 90 pesos). Outlays for the feast in Mexico City totaled some 463 pesos in 1771, for altar candles, musicians, fireworks, sand strewn along the route of the procession (240 pesos), and printed announcements. Guadalupe's feast cost some 319 pesos, for wax, musicians, entertainments, illumination of municipal buildings for vespers, and a sermon (50 pesos, reformed to 32). From records assembled by visitor-general José de Gálvez in 1771, attempting to regularize functions, including feast days, of Mexico City's *ayuntamiento*. "Plan y arreglo de las funciones votivas anuales, que celebra la N.C.," Huntington mssGA 626, box 10; and Pedro Martínez de Salazar y Pacheco to Conde Revillagigedo, "Compendio histórico, político, topográfico, hidráulico, y económico," San Juan del Rio, March 22, 1794, AGN Historia 72 exp. 9, item 49.

84. Alexandro García Arboleya to Viceroy, Teotitlán del Camino Real, October 10, 1804, AGN Epidemias 4 exp. 6; and Juan Pedro de Necoechea to Viceroy, Tehuacán de las Granadas, October 11, 1804, ibid., 180–181.

85. Antonio de Elías Sáenz to Viceroy, Tenancingo, December 22, 1804, AGN Epidemias 4 exp. 1, 14–15.

86. Nicolas Gutierrez to Viceroy, Toluca, December 19, 1804, ibid., 11–12; Nicolas Gutierrez to Viceroy, Toluca, March 6, 1805, ibid., 22r-v; and Nicolas Gutierrez to Viceroy, Toluca, March 12, 1805, ibid., 23r-v.

87. Josef Caballero to Viceroy of New Spain, San Lorenzo, October 15, 1806, AGN IV 5297 exp. 19, 53–54, requesting an explanation for why these demonstrations were not forthcoming in the viceregal capital.

88. Junta Central, Izucar, April 30, 1806, AGMP Expedientes 198 leg. 2278, 349v–350r.

89. By category: 6,772 *españoles* (67.8 percent); 1,300 *indios* (13.4); 818 *mestizos* (8.4); 293 *mulatos* (3.0); 286 *castizos* (2.9); 76 *negros* (0.78); 56 *lobos* (0.58); 42 *moriscos* (0.43); 53 *eclesiásticos* (0.55). "Estado General de las Personas, y Familias, que hay en la Feligresía de Señor San Miguel de México, según resultan del Padrón formado en el Año de 1809, octavo del gobierno del Doctor y Licenciado Don Juan José Guereña, Cura por S.M. de dicha Parroquial," AGN IV 244 exp. 1, and AGN IV 3507 exp 4. These newly classified documents add two years to the register consulted by Francisco Fernández del Castillo in San Miguel's parish archive, *Los viajes de don Francisco Xavier de Balmis*, 141–142 and 195.

90. Balmis to Viceroy, Mexico City, October 30, 1804, AGN Epidemias 4 exp. 13, 355–359; and Balmis to Josef Antonio Caballero, Acapulco, February 5, 1805, AGI Indiferente 1558a, 1034v–1035r.

91. Antonio Serrano to Iturrigaray, Mexico City, November 26, 1804, AGN Epidemias 10 exp. 12, 454–455.

92. José Guereña to Iturrigaray, Mexico City, August 26, 1806, AGN Epidemias 10 exp. 7, 338–341.

93. Plan, Mexico City, April 1, 1805, AGN Epidemias 12 exp. 6, 330v.

94. "Aviso al Público" (printed), AGN IV 5297 exp. 19, 97r.

95. Weber, *Bárbaros*, 119, 315n187, and 31.

96. "Relación del servicio hecho por Don Alexandro García Arboleya en la propagación, y asistencia de la Bacuna en esta Capital," Mexico City, March 10, 1807, AGN IV 4896 exp. 9, 4v.

97. Serrano, though impressed by these shows, sent a notice to the editor of the *Gazeta de México* years later reporting that despite this incentive of *biscochos* for the children, their parents still refused to bring them, and he suggested that alcaldes or primary school teachers be used for this purpose instead. Mexico City, January 20, 1820, AGN IV 5297 exp. 16, 8.

98. Balmis to Caballero, accounting for the Royal Expedition's expenses, Madrid, December 4, 1806, AGI Indiferente 1558a, cited in Ramírez Martín, *La salud del Imperio*, 22n18.

99. Reglamento, signed Bernardo de Bonavía, Durango, September 2, 1804, AGI Indiferente 1558a, 782–783.

100. Junta Central to Teniente Letrado Jose de Peon Valdés, Zacatecas, August 6, 1805, AGN Epidemias 4 exp. 15, 455–457. This expense, if practiced consistently, amounted to 75.5 pesos.

101. Real de Santa María de los Ramos, January 2, 1805, signed José Pablo de la Rosa, AGN IV 5297 exp. 19, 124. A report from Valladolid in the same file shows that, at least briefly, officials there paid a full *real* to each vaccinated child.

102. Manuel Fernandez de los Rios to Intendent Arce, Chalco, July 8, 1808, AGN IV 1717 exp. 18, 4r-v.

103. Licenciado Miguel Dominguez to Viceroy, Querétaro, March 16, 1805, AGN Epidemias 4 exp. 15, 497–498.

104. Estado, Valladolid, May 13, 1808, AHDF 3678 exp. 17, 33.

105. *Gazeta de México* 12, no. 26 (January 1, 1805), 222.

106. For Europe, see the essays in Bensaude-Vincent and Blondel, *Science and Spectacle in the European Enlightenment.*

107. Mauss, *The Gift*, 18. Mauss looked to the rules and conventions of ritual transactions to understand the persuasive (and obligation-inducing) effects of public pageantry. See also Austin, *How To Do Things with Words*; and Bourdieu, *Language and Symbolic Power*.

108. José Miguel Muñoz to Antonio Serrano, Mexico City, August 1810, AGN IV 6177 exp. 15.

CHAPTER 5
Republics of Vaccinators

Epigraph: Bonavía to Justicias de la Provincia, AGI Indiferente 1558a, Durango, August 14, 1804, 780.

1. Suplemento II, *Gazeta de México* 12, no. 12, 99. The first supplement, a report on early successes with vaccination in Mexico City with fluid from Cuba, announced that "with time and practice the same mothers will inoculate their children, and even suffice to observe the entirety of the procedure," 96.

2. Nos el Doctor don Antonio Bergosa, Villa de Etla, December 7, 1804, AGI Indiferente 1558a, 818r. In a preface to the 1801 Spanish edition of the French

work the translator, the physician Pedro Hernández, who had dedicated his life's work to childhood illnesses in the villages around Madrid, addressed parents directly as capable vaccinators with only the simple, accessible publication they held in their hands. See Hernández, *Orígen y descubrimiento de la vaccina*, 11–17.

3. "Nota" following summary of bishop's letter of December 11, n.p., n.d., AGI Indiferente 1558a, 810v–811v; n.p., May 25, 1805, ibid., 811v–812v; and Crown to Obispo de Antequera de Oaxaca, Madrid, July 12, 1805, ibid. There was uncertainty about whether Oaxaca's government had the authority to intervene to prescribe such restrictions, when it was recalled that a royal decree had ordered the creation of *reglamentos* tailored to each place in consultation with Balmis. "S.E. desea saver si el Govierno de Oaxaca tubo facultades para este bando, etc.," written on a slip of paper folded over the file, ibid., 813.

4. Frías Núñez, *Enfermedad y sociedad en la crisis colonial*, 209–212 and 215–223; on the modern features of the expedition, Mark and Rigau-Pérez, "World's First Immunization Campaign"; and Few, *For All of Humanity*.

5. Garner, "Price Trends in Eighteenth-Century Mexico"; Coatsworth, "Obstacles to Economic Growth in Nineteenth-Century Mexico"; and Van Young, *Other Rebellion*, 69–86.

6. Because contemporaries used *inoculación* and *vacunación* interchangeably, or spoke of "inoculación de la vacuna," it can be difficult to discern inoculation with human smallpox when it persisted. In 1814 the district governor of Tehuantepec recorded the provision of medications and food and "la operación de la inoculación" by a practitioner in some dozen pueblos and on two haciendas. Use of human smallpox in this instance is indicated by the omission of reference to a source of vaccine, the elevated mortality rate—66 deaths out of 2,960 operations (2 percent)—and the general scarcity of vaccine during the insurrection. Fr. Nicolas Garcia de Medina to Viceroy, Xalapa de Tehuantepeque, September 24, 1814, AGN Historia 579a exp. 1.2, 5r-v; and Domingo Bermudez, Tehuantepeque, February 4, 1815, ibid., 6–8. For an instance of confusion about whether administrators were actually vaccinating with viable cowpox, see "Relación de los progresos y estado actual en que se halla la vacuna," Guanajuato, June 1, 1815, ibid., 32–34.

7. Cf. Shapin, *Social History of Truth*, chapter 8, esp. 359–360, on "invisible technicians" and the authorship of scientific experiments and knowledge.

8. Flon to Balmis, Puebla, September 4, 1804, AGMP Expedientes 198 leg. 2277/2278, 184–185; and Bando, Puebla, September 20, 1804, AGMP Expedientes 72 leg. 847, 4v.

9. "Estatutos que para la real junta de vacunación," Puebla, October 29, 1804, AGN Epidemias 4 exp. 3 (articles 17 and 19). See also an anonymous review of the statutes, [Puebla], n.d., AGMP Expedientes 78 leg. 848, 50.

10. For instance, see the lists for Cholula, October 1, 1805, AGMP Expedientes 198 leg. 2278, 289–290; Huauchinango, October 5, 1805, ibid., 308–310; and Izucar, August 11, 1805, ibid., 343. Cholula had some of the highest vaccination rates in the region, more than a thousand each month in 1805, according to *estados*. In a less felicitous outcome, Chietla's junta reported discovering that the fluid used to vaccinate 188 children over five days was inert. (A new supply had to be acquired from Izucar.) See Chietla, November 21, 1805, ibid., 259–260.

11. Santiago Tecali, October 21, 1805, AGMP Expedientes 198 leg. 2278, 438.

12. Immediately following the response of Puebla's Junta Central, n.p., [1807], AGMP Expedientes 78 leg. 848, 43. The oversight stemmed from the fact that Tlaxcala was its own province, separate from Puebla's secular jurisdiction.

13. Approximations of population size are from Tanck de Estrada, *Atlas ilustrado de los pueblos de indios*, 158.

14. Bloom, "Early Vaccination in New Mexico," 7–11. For a quarter century, Larrañaga was practitioner at the presidio of Santa Fe, although he was not sole vaccinator in these early campaigns; for more on his career, see Simmons, *Spanish Pathways*, 68–70.

15. For the 1815 registers, Huntington mssRI 70, box 3, signed Josef Larrañaga. Percentages are approximate, calculated from a December 3, 1810, census, in Huntington mssRI 68, box 3. In Nambé, 16 vaccinated children amounts to approximately 7 percent of 236 Indian and non-Indian residents; in the predominantly Spanish villa of Santa Cruz de la Cañada (appearing as Cañada de Cochití), 98 children represent 4 percent of some 2,402; and so on.

16. Several considerations lower the value of the statistical measurement offered here (percentage of total population vaccinated). Only susceptible residents—usually those born since the last smallpox epidemic—could be vaccinated because the fluid would not mature in those who had acquired immunity. Moreover, administrators often moderated the pace to preserve some members of a population for future vaccinations. The *ayuntamiento* of Veracruz illustrated these considerations and complications when answering Balmis's accusations that inhabitants were resisting vaccination. By September 12, 1804, 1,350 persons had been vaccinated from the fluid that arrived in the port from Cuba three months earlier. Because most of the population had been exposed in the epidemic of 1797, it was primarily those born since who lacked immunity, which, according to parish birth registers, amounted to 1,562 children. Subtracting those who died of natural causes and those who left the city with their parents for summer vacation, municipal officials concluded, there was no one left to vaccinate. By this logic 1,350 vaccinations represented the entirety of the available population. See Fernández del Castillo, *Los viajes de don Francisco Xavier de Balmis*, 129.

17. Those with less experience sometimes expressed confusion about the fact that not all were vaccinated at once. When Viceroy Apodaca observed of the reports submitted by Mexico City's corregidor, "[s]on pocos estos niños para una población tan grande," the Crown attorney explained that unvaccinated children were required for future vaccinations. Informed of the reason, the viceroy clarified that his remark was not to be interpreted to mean otherwise. Fiscal to Viceroy, Mexico City, January 16, 1817, AGN Epidemias 14 exp. 3, 67r-v; and Viceroy to Corregidor, Mexico City, January 29, 1817, ibid, 66r-v.

18. Vaccination statistics are from Estado, Valladolid, May 13, 1808, AHDF 3678 exp. 17. Population estimates from Tanck de Estrada, *Atlas ilustrado de los pueblos de indios*, 126.

19. Mazín Gómez, *Entre dos majestades*, chapter 3, and Appendix VII for more on the wealth of the bishopric of Michoacán's *cabeceras* (as measured by rents and salaries).

20. Estado, Valladolid, May 13, 1808, AHDF 3678 exp. 17, 33. This as-

sumes that "Cuyceo" in the summary refers to the former Augustinian *doctrina* of Cuitzeo de la Laguna, north of Valladolid. In the less likely scenario, the 2,210 vaccinations were in Cuiseo and its outlying pueblos, just north of Huetamo.

21. The official attributed the avoidance of a full-blown epidemic to prompt immunization, apparently more effective than care provided in the hospital, which included separate departments of medicine, surgery, and syphilis (*gálico*). José Ygnacio Quiros to Viceroy, Pénjamo, May 31, 1819, AGN IV 4583 exp. 6, 15r; and José Ygnacio Quiros to Viceroy, Pénjamo, August 6, 1819, ibid., 1–2.

22. For instance, separate reports on experiments with this alternative arrived from commander of Interior Provinces Nemesio Salcedo, in Villa de Chihuahua, and the surgeon Alejandro García Arboleya, in partnership with the parish priest of San Miguel, Juan José Guereña, in Mexico City. See AGN IV 5297 exp. 11, 111–114. In 1808, Salcedo instructed the troop surgeon of Santa Fe to employ the same method in the province of New Mexico. See Bloom, "Early Vaccination in New Mexico," 10.

23. Miguel Antonio Arteaga to Ciriaco González Carvajal, Texcoco, September 30, 1807, AGN IV 5297 exp. 19, 40–41.

24. Antolin Orbaneja to Viceroy, Xamiltepec, March 19, 1805, AGN Epidemias 4 exp. 6, 232r; Mora y Peysal to Viceroy, Oaxaca, January 17, 1806, ibid., 232–233; and Antolin Orbaneja to Intendente, Jamiltepec, June 22, 1807, AGN IV 5297 exp. 15, 39r-v.

25. Izquierdo to Viceroy, Oaxaca, January 11, 1805, AGN Epidemias 4 exp. 6, 222–223.

26. Diego de Villasante to Intendente Corregidor, Oaxaca, January 14, 1806, ibid., 231.

27. Fiscal de lo Civil to Iturrigaray, Mexico City, January 31, 1807, AGN Epidemias 10 exp. 7, 356v–357r.

28. Diego de Villasante to Ciriaco González Carvajal, Oaxaca, August 18, 1807, AGN IV 5297 exp. 19, 74.

29. Facultativos de Medicina y Cirugía Juan Bautista Figueroa, José Valerio Fernández, Félix Chazari, Sebastián Espinoza, Gaspar Carranza, Rafael Briones y Juan de Figueroa el hijo, Oaxaca, September 5, 1808, AGN IV 4848 exp. 46, 20; and Antonio María Izquierdo to Viceroy, Oaxaca, September 9, 1808, ibid., 18–19.

30. Juan José Ceruta to Intendant Izquierdo, Teozacualco, July 20, 1807, AGN IV 5297 exp. 15; Emeterio de Cosio to Intendant, Villa de Oaxaca, June 9, 1807, ibid.; and Juan Angel de Yturrios to Intendant, Teposcolula, July 11, 1807, ibid. In the same file are reports from Zimatlán, that Indians have no means to pay a vaccinator's salary; from Quiechapam, of no experts in the vicinity to perform vaccinations; from Chontales, on the complete poverty of Indians, with the district naturally sterile, lacking quality cattle, and with few *gentes de razón* (non-Indians); and from Miahuatlán, on lack of fluid or any "sujeto de inteligencia" to put the method into practice, and pueblos of poor, coarse, and indolent *indios* who "avoid undertaking this beneficial operation."

31. Manuel Ruiz y Parrasar to Intendant, Tehuantepec, July 28, 1807, AGN IV 5297 exp. 15.

32. "Reglamento de orden de S.M. para que se propague y perpetúe la Vacuna

en Nueva España" (printed), Mexico City, October 10, 1810, AHDF 3678 exp. 17, 63–65. See also AGN Historia 530 exp. 1 and AGN Historia 579a exp. 1.

33. Balmis to Viceroy, October 10, 1810, AHDF 3678 exp. 17, 61–62.

34. Balmis to Venegas, Xalapa, July 18, 1811, AGN Epidemias 17 exp. 8, 211r-v. For evidence that they received these salaries from the indicated sources, see Mexico City, November 12, 1812, AGN Epidemias 17 exp. 12, 343. The records of vaccinations submitted by Dancourt and Blanco are remarkable. Beginning in August 1804, the latter vaccinated 6,414 in Campeche and over nine months oversaw propagation of vaccine to another 13,193 adults and children in surrounding districts, where practitioners were instructed in *cabeceras* to continue vaccinations. Benito Perez to Juan Nepomuceno de Cardenas, Mérida, May 4, 1811, AGN Epidemias 17 exp. 12, 333v–334r.

35. Cabildo Metropolitano to Archbishop, Mexico City, December 29, 1810, AHDF 3678 exp. 17, 87–90.

36. Archbishop to Viceroy Venegas, Mexico City, January 24, 1811, ibid., 91–93.

37. Antonio Obispo de Antequera to Viceroy Venegas, Oaxaca, January 1, 1811, ibid., 96–97; and Antonio Obispo de Antequera to José Maria Lazo, ibid., 107–108. Owing to the state of rents the *cabildo eclesiástico* claimed it could not contribute at all. Sala Capitular de Antequera, May 2, 1811, ibid., 109.

38. José María Gómez to Viceroy Venegas, San Luis Potosí, May 30, 1811, ibid., 105.

39. On the political dispute, see Smith, *"Real Expedición Marítima de la Vacuna" in New Spain and Guatemala*, 62–64.

40. Several children had been vaccinated with vaccine found at Cindurio Hacienda in 1804, with results, according to Abad, identical to vaccinations with fluid from Europe. If one cow had viable pox, then others likely did—the implication being not just that Balmis had not completed his task, but that transport of a source from Europe had been unnecessary.

41. Manuel Abad Obispo Electo to Viceroy Venegas, Valladolid, January 25, 1811, AHDF 3678 exp. 17, 120–123. Abad vituperated primarily against Article 13 but also took issue with the following, which called for observations of vaccine's effects on other diseases. He reasoned that such experimentation had to come at the expense of vaccinations, which seemed inappropriate given its demonstrated efficacy against smallpox. Balmis had traveled the globe with vaccinated persons and vaccinators at the Crown's expense, and "has not yet published a single observation on the matter. What can be expected of provincial *facultativos*? Certainly nothing" (ibid., 121v).

42. Melchor Alvarez to Viceroy, Oaxaca, May 10, 1815, AGN Historia 530 exp. 4, 1–3.

43. Melchor Alvarez to Calleja, Oaxaca, August 8, 1815, AGN IV 4848 exp. 16. The intendant received lymph in vitro from Puebla on August 1 and began vaccinations with six "niños robustos" on the seventh. (Mexico City's supply had to be replenished from the same source around this time; see Ayuntamiento to Calleja, Sala Capitular del Ayuntamiento, May 9, 1815, AGN IV 4848 exp. 17.)

44. The bishop pointed triumphantly to a royal *cédula* of December 27, 1802, which listed two responsibilities: (1) pay the expenses of the deceased and aid its

sick members, which primarily compelled members to enlist; and (2) conserve and contribute to sacred worship ("culto divino en la celebración de algunas misas y funciones"). Even before the current "unhappy epoch," the confraternities had met these obligations with difficulty. After forced donations and insurgent occupation, Christian piety had cooled and enlistments and alms were down. Antonio Obispo de Antequera to Felix María Calleja, San Angel, November 4, 1815, AGN Historia 530 exp. 4, 18v–20r.

45. Ibid., 17–18v. For the capital he proposed that a single practitioner be paid 25 pesos a month for weekly sessions in the municipal building and noted that in Mexico City two were paid the same for a larger population.

46. Ayuntamiento to Viceroy, Oaxaca, April 28, 1816, AGN Historia 530 exp. 4, 24–25. In this scheme each pueblo contributing a modest portion would together fund an endowment for a vaccinator.

47. Signed Uribe, Mexico City, November 26, 1816, ibid., 27.

48. Signed José Hipólito Odoardo, Mexico City, January 21, 1817, ibid., 28–29.

49. Balmis to Viceroy, March 1811, AGN IV 5297 exp. 19, 33–34.

50. The distinction between ordinary medical practice and vaccination as an emergency measure—to be performed without compensation in the interest of the public good—was made by the certified surgeon commissioned to vaccinate in Teloloapam, pueblo of *indios* in Real de Minas de Zaqualpam. When requesting payment, he referred to Article 34 of the ordinances for intendants, which designated one quarter of *bienes de comunidad* for the salary of a physician or surgeon, where one existed, and other expenses. Payment was "not so much for vaccination (because this should be done without the least self-interest) as for assistance of the Indians in their other illnesses." Marcelo Alvarez, por Don Francisco Farfán de los Godos, Mexico City, February 20, 1810, AGN IV 5297 exp. 20.

51. Apparently the only document on vaccine to survive the onslaught was the *Instrucción formada para ministrar la vacuna*, published by order of Viceroy Calleja in consultation with Mexico City's Junta Superior de Sanidad, in 1814.

52. Francisco Rendon to Viceroy, Oaxaca, February 24, 1817, AGN IV 4848 exp. 18.

53. Estado, signed by Juan Figueroa, Oaxaca, January 2, 1819, ibid.; Lista, Oaxaca, February 27, 1820, AGN IV 4848 exp. 21, 42–49; Estado, Oaxaca, September 18, 1820, AGN IV 5297 exp. 12, 18–23; and Estado, Oaxaca, February 9, 1821, ibid., 79–84.

54. In Guanajuato, Intendant Fernando Pérez de Marañón reported weekly vaccinations from June 1815, following the smallpox epidemic, through November 1816, when vaccine failed to take in some of the vaccinated children and was lost. He requested a fresh supply from Mexico City's *ayuntamiento* in February 1817. Pérez de Marañón to Apodaca, Guanajuato, February 8, 1817, AGN Epidemias 14 exp. 4, 103; and Pérez de Marañón to Viceroy Venadito, Guanajuato, June 4, 1820, AGN IV 4848 exp. 21, 54, reporting vaccinations in Guanajuato, Silao, and Irapuato.

55. Benito Pérez to Miguel José Monzón, Mérida, May 29, 1804, AGN Epi-

demias 4 exp. 10, 308; and Miguel José Monzón to Benito Pérez, Campeche, July 10, 1804, ibid., 311–312 (emphasis in original).

56. Hernández Sáenz (*Learning To Heal*, 106–108) has argued that in most cases of professional conflict, "personal rivalry or jurisdictional monopoly" rather than national identity (i.e., antagonism between creoles and *peninsulares*) was at stake.

57. Ibid., chapter 2.

58. Ramón de Castro as cited in Rigau-Pérez, "Introduction of Smallpox Vaccine in 1803," 408.

59. Francisco Enriquez del Castillo to Pedro Catani, Tala, January 18, 1805, AGI Indiferente 1558a, 950; and Dr. José María Jaramillo to Pedro Catani, Guadalajara, January 21, 1805, ibid., 952–953.

60. For instance, the remarks of Ciprian Blanco, in Estado, Campeche, December 31, 1814, AGN IV 5297 exp. 18, 12–13.

61. Presidentes Vocales de la Junta de Real Hacienda, Mérida, March 17, 1807, AGN Epidemias 17 exp. 4, 150v–151r; and Benito Pérez to Yturrigaray, Mérida, May 10, 1807, ibid., 164–165. Documentation on Blanco is in AGN Epidemias 17 exp. 6.

62. Mérida's administrator delayed remitting records of vaccination until the risks from fighting had subsided to ensure that they arrived at their destination ("por no exponerlas al extravío que sufren las pérdidas de correos"). They are notable for their detail, consistency, and high numbers of vaccinations: in Campeche and its barrios, Blanco reported 1,681 for 1815 and another 945 in 1816. In the following months, vaccinations migrated to Mérida, its barrios, and dozens of Indian pueblos. Estado, Campeche, December 31, 1816, AGN Epidemias 14 exp. 9, 247r; Estado, Campeche, July 1, 1815, AGN IV 4848 exp. 25, 3r; and Estado, Campeche, December 30, 1815, AGN IV 5297 exp. 18, 3r.

63. Miguel de Castro Araez to Viceroy, Mérida, March 17, 1817, AGN IV 4848 exp. 25.

64. Short of an assumption of collusion among corrupt administrators throughout the region, these lists can be taken as reliable evidence of practice: names and ages of children are indicated in every case, and the file is full of certifications by priests and caciques (writing in Maya) asked to verify the practitioner's work and thus authorize payment of communal funds. Vaccination numbers by location are: Tekanto, 1,102; Citicum, 190; Kimbilá, 260; Bokolá, 435; Tepakam, 350; Teya, 600; Kamcabchen, 59 (from Partido de la Costa, December 23, 1817, to January 4, 1818, AGN IV 1997 exp. 2); Tekal, 1,273; Izamal, 1,052; Pixila, 384; Sudul, 1,284; Xanaba, 240; Kantunil, 683; Sitilpech, 884 (May 22, 1818, AGN IV 1997 exp. 3).

65. Yturrigaray to Intendente Arce, Mexico City, May 21, 1808, AGN IV 1717 exp. 18.

66. The physician had already performed 1,295 vaccinations in Texcoco and its barrios, mostly of children, and in Ixtapa, Ocopulco, Nexquipayac, and Tesoyuca over the course of forty days the previous year. Lista, Texcoco, May 30, 1807, AGN IV 6172 exp. 16, 30–39; and Manuel Fernandez de los Rios to Intendant, Chalco, July 8, 1808, AGN IV 1717 exp. 18.

67. Juan Sanchez de Movellan to Intendant, Tecpam, July 16, 1808, AGN IV

1717 exp. 18, 30–31; and Tomás Arnaldo Escobar to Intendant, Tlalchapa, July 20, 1808, ibid.

68. Francisco Menendez Valdez to Intendant, Santiago Tianquistenco, July 9, 1808, ibid.; Antonio Enriques de Otero to Intendant, San Christobal Ecatepec, July 9, 1808, ibid.; Francisco de la Vega to Intendant, Yahualica, July 19, 1808, ibid.; and Manuel Guemes y Sierra to Intendant, Huejutla, July 19, 1808, ibid.

69. In New Mexico, surgeon Cristóbal Larrañaga received a *real* for each of the 3,610 persons vaccinated in 1805, amounting to some 451 pesos, paid from donations and the sale of gunpowder. Jones, *Los Paisanos*, 140–141; and Cramaussel, "La lucha contra la viruela en Chihuahua," 112–118, on salaries in Villa de Chihuahua (Nueva Vizcaya), where 130 pesos yearly were paid to the first two individuals charged with propagating vaccination (until 1814), and 25 pesos monthly to the third (beginning in 1817).

70. Esteban Melgar to Intendant, Teotitlan del Valle, July 20, 1807, AGN IV 5297 exp. 15.

71. "Plan que manifiestan ... los comisionados de la vacuna, para la segura conservación del fluido vacuno en esta Capital," Mexico City, April 1, 1805, AGN Epidemias 12 exp. 6, 330v.

72. On the licensing process and obstacles in Mexico City, see Lanning, *Royal Protomedicato*, 282–286 and 290–297.

73. Reglamento, signed Bernardo de Bonavía, Durango, September 2, 1804, AGI Indiferente 1558a, 782–783.

74. Nemecio Salcedo to Joseph Antonio Cavallero, Hacienda de Encenillas, October 9, 1804, ibid., 758–760.

75. Cramaussel, "La lucha contra la viruela en Chihuahua," 112–118. Remarkable rates were reported in the first month in Chihuahua: 965 children vaccinated between July 6 and July 27, 1804, or the vast majority of the 1,089 children born in the previous four years, according to parish registers. As elsewhere, struggles to maintain a viable source of vaccine in Nueva Vizcaya ensued, with *alcaldes de barrio* and *regidores* charged with neglect in obliging parents to bring their children during the insurgency years, flagging interest and military upheaval, lost fluid in 1817, and again in 1829–1830 and 1836.

76. Domingo Lasquelty to Intendant, Huajuapan, July 1, 1807, AGN IV 5197 exp. 15.

77. Jose Joaquin Duarte to Intendente Corregidor Antonio de Riaño, Acámbaro, March 22, 1805, AGN Epidemias 4 exp. 15, 486.

78. Jose María de Zenea to Yturrigaray, Tacuba, June 17, 1807, AGN IV 3885 exp. 10, 2v–3r. As so often, the official stressed the impoverishment and remoteness of the village: "there is not a single dwelling where a hospital could be established."

79. María de Zenea to Gonzalez Carvajal, Tacuba, July 13, 1807, AGN IV 3885 exp. 10; Zenea to Gonzalez Carvajal, Tacuba, July 15, 1807, ibid.; and Zenea to Gonzalez Carvajal, Tacuba, July 19, 1807, ibid., 20v. A makeshift infirmary was established in Tecamachalco under the supervision of a physician from the capital, José de Dios Salazar.

80. Guatemala City's vaccination board, for instance, had its final session in

July 1817, after twelve years in operation. Smith, *"Real Expedición Marítima de la Vacuna" in New Spain and Guatemala*, 56.

81. Manuel Merino to Viceroy Apodaca, Valladolid, March 10, 1817, AGN Epidemias 14 exp. 3, 62–63; Merino to Viceroy, Valladolid, May 2, 1817, AGN Epidemias 14 exp. 6, 126; Merino to Viceory, Valladolid, June 17, 1817, AGN Epidemias 14 exp. 10, 231; Merino to Viceroy, Valladolid, November 22, 1817, AGN Epidemias 14 exp. 8, 178; and Merino to Viceroy, Valladolid, February 4, 1818, AGN IV 4583 exp. 10.

82. As Merino explained to Viceroy Venadito, Valladolid, October 18, 1820, AGN IV 4848 exp. 21, 103r-v.

83. Francisco Xavier de Arvelo y Suarez to Yzquierdo, Tlacolula, October 10, 1807, AGN IV 4957 exp. 47, 2r-v.

84. Juan Antonio de Laguno to Intendant, Villa Alta, June 20, 1807, AGN IV 5297 exp. 15.

85. "La Junta central de Zacatecas en Oficio de 28 de Enero de [1]806 dice" (on a slip of paper), AGN IV 5297 exp. 19, 139. Originally a salary of 30 pesos was reported, perhaps indicating that the "maestro sangrador" had received a reduction in payment or had been replaced by a more economical vaccinator.

86. Hernández Sáenz, *Learning To Heal*, chapter 4 and 252–254.

87. In 1767, Thomas Peña, a forty-eight-year-old *mulato curandero* from Tlaxcala, was condemned by the widow and owner of Tebue Hacienda (Valley of Toluca) for healing among workers on her estate. Testimonies describe him sucking various objects from affected parts of the bodies of Indian and *mulato* workers after declaring the illness the result of witchcraft. He thus offered plausible expectations for disease and suffering, while methods of sucking, blowing, rubbing, and use of a range of herbs and potions connected him to other informal healers in colonial Mexico. Bancroft Library, M-M 96/95, vol. 9 exp. 8. For summaries of trials of healers that featured similar mechanisms of extraction, see Quezada, *Enfermedad y maleficio*, 82–93.

88. *Mercurio volante*, no. 6 (November 25, 1772), 64.

89. Shapin, "Trusting George Cheyne," 293–294.

90. Pedro Fessar to Governador de Tequisistlan, Tehuantepec, June 9, 1796, AGN Historia 531 exp. 3, 172–173; and, at top, "Ocurrencias del Pueblo de Tequisistlan," July 7, 1796, AGN Epidemias 12 exp. 3, 136–138.

91. Fessar to Mora y Peysal, Tehuantepec, June 12, 1796, AGN Historia 531 exp. 3, 177–178; and Fessar to Mora y Peysal, Tehuantepec, June 7, 1796, ibid., 163–164. The same reason was given for Santa Maria Chimalapa: Fessar noted that no women from that pueblo had been seen in Villa de Tehuantepec, for him a clear sign of their rusticity. For Guichicobi, see also the vivid remarks of its officials, "Comparecencia de la república ante el subdelegado," Santa Maria Petapa, May 20, 1796, AGN Historia 531 exp. 3, 144r–145v.

92. Machuca, "La viruela de 1795–1797 en Tehuantepec, Oaxaca," 67–70.

93. Fessar to Mora y Peysal, Tehuantepeque, July 7, 1796, AGN Epidemias 12 exp. 3, 140; and Sennhauser, "Política sanitaria y lucha social en tiempos de viruelas," 64–65.

94. Juan de Yriarte to Subdelegado, San Juan Guichicobi, July 7, 1796, AGN Epidemias 12 exp. 3, 146. The new commission would not have been easily distin-

guishable from the harsh isolation measures recently experienced. Melo tellingly reported that one barrio—entering from the Villa—had been most resistant, while on the other side in the *barrio mayor* toward Sarabia, where smallpox had not struck, residents were allowing inoculation. Where measures to isolate children were implemented, moreover, the women healers were less likely to have been associated with them. Rafael Melo to Fessar, Guichicobi, June 6, 1796, AGN Historia 531 exp. 3, 146v–148.

95. *Gazeta de México* 10, no. 2 (November 11, 1799).

96. For instance, the subdelegate of Chontales and Huamelula received a copy with strict orders that the part on inoculation be practiced voluntarily, and the parishes of Villa Alta received copies in July 1797. Intendant to Subdelegate of Huamelula, Oaxaca, May 28, 1796, AGN Epidemias 12 exp. 3, 111–113; and AHJO VA Civil 31 exp. 14, 26–28.

97. "Señores Curas propios, Interinos, Coadjutores, Vicarios de pie fixo, y R.R. P.P. Ministros," signed Alonso Arzobispo de Mexico, Tacubaya, October 6, 1797, AGN BN 873 exp. 195; and Milpa Alta, dated December 27, 1797, AGN BN 754 exp. 3.

98. Cooper, *Epidemic Disease in Mexico City*, 117–118, reviewed only one of these circulars and dismissed its impact, citing the late arrival of the pamphlet in parishes.

99. See the pamphlet titled *Método claro, sencillo y fácil*. In republican Nuevo Leon, practitioners were so scarce that a guide for inoculation with human smallpox, by lancet or needle, appeared in the state's *Gazeta Constitucional* as late as February 11, 1830. Nearly identical to the 1797 instruction, the article explained that the detailed description had been written with the "greatest clarity" so that poor Indians (*los infelices indios*), presumably lacking access to vaccine fluid, might perform inoculations in "abandoned villages" without trained physicians, magistrates, or priests. García Flores, "Morbilidad y vulnerabilidad en una epidemia de viruela," 51.

100. Razzell, *Conquest of Smallpox*, 49–50 and 56–82.

101. Suplemento II, *Gazeta de México* 12, no. 12 (May 26, 1804).

102. The intendancies split the total cost of 680 pesos, 6 *reales*. Balmis to Señores Intendentes, Mexico City, July 4, 1810, AGN IV 6177 exp. 17, 5; Circular to Subdelegates, Mexico City, July 7, 1810, AGN IV 4062 exp. 27, 9–10; Balmis to Viceroy Venegas, Mexico City, January 10, 1811, AGN IV 6177 exp. 19, 7–8; and Joseph María Lassos to Viceroy, Oaxaca, March 22, 1811, ibid., 22.

103. *Estatutos, que la Real Junta Central Filantrópica General de Vacunación Pública de San Carlos de la Ciudad de la Puebla*, articles 24 and 25.

104. Bonavía to Justicias de la Provincia, Durango, August 14, 1804, AGI Indiferente 1558a, 780.

105. José María Victorino Cervantes to Viceroy, passed to the Protomedicato on December 25, 1804, AGN Epidemias 4 exp. 1, 16. The response was that the surgeon should obtain fluid from the capital and begin operations.

106. Manuel de Ortega to Intendente Izquierdo, Miahuatlan, July 14, 1810, AGN IV 5297 exp. 17; and Manuel de Ortega to Intendente, Miahuatlan, September 15, 1810, ibid., 8–9.

107. It was not uncommon for testimony about race to be brushed aside

when licensing phlebotomists in particular. Hernández Sáenz, *Learning To Heal*, 184–185.

108. Junta de Vacuna, Acatlan, November 6, 1805, AGMP Expedientes 198 leg. 2277/2278, 497.

109. Ayuntamiento to Calleja, Mexico City, February 18, 1814, AGN Historia 530 exp. 3, 4–6.

110. Estado signed Alejo Dancourt, Mérida, April 10, 1817, AGN Epidemias 14 exp. 10, 248–249.

111. October 3, 1814, AGMP Expedientes 78 leg. 885, 268r–269r; and October 10, 1814, ibid., 269v–270v.

112. Signed by junta members, Santiago Tecali, October 21, 1805, AGMP Expedientes 198 leg. 2278, 438.

113. One historian argues that beyond Mexico City a blurring of professional boundaries between practitioners of medicine "was accepted as a way of life"; see de Vos, "Art of Pharmacy in Seventeenth- and Eighteenth-Century Mexico," 63.

114. Voekel, *Alone before God*, chapter 7, especially 172–176, sees an Enlightenment campaign against superstitious healers and *parteras* (midwives) in particular, whose prosecution by the establishment widened the gap between authorized (male) and local (Indian and female), bolstered licensed male practitioners, and helped professionals "rise on the officially rebuked backs of the undocumented." Voekel also acknowledges that most of the population continued to place their trust in these healers. In Brazil, where regulation was similarly inadequate, there were stark differences between the assessment of the medical licensing body (*Fisicatura-mor*), which typically devalued the abilities of the few *curandeiros* it licensed, and patients who esteemed their knowledge of ailments more highly than that of their physician and surgeon counterparts. See Salgado Pimenta, "Barbeiros-sangradores e curandeiros no Brasil (1808–28)."

115. Hernández Sáenz, *Learning To Heal*, 106. Barrera was allowed to practice owing to a shortage of practitioners during an epidemic outbreak.

116. See Chapter 2 in this volume.

117. Fr. Joseph Venavides to Francisco Lacoma, Mexico City, August 1, 1795, AGN Historia 140 exp. 6, 77–78.

118. Francisco Lacoma to José Venavides, Izucar, August 12, 1795, ibid., 81–82.

119. Following the discussion of the source in Taylor, *Magistrates of the Sacred*, 152–166.

120. Cited in ibid., 158.

121. On late colonial conceptions of parish priests and their relationship to secular authority, see ibid., chapters 7 and 16.

122. Ibid., 159.

123. Issued in Valladolid, November 19, 1785, reprinted in *Gazeta de México*, no. 52 (December 6, 1785).

124. For example, see testimonials pertaining to Diego José Teruel's "merits" as pastor of San Juan del Rio and Tequisquiapam, 1786, Tulane VEMC leg. 73 exp. 30. Issues of the *Gazeta de México* from these years make repeated mention of these efforts.

125. Marqués de Branciforte to Archbishop of Mexico, Orizaba, October 23, 1797, AGN BN 754 exp. 1, 2r.

126. García Flores, "Morbilidad y vulnerabilidad en una epidemia de viruela," 55.

127. See Chapter 4 in this volume.

128. González del Campillo, *Exhortacion que el Ilustrísimo Señor Don Manuel Ignacio González del Campillo*, 24: "el influxo que vuestras palabras y exemplo tienen en la opinion pública."

129. Ibid., 25.

130. Nos el Doctor Don Antonio Bergosa, December 7, 1804, AGI Indiferente 1558a, 820v.

131. "Soi un Sacerdote y por tanto no puedo ni debo desear mal a nadie," Tehuacan, December 27, 1804, AGN Epidemias 4 exp. 3, 106r. The matter of cost surfaced when Puebla's vaccination junta requested permission to use communal funds for this expense. See Junta Central to Crown, Puebla, January 27, 1805, ibid., 109–125.

132. Arboleya to Viceroy, Oaxaca, October 26, 1804, AGN Epidemias 4 exp. 6, 192–194; and Joaquin Freiria y Sotomayor to Intendant Izquierdo, Teotitlan del Camino Real, June 20, 1807, AGN IV 5297 exp. 15.

133. José Ygnacio Garcés to Viceroy, Toluca, n.d., AGN Epidemias 4 exp. 1, 24–25. For attributions of success to the parish priest, see, for Tepotzotlán, Francisco Fugairon to Josef de Cuevas, n.p., June 23, 1807, AGN IV 5297 exp. 19, 109.

134. Juan de Pimentel y Sotomayor to Intendant Izquierdo, Zoyaltepec de Teutila, June 28, 1807, AGN IV 5297 exp. 15, 29.

135. Certificación, Guadalajara, January 16, 1815, Tulane VEMC leg. 71 exp. 30, with other documents assembled when José de la Cruz presented for a vacant post in Monterrey's cathedral chapter.

136. Begun in 1827 or 1828 (with the second volume actively filled in two years after the first, in 1829 or 1830), they are ongoing summaries from the original *relaciones de méritos* of priests in the archbishopric, with biographical details, dates and places of work, conduct, and services. See AHAM Siglo XIX 110,1, entries for Juan de German, Joaquin Huarris [*sic*], José Rafael Melgarejo, Porfirio Agustín Madrid, and José Crecencio Villegas; and AHAM Siglo XIX 111,1, entry for Manuel Cruz Manjarres.

137. Signed José Hernandez, Oaxaca, June 11, 1829, AGEO Gobernación, Juntas y Consejos, Sanidad, Hospitales, leg. 1 [1829].

138. Carbajal López, "La epidemia de viruela de 1830–1831," 19–21. This reading departs from the author's suggestion that prayer and spiritual aid were at odds with vaccination.

139. Brading, *Miners and Merchants*, 28 and 43–44; and Weber, *Bárbaros*, for the frontiers of Spanish America.

140. Taylor, *Magistrates of the Sacred*.

141. Izquierdo to Viceroy, Oaxaca, October 19, 1804, AGN Epidemias 4 exp. 6, 187; and Diego de Villasante to Intendente Corregidor, Oaxaca, November 8, 1805, ibid., 228–229. For Querétaro, where corregidor Miguel Dominguez vo-

lunteered to vaccinate his children first, see Dominguez to Iturrigaray, Querétaro, October 29, 1804, AGN Epidemias 4 exp. 2, 43.

142. Occasionally they nearly demanded it. In July 1804 one of the carriers who traveled aboard the *Nuestra Señora de la O*, José Angel de Zumarán, wrote the viceroy reminding him of his role in transporting vaccine to Veracruz. Zumarán expressed disappointment that his name had not appeared in the recent supplement to the gazette on vaccination's propagation in Mexico City (discussed in the Introduction in this volume), and pointed out that, without him, vaccine would never have arrived. Zumarán requested that the viceroy order a revision of the supplement. Zumarán to Viceroy, Veracruz, July 7, 1804, AGN Epidemias 12 exp. 6, 299–300.

143. By the end of the year, 2,448 vaccinations had been performed in the district. Antonio de Elías Sáenz to Iturrigaray, Tenancingo, October 10, 1804, AGN Epidemias 4 exp. 1, 4–5; Iturrigaray to Elías Sáenz, Mexico City, October 27, 1804, ibid., 7; Balmis to Viceroy, Mexico City, November 3, 1804, ibid., 9; Elías Sáenz to Viceroy, Tenancingo, February 23, 1805, ibid., 20; and Francisco Sáenz de Sizilia to Viceroy, Tenancingo, November 30, 1805, ibid., 28.

144. This raised the matter of converting symbolic capital into material support, which royal administrators considered at length (see Chapter 1 in this volume for Guevara's reflections on monuments designed to commemorate and encourage charitable giving).

145. Pedro Arzobispo to Ramon Gutierrez del Mazo, Mexico City, April 6, 1820, AGN IV 5424 exp. 26. The archbishop mentioned interactions with the subdelegates of Huejutla, Metztitlán, and Yahualica.

146. The content of the intendant's letter is inferred from the responses, collected and filed under "viceregal miscellany" in Mexico's national archive and cited below.

147. Francisco Menéndez Valdez to Gutierrez, Mextitlan, April 16, 1820, AGN IV 5572 exp. 5, 24–25.

148. Martin Martinez to Gutierrez, Actopan, April 25, 1820, ibid., 13.

149. Elías Sáenz to Gutierrez, Texcoco, April 28, 1820, AGN IV 5353 exp. 39, 3.

150. Licenciado Manuel Neyra to Gutierrez, Cadereyta, April 26, 1820, AGN IV 5572 exp. 5, 27.

151. José Joaquin Abalia to Gutierrez, Toluca, April 22, 1820, ibid., 20–21.

152. Nicolas de Arias to Gutierrez, Lerma, April 21, 1820, ibid., 2.

153. Manuel de Valdivieho to Gutierrez, Otumba, April 22, 1820, ibid., 5.

154. Miguel Avalesi to Gutierrez, Cuernavaca, April 29, 1820, ibid., 36–37.

155. Manuel de la Hoz to Gutierrez, Huichapan, April 27, 1820, ibid., 14–15.

156. José María Marin to Gutierrez, Quautitlan, April 22, 1820, ibid., 18–19.

157. José Horabuena to Gutierrez, Zumpango, May 8, 1820, ibid., 31.

158. Manuel de la Torres to Gutierrez, Zempoala, May 5, 1820, ibid., 28–29.

159. Rafael Zevallos to Gutierrez, Coatepec-Chalco, June 19, 1820, AGN IV 5424 exp. 26, 3–4.

160. Puebla served as a reservoir for surrounding regions, sending lymph not only to Mexico City and Oaxaca in 1820, but also Amozoc, Atlixco, Cholula, Córdoba, Orizaba, Tehuacán, Tepeaca, and Xalapa. The records documenting periodic vaccination sessions in the insurgency years in cities like Puebla and

Mexico City confirm practice but mask many of the struggles and disagreements behind the scenes. For Mexico City the records are scattered throughout the following boxes in AGN IV 5297 exps. 10, 11, 12, 13 (the record ends chronologically here, with thirty-seven vaccinations on August 8, 1821), and 18; AGN IV 6408 exp. 6; AGN IV 4833 exps. 8 and 9; AGN IV 4848 exps. 14, 19, 20, and 21; AGN IV 4984 exps. 39 and 42; AGN IV 4583 exp. 5; AGN IV 4394 exp. 6; AGN IV 4376 exp. 62; AGN IV 4973 exp. 24, along with bound records from 1816–1817 in AGN Epidemias vol. 14. For Puebla, see AGN IV 5297 exps. 10, 11, 12, and 13; and AGN Epidemias vol. 14 exp. 9.

161. Pedro Boho to Superintendente de la Hacienda Pública, Mérida, October 10, 1820, AGN IV 4848 exp. 21, 116.

162. Manuel de la Concha to Venadito, Mexico City, October 18, 1820, AGN IV 4984 exp. 41; and Junta Municipal de Sanidad to Venadito, Acapulco, February 16, 1821, AGN IV 4376 exp. 61.

163. For studies with these parameters, see Few, *For All of Humanity*; Mark and Rigau-Pérez, "World's First Immunization Campaign"; Rigau-Pérez, "Introduction of Smallpox Vaccine in 1803"; and Warren, *Medicine and Politics in Colonial Peru*.

164. See Warren, *Medicine and Politics in Colonial Peru*, chapter 2, showing how the rivalries and ambitions of these medical men shaped movements for reform in Peru.

165. Certificación, Huajuapan de Leon, January 18, 1834, AHJO Huajuapan Criminal 14 exp. 1, 2. The healer appears more interested in the victim's life in this instance than in legal formalities. (It is rare for the nature of the expert's training to be expressly indicated.)

166. Hernández Sáenz, *Learning To Heal*, 207 and 210–211.

CHAPTER 6

Medicine's Malcontents

Epigraph: Junguera to Gonzalez del Campillo, Tlatlauquitepec, August 18, 1806, AGMP Expedientes 198 leg. 2278.

1. José Barreyro y Quijano to José Antonio Caballero, Acapulco, February 16, 1805, AGI Indiferente 1558a, 978–979; and Balmis to José Antonio Caballero, Acapulco, February 5, 1805, ibid., 1033v–1034r.

2. Porter, introduction to *Patients and Practitioners*, 3. For an example of the kinds of "narrations of illness" that literate sources have provided for preindustrial England, see Porter and Porter, *In Sickness and in Health*.

3. See Certeau, *Practice of Everyday Life*, 8, on the tendency to conflate authority conferred by "social *place*" and "technical *discourse*" (emphasis in original). Hernández Sáenz, *Learning To Heal*, observes that the medical elite in eighteenth-century Mexico continued to make authoritative claims on the basis of social position even after the empirical grounds of their knowledge shifted, in part because the profession's racial privilege (*limpieza de sangre*) persisted.

4. Porter, *Bodies Politic*, 22–26.

5. In this case the government approved the destruction of those used in contravention of prohibitions, while acknowledging licit uses and the considerable cost in money or labor of their construction. Pedro Marin to Viceroy, Orizava, November 8, 1797, AGN Epidemias 5 exp. 3, 274r-v; Cabildo to Branciforte, Orizava, November 9, 1797, AGN Epidemias 5 exp. 6, 423–425; and Viceroy to Ayuntamiento, Orizava, November 27, 1797, ibid., 427.

6. In addition to seminal articles by Gluckman, "Gossip and Scandal," and Abrahams, "Performance-Centered Approach to Gossip," on the ways intimacy or solidarity is produced between those who share rumors, see Tackett, "Conspiracy Obsession in a Time of Revolution"; Farge, *Subersive Words* (stressing social context and the consequences of reports of conspiracies or kidnapping for authorities); Farge and Revel, *Vanishing Children of Paris*; and Van Young, *Other Rebellion*, chapters 14 and 18 (on the oral culture of Mexico's insurgency period). On rumors and medicine, see Arnold, *Colonizing the Body*, 218–226; Sutphen, "Rumoured Power"; Durbach, *Bodily Matters*, chapter 5; and White, *Speaking with Vampires*, chapter 2.

7. See Guha, "On Some Aspects of the Historiography of Colonial India"; Guha, "Prose of Counter-Insurgency"; Spivak, "Can the Subaltern Speak?"; and Frederick Cooper's challenge to subaltern studies in "Conflict and Connection." Cooper asks whether "the theorist [can] listen," and although he was addressing the oral sources upon which his fellow Africanists have relied in writing history, I take it as a provocation to consider the oral forms and paralinguistic dimensions of peasant knowledge.

8. Lomnitz, *Deep Mexico, Silent Mexico*, chapter 7.

9. Lévi-Strauss, *Raw and the Cooked*, 3.

10. Josef Manuel Vayeto to Viceroy, Mexicaltzingo, October 7, 1773, AGN IV 5531 exp. 70, 1.

11. Miguel Dávila Galindo to Viceroy, October 19, 1773, ibid., 65–66.

12. Luis Fernando de Hoyos to Viceroy, October 10, 1773, ibid., 6; and Antonio de Arroyo to Peramas, October 15, 1773, ibid., 49–50r. The Protomedicato hesitated when informed of the need for an attending physician, inquiring about cost of care, availability of pharmaceuticals and a bleeder, and the possibility of deep burials, as the practitioner would have no use without these things. The royal attorney expressed amazement that, with so many physicians in the capital, one had not been sent right away. Fiscal to Viceroy, Mexico City, October 11, 1773, ibid., 11–13.

13. Manuel Gómez to Secretario de Cámara Josef del Valle, October 12, 1773, ibid., 24; José Manuel Vayeto to Melchor de Peramas, October 13, 1773, ibid., 37; and "Este es traslado de una carta que reciví oi, del Médico de Santa Marta," October 14, 1773, ibid., 34.

14. Manuel Gómez to Corregidor, October 14, 1773, ibid., 38r; Manuel Gómez to Corregidor, October 15, 1773, ibid., 44; and Josef Manuel Vayeto to Melchor de Peramas, October 17, 1773, ibid., 59.

15. Miguel Dávila Galindo to Viceroy, October 19, 1773, ibid., 66v; and Ignacio Segura and Juan Bermudes to Viceroy, October 21, 1773, ibid., 79.

16. "Exhortación, a los Párrocos para que cuiden, que los Naturales sepan, y

practiquen las Reglas, que se señalen," in Lorenzana y Buitrón, *Cartas pastorales, y edictos*, 42–48, quote on 44.

17. Ibid., especially items II and VI–VIII.

18. Underlying this was the assumption that priests in parishes, rather than the viceregal government, would reform these medical and hygienic habits, which also guided the establishment of schools for instruction in Spanish language in the following years. Lorenzana's language policy, with its disparagement of American priests fluent in regional dialects, was widely perceived as an assault not only on indigenous languages but on the creole clerics who had overseen and encouraged their use. On the royal *cédulas*, viceregal orders, and strident defense of indigenous languages on the part of creole Americans at home and abroad, see Tanck de Estrada, *Pueblos de indios y educación en el México colonial*, 168–187.

19. See Bartolache, *Instrucción que puede servir*; and Moreno, *Ensayos de historia de la ciencia y la tecnología,* 193–199. Francisco Gil's method for treating smallpox drew on this intellectual tradition when it advised that physicians and surgeons prescribe fruits to give the blood a healthy disposition and protect against infection; see *Extracto de la obra publicada en Madrid el año pasado de 1784 con el título de Disertación Físico-Médica*, Article 18.

20. Miguel Dávila Galindo to Viceroy, December 7, 1773, AGN IV 5531 exp. 70, 212–213.

21. Vayeto to Peramas, October 28, 1773, ibid., 104–105.

22. Protomedicato to Viceroy, October 30, 1773, ibid., 106; and Protomedicato to Viceroy, December 9, 1773, ibid., 216. Its medical experts unhelpfully put forth the view, likely suggested by one of the attending physicians, that residents were faking their illness.

23. For the debate on the origins of the humoral tradition in Mexico (whether European or pre-Hispanic) between historian Alfredo López Austin and anthropologist George Foster, see López Austin, *Human Body and Ideology*, 267–282; and Foster, "Hippocrates' Latin American Legacy," 3–19. What they more or less agreed on was the significance attached to hot and cold properties of body parts, plants, foods, places, seasons, and states, with illness implying a physiological or moral disequilibrium that increased the patient's vulnerability.

24. The author of Tlaxcala's prolix *relación geográfica*, for instance, concluded his detailed description of the steam baths used by pregnant women with this: "Likewise they use these baths for the sick, and they are of great benefit, as some of our Spaniards use them, and find them beneficial." Muñoz Camargo, *Relaciones geográficas de Tlaxcala*, 37. Fields, *Pestilence and Headcolds*, 128–129 and 141–142, argues for the early convergence of practices on the basis of remarks made about indigenous bathing practices in these reports.

25. Misión de los Ures, Sonora, November 25, 1770, Huntington Library, mssHM 4055.

26. The endorsement appeared in a supplement to the *Gazeta de México* 6, no. 79 (November 19, 1794), "Carta de don Gabriel de Ocampo . . . sobre las virtudes de los Baños del Peñol." Several "quasi-miraculous" cures reportedly ensued when a charitable merchant from Mexico City arranged to have more than four hundred sick poor taken there over four days in November 1796; see *Gazeta de México* 8, no. 26 (December 7, 1796).

27. Rosenberg, *Explaining Epidemics*, 26. On the stability of medical advice in Europe, see Shapin, "Philosopher and the Chicken." Hernández Sáenz, *Learning To Heal*, 43–44 and passim, stresses the primitive state of medicine and the fact that the medical profession was coming to terms with the limited effectiveness of its treatments, with little to offer the public that might not be found in homemade remedies or the repertoires of local healers.

28. Dávila Galindo to Viceroy, October 26, 1773, AGN IV 5531 exp. 70, 99.

29. The priest and physician had together decided on a course of purges, which required careful monitoring of the patients' diets and were carried out in the priest's quarters. Dávila Galindo to Viceroy, October 22, 1773, ibid., 86r-v; and Dávila Galindo to Viceroy, October 26, 1773, ibid., 99v.

30. Protomedicato to Bucareli, October 30, 1773, ibid., 106.

31. Vayeto to Crown, November 6, 1773, ibid., 137.

32. Dávila Galindo to Viceroy, December 5, 1773, ibid., 212v. On the presence of blood altering the sense of self in pre-Columbian rituals, a sensation sometimes heightened by intoxication with pulque or another local beverage, see Clendinnen, "Ways to the Sacred," 117–119 and 123–125.

33. Fiscal to Viceroy, October 31, 1773, AGN IV 5531 exp. 70, 107; and Antonio de Arroyo to Viceroy, December 22, 1773, ibid., 237–239.

34. Most of the documentation on these episodes is in AGN Epidemias 7.

35. Signed by subdelegate, priest, and two *testigos*, San Pedro Azcapotzaltongo, May 6, 1793, AGN Epidemias 7 exp. 7, 287r-v (followed by four responses from *regidores* and other officials of republic, in some instances thanking the subdelegate for the medical supplies).

36. Morel to Bonavia, Mexico City, May 24, 1793, ibid., 302–303; and Morel to Bonavia, Mexico City, November 8, 1790, ibid., 201.

37. Julian Chrisostomo Quintana to Viceroy, San Pedro Azcapotzaltongo, July 11, 1793, ibid., 318.

38. Julian Chrisostomo Quintana to Viceroy, San Pedro Azcapotzaltongo, May 23, 1793, ibid., 309–310: "se ausentaran de sus Pueblos, se escondieran en los bosques, y varrancas en donde perecerian seguramente sin auxilio temporal ni espiritual."

39. Dated December 23, 1805, AGN IV 4062 exp. 9.

40. Explaining illness through personification recalls the furious divinities of the Nahua pantheon believed responsible for the infirmities of humankind; see Aguirre Beltrán, *Medicina y magia*, 43–45.

41. Dr. José Rafael Valdés de Anaya to Viceroy, Parish of Tizayuca, January 23, 1806, AGN IV 3885 exp. 4, 36–39; and Valdés to González Carvajal, ibid., 40.

42. Anastasio Bustamante to García Jove, San Bartolome Quautlalpan, December 17, 1805, AGN IV 1815 exp. 4, 14–15, where he confirmed that the sickness had carried off more than half of the population. These were common medicaments during the outbreak: another physician's list included tartaric, sulfuric acid, quinine, mustard, vinegar, common salt, lime cough syrup (*jarabe de limón*), camphor, and canker weed. See Patricio Yeper to García Jove, Tultitlán, December 19, 1805, ibid., 22–23.

43. Anastasio Bustamante to García Jove, San Bartolome Quautlalpan, January 28, 1806, AGN IV 3885 exp. 4, 21–22. He added that those who did not live

like Indians, but instead "like those commonly called *de razón*," resisted succumbing to infection, along with other castes.

44. Indigenous governance was a complicated affair. Upon marrying, a male villager typically received a distribution of land to maintain his family and the right to vote in elections for *república* officials, which a royal official, priest, or other (European) outsider witnessed. The new governor or alcalde, along with one or more *regidores* to assist them, depending on the size of the population, together represented the community, oversaw distribution of resources, collected tribute, and mediated with the world beyond. Those who were not village elders or *principales* might still influence village politics, occasionally vote in elections, and carry weight in formal petitions to courts and other juridical institutions. For descriptions of elections in central Mexico, see Guarisco, *Los indios del valle de México*, 83–91.

45. Junta de Sanidad to Vicente Ramon Jaen, Mexico City, December 22, 1805, AGN IV 1815 exp. 4, 43r–v; and Vicente Ramon Jaen to González Carvajal, San Bartolome Quautlalpam, January 20, 1806, AGN IV 3885 exp. 4, 17–18.

46. Anastasio Bustamante to García Jove, San Bartolome Quautlalpam, January 13, 1806, AGN IV 1815 exp. 4, 57–58.

47. José Osorio to González Carvajal, Tlaquilpan, December 20, 1806, AGN IV 3885 exp. 8; Francisco Veyra Pardo to González Carvajal, Zempoala, January 3, 1807, ibid.; José Osorio to González Carvajal, Tlaquilpan, January 19, 1807, ibid.; and José Osorio to González Carvajal, Tlaquilpan, February 4, 1807, ibid.

48. Certificación, signed Manuel Lopez Escudero, cura por S.M. y Juez Ecco. del Pueblo de San Juan Baptista, October 31, 1807, AGN IV 1860 exp. 3, 20r.

49. Antonio María Campos to González Carvajal, Juanico, January 8, 1807, AGN IV 1860 exp. 7, 27–28.

50. "Relacion del estado del Pueblo de Tecamachalco, quando se puso el Hospital, en 23 de Junio anterior," signed José María de Zenea, Tacuba, August 14, 1807, AGN IV 3885 exp. 10, 44.

51. "Razon de lo q^{e} voy subministrando al Sor. D. Mariano Jose de Car[r]anza," Tesoyuca, December 17, 1806, AGN IV 2784 exp. 16, 27–28; and "Lista de los q^{e} murieron en la $admist^{n}$ de Tesoyuca en el año de 1806," January 8, 1807, ibid., 29–30. Generalizations here are based on a review of expense lists for provisional hospitals, in AGN IV 3885 exp. 7 (Ayutla, 1807), AGN IV 3885 exp. 10 (Tecamachalco, 1807), and AGN IV 1860 exp. 6 (Tultitlan, 1806). By comparison, in the 1797 smallpox epidemic, of 127,899 pesos spent by charitable societies in the eight sectors of Mexico City, 35.8 percent went toward foodstuffs, 28 percent toward clothing and shelter, 18.4 percent toward medications, and 17.7 percent to pay physicians and barbers. "Resumen General," Mexico City, February 17, 1798, AGN BN 1024 exp. 1.

52. Antonio María Campos to González Carvajal, Juanico, January 8, 1807, AGN IV 1860 exp. 7, 27–28v.

53. Antonio José Romo to Conde de la Cadena, Tochimilco, September 24, 1807, AGMP Expedientes 198 leg. 2277/2278, 448. A census showed 1,350 Spaniards and *castas* and 1,870 *indios* in the head town (ibid., 451).

54. On the importance of bodily presentation and comportment in establish-

ing the authority and scholarly knowledge of English physicians and surgeons, see Lawrence, "Medical Minds, Surgical Bodies," 156–201.

55. Josef Antonio Frera to Arzobispo Francisco Xavier de Lizana, Quautitlan, January 13, 1806, AGN IV 3885 exp. 4, 11–13.

56. Dr. José Rafael Valdés de Anaya to Viceroy, Parroquia de Tizayuca, January 23, 1806, ibid., 36–39; for the original commission, see Junta de Sanidad, Mexico City, January 9, 1806, AGN IV 1815 exp. 4, 55–56.

57. Junta de Sanidad, Mexico City, January 3, 1806, ibid., 53–54.

58. In 1813, when Mexico City's *ayuntamiento* tried to determine the cause of a new outbreak, a consulting surgeon traced it to Cuautitlán and its environs, where, instead of allowing outside assistance, inhabitants "bled themselves and drank *aguardiente*, and other harms of this nature," which allegedly caused the epidemic to propagate to other pueblos and eventually to the capital. Rafael Sagaz, Mexico City, September 2, 1813, AGN Epidemias 13 exp. 6, 238v.

59. The priest ministering in Santa Marta in 1773, for instance, remarked that poor villagers in particular could not discern good from bad; if left in their homes, Hippocrates himself would be unable to prevent the epidemic's spread. Miguel Dávila Galindo to Viceroy, December 7, 1773, AGN IV 5531 exp. 70, 212–213.

60. Aguirre Beltrán, *Medicina y magia*, 41.

61. Nicolas Junguera to Manuel Ignacio Gonzalez del Campillo, Tlatlauquitepec, August 18, 1806, AGMP Expedientes 198 leg. 2278, 375–378; and for the response of Santiago Yaonahuac's governor, beginning "Amado Padre y Señor," see ibid., 379r.

62. José Rodrigo Valdés to Riaño, San Juan Bautista de Apaseo, March 23, 1805, AGN Epidemias 4 exp. 15, 490; and José Manuel de Septién y Primo to Riaño, San Luis de la Paz, March 28, 1805, ibid., 492r, where official, parish priest, and *vecindario decente* together covered the expense of transporting vaccine from Celaya.

63. Domingo González de Ossio to Riaño, Salvatierra, March 23, 1805, ibid., 489. Undaunted, the town's physician accompanied several children to Celaya to bring back fluid, which was paid for by a "pious" resident (to ensure that no cost be incurred by the royal treasury or communal funds for this "humanitarian" undertaking).

64. José Ramon de Huerta to Juan Antonio de Riaño, Chamácuaro, March 21, 1805, ibid., 485.

65. Manuel de Urodea y Duque to Riaño, Yuririhapúndaro, March 29, 1805, ibid., 493r. Children would again be sent for vaccination in Celaya, with expenses (10 pesos) once more paid by the official and the town's merchants and businessmen ("los vecinos de este comercio").

66. Yldefonso Rafael de Rocas to Intendant Izquierdo, Nochistlan, June 20, 1807, AGN IV 5297 exp. 15, 18.

67. Manuel de Ahedo to Intendant Arce, Mexicalcingo, July 8, 1808, AGN IV 1717 exp. 18, 51r: "que aquella operación era como una marca del Rey con que se señalaban."

68. By the time these complaints were recorded, events unfolding in Europe had led to the abdication of Charles IV and his replacement by Ferdinand VII. New of this had not yet arrived in the region, however; as far as members of the

community knew, it was business as usual, and any critique leveled reflected a preexisting colonial dynamic. On rumors of the monarch's return, see Van Young, *Other Rebellion*, chapter 18, calling the phenomenon "naïve monarchism."

69. By then the Bourbons had abolished the branding even of enslaved Africans arriving in Spanish ports, as publicly announced in *Gazeta de México* 2, no. 14 (July 25, 1786).

70. Paraphrasing Clendinnen, "Ways to the Sacred," 114–115.

71. Francisco Hevia to Viceroy, Veracruz, November 12, 1817, AGN Epidemias 14 exp. 8, 194. Sobreviñas witnessed numerous successes as well: the volume in which this report is nestled is full of registers submitted by him, with the results of dozens of sessions in outlying villages, in addition to the district seat of Acayucan, with claims that everyone in Moloacan and Ixhuapan (both "small pueblos") had been vaccinated.

72. Aguirre Beltrán, *Regiones de refugio*, and for an application of the concept in the Yucatán, see Farriss, *Maya Society under Colonial Rule*, 72–79.

73. In this case, the procurator cited a provision in the Laws of the Indies "that in the event that Indians suffer *contagio de peste* and mortality" or sterility, they be granted relief in their time of need; his charges had suffered both, and it was only fitting, he argued, that their debt be forgiven. Procurador Mariano Perez de Tagle, on behalf of *común de naturales* of Tixtla and Zimpantzingo, to Fiscal, January 23, 1779, AGN Epidemias 13 exp. 5, 120r-v (followed by statements from priests and village leaders blaming illness on irregular eating habits).

74. On migration as protest, and a reminder that flight was not always to sparsely settled areas, see Taylor, *Magistrates of the Sacred*, 374–376. During the insurgency, rebels took advantage of the refuge afforded by terrain to oppose royalist-controlled head towns, forming shadow communities (*cantones*) that acquired formal physical, commercial, and political dimensions. Ducey, "Village, Nation, and Constitution," 472–474.

75. Miguel Antonio de Arteaga to Gonzalez Carvajal, Texcoco, April 19, 1807, AGN IV 6172 exp. 16, 18–19; and Lista, Texcoco, May 30, 1807, ibid., 30–39.

76. Thompson, "Moral Economy of the English Crowd," 115.

77. Reglamento, Mexico City, September 5, 1804, AHDF 3678 exp. 17, 18–26, translated in Cook, "Francisco Xavier Balmis," Appendix II, 95–99. Nearly identical language appeared in Article 14 of Acapulco's statutes, see Reglamento, Acapulco, February 5, 1805, AGI Indiferente 1558a, 982–985v. In Guatemala physicians were instructed to experiment on dogs to determine whether the procedure might reduce cases of rabies; see Reglamento, signed Antonio Gonzalez Saravia, Guatemala, January 25, 1805, ibid., 1258–1275.

78. Phelipe Diaz de Ortega to Balmis, Valladolid, January 16, 1805, ibid., 1051r.

79. Balmis to Caballero, Acapulco, February 5, 1805, ibid., 1031–1036.

80. Antonio Obispo de Antequera to Felix María Calleja, San Angel, November 4, 1815, AGN Historia 530 exp. 4. See also AGN Epidemias 14 exp. 2.

81. Vicente Ferrer, Spanish philosopher and vocal opponent of inoculation in the 1780s, supported his views on the threat of infection by reproducing a report from the pages of the *Gazeta de Madrid*, according to which enslaved black deserters fleeing plantations in the wars of American Independence had been caught

and inoculated by the English and sent into the American army to infect it. The authors of a critical edition of Ferrer's work suggest that in Spain, as in England and France, few who weighed the benefits against the risks of inoculation tried to remain objective, frequently drawing on public knowledge, as manifest in such rumors, without much interest in whether any factual basis might be verified; see León Sanz and Barettino Coloma, *Vicente Ferrer Gorraiz Beaumont y Montesa*, 244–245. On reports in the American colonies that the British were waging biological warfare, see Fenn, *Pox Americana*, 88–92.

82. Sala Capitular to Viceroy, San Luis Potosí, July 21, 1804, AGN Epidemias 4 exp. 9, 292–293.

83. For the official's assessment that the efforts of the intendant were insufficient to attract these parents, see ibid., 285–286.

84. Owensby, *Empire of Law and Indian Justice in Colonial Mexico*, 72 and 302.

85. Farge, *Subversive Words*, 9, suggests that only with difficulty did actors of any stripe in Paris remain indifferent to what ordinary people said, no matter the scorn sometimes heaped upon vulgar opinion.

86. For extended comments on the unique socioethnic composition of the port and the need to vary practice, see the *reglamento* for vaccine that Balmis composed for Acapulco following this episode. Reglamento, Francisco Xavier de Balmis to Governor Jose Barreyro, Acapulco, February 5 1805, AGI Indiferente 1558a, 982–985v (especially Article 6); and Juan Molina to Governor Barreyro, Acapulco, March 18, 1805, ibid., 991.

87. Ramon Maseras y Mazo to Gutiérrez del Mazo, Mexicalcingo, May 4, 1820, AGN IV 5353 exp. 39.

88. Nicolas Junguera to Manuel Ignacio Gonzalez del Campillo, Tlatlauquitepec, August 18, 1806, AGMP Expedientes 198 leg. 2278, 375–378.

89. Manuel María de Ortega to Intendant, Miahuatlan, September 15, 1810, AGN IV 5297 exp. 17, 8v–9r.

90. Certeau, *Practice of Everyday Life*, 37–38, following Freud and sociolinguists' "ethnographies of speaking."

91. Hearsay was admissible evidence in royal and ecclesiastical courts, before tribunals of the Inquisition, and in legal and territorial disputes. Proceedings to confirm the purity of blood of a candidate for official posts often asked familiars to attest to public reputation and lineage, things most often gleaned by word of mouth. Confirmations of the miraculous repute of a saint image might involve lengthy oral testimonies that related what had been said and heard, if not necessarily seen. On oral testimony in blood purity proceedings, see Martínez, *Genealogical Fictions*, chapter 3.

92. Geertz, *Interpretation of Cultures*, 5: "man is an animal suspended in webs of significance he himself has spun."

93. There is a regrettable lack of comparable studies for the period prior to 1850. For Navajo reservations in New Mexico after 1863, see Trennert, *White Man's Medicine*, especially 32–34, 43–52, and 107–117; and Lambert, "Plural Traditions?", 191–211.

94. Cf. Foucault, "Politics of Health in the Eighteenth Century," 166–182, for a narrative of medical reform that posits a "surplus of power" bestowed on the

eighteenth-century physician in consequence of his growing influence as social observer, reformer, and hygienist.

95. "He who makes two consecutive visits to a home without ordering anything other than good regimen or some simple, common, domestic medicine," Bartolache warned in his periodical, "need do no more to earn his dismissal, and another is called who better knows the medicinal jungle." *Mercurio volante*, no. 12 (January 13, 1774), 122–123.

CONCLUSION

1. Ross, "Mexico's Superior Health Council and the American Public Health Association."

2. Consejo Superior de Salubridad, "Iniciativa para celebrar el primer centenario del descubrimiento de la vacuna," 7.

3. Municipal legislation in 1882 mandated vaccination before the age of six months and was extended to the entire republic at the turn of the century. McCaa, "Revisioning Smallpox in Mexico City-Tenochtitlán, 1520–1950," 460–463. On the diversity of practice during the Porfiriato, see Carrillo, "Por voluntad o por fuerza."

4. Dr. Daniel Escobar to Mitra, Mexico City, July 13, 1889, AHAM Labastida y Dávalos 202 exp. 56.

5. Chowning, "Convent Reform, Catholic Reform, and Bourbon Reform"; Arrom, *Containing the Poor*; Larkin, *Very Nature of God*, especially 188–215; and Voekel, *Alone before God*.

6. For the strenuous combined efforts of the surgeon and the intendant governor of Durango, see the certifications of Felix Garda y Ferraris's commission, Sombrerete, August 10, 1803, AGN IV 5297 exp. 19; Durango, September 3, 1803, ibid.; and Bonavia to Cavallero, Durango, November 15, 1804, AGI Indiferente 1558a, 778–779. On the island of Puerto Rico, early vaccinations with fluid obtained from Saint Thomas led to vigorous protest from Balmis, initiating a pattern of conflict seen in New Spain; see Rigau-Pérez, "Introduction of Smallpox Vaccine in 1803." In Guatemala the search for cowpox began when news of Jenner's discovery arrived in 1800 and yielded success by the time of the arrival of a subsidiary expedition under Francisco Pastor, in August 1804; see Smith, *"Real Expedición Marítima de la Vacuna" in New Spain and Guatemala*, 49–54; and Ramírez Martín, *La salud del Imperio*, 51 and 138–143.

7. Navarro García, "Análisis de los documentos esenciales sobre la Real Expedición de Balmis-Salvany," 74. The debate can be traced through seminal works on the expedition, beginning with Sherburne F. Cook, "Francisco Xavier Balmis," who formulated the thesis that the efforts of viceroys, intendants, physicians, and governors to vaccinate in advance of the expedition represented an attempt at sabotage, following the vituperative complaints of Balmis. Ramírez Martín, *La mayor hazaña médica de la colonia* and *La salud del Imperio*, rely primarily on Spanish archives and published sources and view Balmis and Salvany as primary agents who, with indispensable support from civil, military, and ecclesiastical officials, put into practice "objetos previstos" (*La salud del Imperio*, 12–13). Studies

that stress local initiatives prior to the expedition's arrival and the colonial networks that made propagation possible include Smith, *"Real Expedición Marítima de la Vacuna" in New Spain and Guatemala*; Fernández del Castillo, *Los viajes de don Francisco Xavier de Balmis*, especially 97–119 and 128–129; Aceves Pastrana and Morales Cosme, "Conflictos y negociaciones en las expediciones de Balmis"; and Smith, "Balmis en la Nueva España," 125–127.

8. Smith, *"Real Expedición Marítima de la Vacuna" in New Spain and Guatemala*, 21–22; and Ramírez Martín, *La salud del Imperio*, 196 and 186–188.

9. Balmis to Caballero, Madrid, February 12, 1807, AGI Indiferente 1558a, 1413r-v and 1414v–1415r; and Reglamento, n.p., n.d. (submitted to the Spanish crown on February 12, 1807), ibid., 1422–1427, Article 5. Mexico City's regulations stipulated that the vaccine clinic should be central and clean, as distinct from hospitals and hospices, which must be avoided, "for the mothers do not want their children vaccinated except from the healthiest carriers, robust and of good appearance, as I have seen elsewhere." Cook, "Francisco Xavier Balmis," Appendix II, 99–101. Durango's intendant composed a *reglamento* for Provincias Internas that made a change suggested by Balmis, that a house rather than hospital be designated for vaccinations. Bonavia to Cavallero, Durango, November 15, 1804, AGI Indiferente 1558a, 778–779.

10. For Colombia the analysis of Marcelo Frías Núñez balances private initiative against that of the Crown and the considerable role of José Celestino Mútis, the physician whose guiding hand was evident in immunization campaigns from 1782 up to the Royal Vaccination Expedition and who presents a strong case for continuity and local innovation. Frías Núñez, *Enfermedad y sociedad en la crisis colonial*, especially 231–232.

11. Received April 12, 1813, AGN Epidemias 13 exp. 6, 242–243.

12. "Reglamento de S.M. para perpetuar en Indias la Vacuna," AGI Indiferente 1558a, articles 15 and 19. The clause prohibiting unauthorized persons from operating to avoid spurious vaccinations appears in regulations issued for several provincial capitals.

13. See Schiebinger, *Secret Cures of Slaves*, especially 89–99, on the control of slave masters over the provision of medicine in the British and French Caribbean in this period.

14. Following E. P. Thompson, Alfonso Zarzoso (in "¿Obligación moral o responsabilidad política?") highlights both types of "moral obligation" during epidemics in Cataluña in the 1720s.

15. For Russia, the historian John Alexander concluded that "building a comprehensive system of sanitary surveillance remained an aspiration, constantly postponed by practical difficulties, financial constrains, and conflicting priorities." See Alexander, *Bubonic Plague in Early Modern Russia*, 33–34.

16. Ibarra, "De tareas ingratas y épocas difíciles," 340–342. Bourbon policies fueled this perception on the part of prelates and priests, even as religious paradigms of governance flourished in the political economy and regalist jurisprudence of ministers and officials.

17. The procedure was intended to save the soul of the fetus by baptism and, if possible, its life. In Mexico the viceroy and archbishop formally endorsed the practice in 1772, when instructions were made available that encouraged priests

to perform it themselves when no surgeon was available; see Lanning, *Royal Protomedicato*, 309–313; Rigau-Pérez, "Surgery at the Service of Theology"; and Warren, "Operation for Evangelization," on how caesarean sections enlaced surgical instruction with soteriology and matters of evangelization in 1780s Peru, "entailing a religious reclaiming of medical expertise," 650. Few, *For All of Humanity*, 98 and 114, shows that incidences of rural caesarean operations in Guatemala were not uncommon and interprets the broader interest in the fetus as a process of biomedicalization, which "dissolved the autonomy of women over matters of birth."

18. *Relación de méritos del bachiller Julian Antonio Monroy* [printed], 1828 [1838], AHAM Siglo XIX 20 exp. 6, 3–6. Notable in these *relaciones* from the Mexican republic is the significance of the epidemic of 1812–1814 for those who lived and worked through it, perhaps amplified by reigning conditions of poverty, warfare, and political uncertainty. In addition to the references to vaccine in résumés (discussed in Chapter 5), see AHAM Siglo XIX caja 110, 1, Felix de Osores, citing support of schools in Querétaro and the sick in smallpox outbreaks of 1802–1803 and 1813–1814, and Pedro María Solano, citing useful works "in times of *peste*." Additional references to pastoral service in times of pestilence, including 1813 and 1814, are in AHAM Siglo XIX caja 111, 1: Miguel Balbuena, José Ildefonso Castillo, José Francisco Cisneros, José Ignacio Camacho y Davila, José Camilo Escobar, Manuel Rivera, and José Francisco Lezo y Trejo, who was *vicario* in the *peste* of 1813 and learned Nahuatl (*el idioma Mejicano*) to better assist parishioners, "which today he speaks perfectly." For the cholera outbreak of 1833, see the printed *relación* of Francisco Orive y Figueroa, 1838, AHAM Siglo XIX 44 exp. 43.

19. On these blinds spots see Cañizares-Esguerra, introduction to *Science in the Spanish and Portuguese Empires*, 1–5.

20. Voekel, *Alone before God*, 9–10, 189, 197, 199–201, 205–208, and especially 184.

21. Warren, *Medicine and Politics in Colonial Peru*, 218–219, notes that in Peru the Catholic Church looked more stable and reliable than medical institutions, which presumably compelled José de San Martín, Peru's "liberator" and first president, to place vaccine formally in the hands of priests. In the following decades, Peru's republican governments granted the church a major role in vaccination's administration at the same time that it was losing control over hospitals and other charitable institutions. Warren, "Piety and Danger," 176–179.

22. On the politics of state and religion in the 1810s and 1820s, see Connaughton, "Transiciones en la cultura político/religiosa mexicana" and "Most Delicate Balance." See also O'Hara, *A Flock Divided*, on how corporate religious identities and politics in Mexico City were reiterated as a consequence of Bourbon reforms.

23. Connaughton, *Clerical Ideology in a Revolutionary Age* and "Los curas y la feligresía ciudadana en México." For years (1823–1840) Mexico lacked an archbishop (the Vatican declined to appoint one so long as the newly independent nation refused to make amends to Spain).

24. Daniela Bleichmar has proposed modifying the model of scientific practice put forth by philosopher Bruno Latour, in which raw data are standardized and

accumulated at a stable center of processing. Natural historians in places like Bogotá, Lima, and Mexico City, she notes, were at the nodes of networks and pursued trajectories that "were multiple, overlapping, and highly sensitive to local interests, emphases, and interpretations." Bleichmar, *Visible Empire*, 141–142.

25. Reviewing Scott's work, Venezuelan anthropologist Fernando Coronil insisted that the combination of "multiple modalities of knowledge" is a feature of all states. See Coronil, "Smelling Like a Market," 127.

26. José María Marin to Ramón Gutiérrez del Mazo, Quautitlan, April 18, 1818, AGN IV 5297 exp. 10, 78–79; Gutiérrez del Mazo to Apodaca, Mexico City, April 18, 1818, ibid.; and Gutiérrez del Mazo to Apodaca (quoting the subdelegate's letter), Mexico City, July 7, 1818, ibid., 97. The items in this dossier were forwarded to the gazette.

27. Estado, signed Pedro Martinez and Manuel de Abréu, Zacatecas, January 1, 1820, AGN IV 4376 exp. 63, 11r (under "Observaciones"); and Estado, signed Martinez and Abréu, Zacatecas, August 1, 1820, ibid., 35r.

28. These episodes are recounted in Agostoni, "Estrategias, actores, promesas y temores."

29. Miguel Angel Gutiérrez, "Iglesia Saca Cristo de la Salud a Calles de México por Influenza," *Reuters*, April 27, 2009.

30. For instance, David Luhnow, Jose de Cordoba, and Ana Campoy, "Mexico's High Death Rate Poses Key Question on Virus," *Wall Street Journal*, April 29, 2009, A6; and Tim Padgett, "Living with Swine Flu: Mexico City under the Cloud," *Time*, May 2, 2009. Historians, physicians, and journalists continue to insist that religious people in the past brought primarily fatalism, fear, ignorance, and superstition to modern techniques like vaccination, until the moment at the end of the nineteenth century when a modern worldview premised on empiricism and rationalism prevailed and allowed scientific medicine to supersede outdated ways of succumbing to disease. For a recent formulation of this thesis, see Bliss, *Making of Modern Medicine*, especially chapter 1. The transference of faith from priests to doctors, religion to science, is rarely so clear-cut or all encompassing, and people in the past not so fatalistic.

Bibliography

ARCHIVAL SOURCES

Archivo General de Indias, Seville (AGI)
- Audiencia de México
- Indiferente General (Indiferente)

Archivo General de la Nación, Mexico (AGN)
- Bienes Nacionales (BN)
- Criminal
- Epidemias
- General de Parte
- Historia
- Hospitales
- Indiferente Virreinal (IV)
- Templos y Conventos
- Tributos

Archivo General del Estado de Oaxaca (AGEO)
- Alcaldías Mayores
- Obispado

Archivo General Municipal de Puebla (AGMP)
- Expedientes

Archivo Histórico del Arzobispado de México (AHAM)
- Base Colonial
- Base Pelagio Antonio de Labastida y Dávalos
- Base Siglo XIX

Archivo Histórico del Distrito Federal (AHDF)

Archivo Histórico Judicial de Oaxaca (AHJO)
- Huajuapan Criminal
- Teposcolula Civil
- Villa Alta (VA) Civil
- Villa Alta (VA) Criminal

Archivo Municipal de Guadalajara (AMG)
- Asuntos Eclesiásticos (AE)
- Ayuntamiento (AY)

Bancroft Library, University of California–Berkeley
- Mexican Manuscripts (M-M)

Benson Latin American Library, University of Texas–Austin
Mariano Riva Palacio Papers
The Huntington Library, San Marino, California
José de Gálvez Papers (mssGA)
Mexican Manuscripts (mssHM)
William G. Ritch Collection (mssRI)
Instituto Nacional de Antropología e Historia, Mexico (INAH)
Papeles Sueltos
Zaachila
Tulane University, Latin America Library
Viceregal and Ecclesiastical Mexican Collection (VEMC)

PUBLISHED PRIMARY SOURCES

Acuña, René, ed. *Relaciones geográficas del siglo XVI*. 3 vols. Mexico City: Universidad Nacional Autónoma de México (UNAM), 1984.

Alzate y Ramírez, José Antonio de. *Gacetas de literatura de México*. 4 vols. Puebla, Mexico: Hospital de San Pedro, 1831.

———. *Gazeta de literatura*. 3 vols. Mexico City: Don Felipe de Zúñiga y Ontiveros, 1788–1795.

———. *Memorias y ensayos*, ed. Roberto Moreno. Mexico City: UNAM, 1985.

———. *Obras I. Periódicos*. Mexico City: UNAM, 1980.

Amar, José. *Instrucción curativa de las viruelas, dispuesta para los facultativos y acomodada para todos*. Madrid: D. Joachin Ibarra, 1774.

Bartolache, José Ignacio. *Instrucción que puede servir para que se cure a los enfermos de las viruelas epidémicas que ahora se padecen en México, desde fines del estío, en el año corriente de 1779*. Mexico City: Zúñiga y Ontiveros, 1779.

———. *Mercurio volante (1772–1773)*, ed. Roberto Moreno. Mexico City: UNAM, 1979.

Cabrera y Quintero, Cayetano. *Escudo de armas de México*. Mexico City: Instituto Mexicano del Seguro Social, 1981 [1745].

Campomanes y Sorriba, Pedro Rodríguez. *Discurso sobre el fomento de la industria popular*. Madrid: D. Antonio de Sancha, 1774.

Condamine, Charles Marie de la. *Mémoire sur l'inoculation de la petite vérole: Lu a l'assemblée publique de l'Académie Royale des Sciences, le mercredi 24 avril 1754*. Paris: Chez Durand, 1754.

Consejo Superior de Salubridad. "Iniciativa para celebrar el primer centenario del descubrimiento de la vacuna." *Boletín del Consejo Superior de Salubridad* (May 22, 1896).

Echeverría y Veitia, Mariano Fernández. *Baluartes de México*. 1754. Reprint, Mexico City: Imprenta de A. Valdés, 1820.

Esquivel Navarrete, Joseph. *Sermón eucarístico por la felicidad que logró la ciudad de Durango en la epidemia de viruelas del año de mil setecientos noventa y ocho*. Mexico City: Imprenta Madrileña de Joseph Fernández Jáuregui, 1799.

Estatutos, que la Real Junta Central Filantrópica General de Vacunación Pública de San Carlos de la Ciudad de la Puebla, ha dictado para el establecimiento y gobierno de las foráneas que han de erigirse en toda la Diócesis y Provincia. Puebla, Mexico: D. Pedro de la Rosa, 1805.

Esteyneffer, Juan de. *Florilegio medicinal, de todas las enfermedades: Sacado de varios, y clasicos authores, para bien de los pobres....* Mexico City: Herederos de Juan Joseph Guillena Carrascoto, 1712.

Extracto de la obra publicada en Madrid el año pasado de 1784 con el título de Disertación Físico-Médica...compuesta por Don Francisco Gil, Cirujano del Real Sitio y Monasterio de San Lorenzo. Mexico City, 1788.

Farfán, Agustín. *Tractado brebe de medicina, y de todas las enfermedades....* Mexico City: Casa de Pedro Ocharte, 1592.

Ferrer Gorraiz Beaumont, Vicente. *Juicio, o dictamen, sobre el proceso de la inoculación, presentado al tribunal de los sabios, para que la juzguen....* Pamplona, Spain: Imprenta de Joseph Longas, 1785.

Florencia, Francisco de, and Juan Antonio de Oviedo. *Zodíaco mariano.* Mexico City: Consejo Nacional para la Cultura y las Artes, 1995.

Florescano, Enrique, ed. *Fuentes para la historia de la crisis agrícola de 1785–1786.* 2 vols. Mexico City: AGN, 1981.

Gálvez, José de. *Informe sobre las rebeliones populares de 1767*, ed. Felipe Castro Gutiérrez. Mexico City: UNAM, 1990.

Gazeta de Madrid. Madrid: Imprenta Real, 1806.

Gazeta de México. 14 vols. Mexico City: Don Manuel Antonio Valdés, 1784–1809.

Gil, Francisco. *Disertación físico-médica, en la qual se prescribe un método seguro para preservar a los pueblos de viruelas hasta lograr la completa extinción de ellas en todo el reyno.* Madrid: D. Joaquin Ibarra, 1784.

González del Campillo, Manuel Ignacio. *Exhortacion que el Ilustrísimo Señor Don Miguel Ignacio González del Campillo, obispo electo de la Puebla, hace a sus diocesanos para que se presten con docilidad a la importante práctica de la vacuna.* Mexico City: Don Mariano Joseph de Zúñiga y Ontiveros, 1804.

González-Polo, Ignacio, ed. *Reflexiones y apuntes sobre la Ciudad de México (fines de la colonia).* Mexico City: Departamento del Distrito Federal, 1984.

Hernández, Pedro, trans. and ed. *Orígen y descubrimiento de la vaccina....* Madrid: La Oficina de Don Benito García, y Compañía, 1801.

Instrucción formada para ministrar la vacuna, como único preservativo del contagio de las viruelas, y en efecto de su fluido inocular con el pus de esta; del modo de conocer y distinguir las calidades de las naturales, y el método de curarlas. Mexico City: Don Mariano Ontiveros, 1814.

Instrucción para ministrar la vacuna en las poblaciones donde no hubiere facultativos. Mexico City: Consejo Superior de Salubridad, 1854.

López, Gregorio. *Tesoro de medicinas, para diversas enfermedades.* Mexico City: Francisco Rodriguez Lupercio, 1674.

López de Hinojosos, Alonso. *Summa, y recopilacion de Chirugia, con un Arte para sangrar muy útil y provechosa.* Mexico City: Antonio Ricardo, 1578.

Lorenzana y Buitrón, Francisco Antonio. *Cartas pastorales, y edictos.* Mexico City: Imprenta del Superior Gobierno, 1770.

Mather, Increase. *Several Reasons Proving That Inoculation or Transplanting the*

Small Pox, Is a Lawful Practice, and That It Has Been Blessed by God for the Saving of Many a Life. Boston: S. Kneeland, 1721.

Menós de Llena, Jaime. *Memoria contra la inoculación, sacada de las dudas y disputas entre los autores excitadas acerca de la utilidad, o daños causados por la inoculación de las viruelas....* Manresa, Spain: Ignacio Abadal, 1785.

Método claro, sencillo y fácil que para practicar la Inoculación de viruelas presenta al Público el Real Tribunal del Protomedicato de esta N.E. por Superior orden del Exmo. Señor Marqués de Branciforte Virrey de este Reyno. Mexico City, 1797.

Moreau de la Sarthe, Jacques Louis. *Tratado histórico y práctico de la vacuna*, trans. Francisco Xavier de Balmis. Madrid: Imprenta Real, 1803.

Muñoz Camargo, Diego. *Relaciones geográficas de Tlaxcala*, ed. Rene Acuña. 2nd edition. San Luis Potosí, Mexico: El Colegio de San Luis, 1999.

Núñez de Haro y Peralta, Alonso. *Nos el Dr. D. Alonso Nuñez de Haro y Peralta, por la gracia de Dios.... Por quanto esta N.C. con vivos deseos de socorrer a este público en la presente calamidad de viruelas que le aflixe....* [Mexico City], November 8, 1779.

O'Scanlan, Timoteo. *Ensayo apologético de la inoculacion, o demostracion de lo importante que es al particular, y al Estado*. Madrid: Imprenta Real, 1792.

———. *Practica moderna de la inoculacion: Con varias observaciones y reflexiones fundadas en ella, precedidas de un discurso sobre la utilidad de esta operacion, y un compendio historico de su origen, y de su estado actual, particularmente en España*. Madrid: Imprenta de Hilario Santos, 1784.

Parets, Miquel. *A Journal of the Plague Year: The Diary of the Barcelona Tanner Miquel Parets*, trans. James Amelang. New York: Oxford University Press, 1991.

Prieto, Guilliermo. *Memoria de mis tiempos*. 2 vols. Mexico City: Viuda de C. Bouret, 1906.

Real Cédula sobre diezmos en el pleyto contra las jesuitas. Mexico City, 1736.

Recopilación de leyes de los reinos de las Indias. 3 vols. Madrid: Centro de Estudios Políticos y Constitucionales, 1998 [1681].

Reglamento formado por la Junta Superior de Sanidad del Estado de México, para que se propague y perpetúe la vacuna en todos los Pueblos de la comprensión de aquel. Tlalpam [Mexico City]: Juan Matute y González, 1829 [November 8, 1824].

Riva Fernández, Amanda de la, ed. *Guía de las actas de Cabildo*. Vol. 5. Mexico City: Departamento del Distrito Federal, 1970.

Rodríguez Campomanes y Sorriba, Pedro. *Discurso sobre el fomento de la industria popular*. Madrid: D. Antonio de Sancha, 1774.

Sahagún de Arévalo, Juan Francisco. *Gacetas de México*. 3 vols. Mexico City: Secretaría de Educación Pública, 1950.

Tissot, S.A.D. *Aviso al pueblo acerca de su salud, o Tratado de las enfermedades mas frequentes de las gentes del campo*, trans. Juan Galisteo y Xiorro. Madrid: Imprenta de Pedro Marín, 1790.

Torre Villar, Ernesto de la, ed. *Instrucciones y memorias de los virreyes novohispanos*. Mexico City: Editorial Porrúa, S.A., 1991.

Velasco Ceballos, Rómulo, ed. *La cirugía mexicana en el siglo XVIII*. Mexico City: Archivo Histórico de la Secretaría de Salubridad y Asistencia, 1946.

———. *Visita y reforma de los hospitales de San Juan de Dios de Nueva España*. Vol. 2. Mexico City: Archivo Histórico de la Secretaría de Salubridad y Asistencia, 1945.

Venegas, Juan Manuel. *Compendio de la medicina: O Medicina práctica, en que se declara laconicamente lo mas útil de ella, que el autor tiene observado en estas regiones de Nueva España, para casi todas las enfermedades que acometen al cuerpo humano, dispuesto en forma alfabética*. Mexico City: Felipe de Zúñiga y Ontiveros, 1788.

SECONDARY SOURCES

AHR	*The American Historical Review*
BHR	*Bulletin of the History of Medicine*
HAHR	*Hispanic American Historical Review*

Abrahams, Roger D. "A Performance-Centered Approach to Gossip." *Man* 5:2 (1970): 290–301.

Aceves Pastrana, Patricia. "Átomos y luces en los periódicos de Alzate y Ramírez." In *Periodismo científico en el siglo XVIII: José Antonio de Alzate y Ramírez*, ed. Aceves Pastrana. Mexico City: Universidad Autónoma Metropolitana (UAM)–Xochimilco, 2001.

———, ed. *Medicina, minería e inquisición en la Nueva España: Esteban Morel, 1744–1795*. Mexico City: UAM–Xochimilco, 2002.

———, ed. *Periodismo científico en el siglo XVIII*.

———. *Química, botánica y farmacia en la Nueva España a finales del siglo XVIII*. Mexico City: UAM–Xochimilco, 1993.

Aceves Pastrana, Patricia, and Alba Morales Cosme. "Conflictos y negociaciones en las expediciones de Balmis." *Estudios de historia novohispana* 17 (1997): 171–200.

Achim, Miruna. "From Rustics to Savants: Indigenous *Materia Medica* in Eighteenth-Century Mexico." *Studies in History and Philosophy of Biological and Biomedical Sciences* 42 (2011): 275–284.

———. *Lagartijas medicinales: Remedios americanos y debates científicos en la Ilustración*. Mexico City: UAM–Cuajimalpa, 2008.

———. "Making Lizards into Drugs: The Debates on the Medical Uses of Reptiles in Late Eighteenth-Century Mexico." *Journal of Spanish Cultural Studies* 8:2 (July 2007): 169–191.

Agostoni, Claudia. "Estrategias, actores, promesas y temores en las campañas de vacunación antivariolosa en México: Del Porfiriato a la Posrevolución (1880–1940)." *Ciência y saúde colectiva* 16:2 (2011): 459–470.

Aguirre Beltrán, Gonzalo. *Medicina y magia: El proceso de aculturación en la estructura colonial*. Mexico City: Instituto Nacional Indigenista, 1963.

———. *Regiones de refugio: El desarrollo de la comunidad y el proceso dominical en mestizo América*. Mexico City: Instituto Indigenista Interamericano, 1967.

Alexander, John T. *Bubonic Plague in Early Modern Russia: Public Health and Urban Disaster*. Baltimore, MD: Johns Hopkins University Press, 1980.

Anderson, Benedict. *Imagined Communities: Reflections on the Origin and Spread of Nationalism*. London: Verso, 1991.

Arnold, David. *Colonizing the Body: State Medicine and Epidemic Disease in Nineteenth Century India*. Berkeley: University of California Press, 1993.

Arrom, Silvia. *Containing the Poor: The Mexico City Poor House, 1774–1871*. Durham, NC: Duke University Press, 2001.

Austin, John. *How To Do Things with Words*. Cambridge, MA: Harvard University Press, 1962.

Austin Alchon, Suzanne. *Native Society and Disease in Colonial Ecuador*. New York: Cambridge University Press, 1991.

Ávila, Alfredo. "De las independencias a la modernidad: Notas sobre un cambio historiográfico." In *Conceptualizar lo que se ve: François-Xavier Guerra, historiador, homenaje*, ed. Erika Pani and Alicia Salmerón. Mexico City: Instituto Mora, 2004.

Bailey Glasco, Sharon. *Constructing Mexico City: Colonial Conflicts over Culture, Space, and Authority*. New York: Palgrave Macmillan, 2010.

Baker, Keith M. "Defining the Public Sphere in Eighteenth-Century France: Variations on a Theme by Habermas." In *Habermas and the Public Sphere*, ed. Craig Calhoun. Cambridge, MA: MIT Press, 1992.

Barona, Josep Lluís, Javier Moscoso, and Juan Pimentel, eds. *La Ilustración y las ciencias: Para una historia de la objetividad*. Valencia, Spain: Universitat de València, 2003.

Barrera, Antonio. "Local Herbs, Global Medicines: Commerce, Knowledge, and Commodities in Spanish America." In *Merchants and Marvels: Commerce, Science, and Art in Early Modern Europe*, ed. Pamela H. Smith and Paula Findlen. New York: Routledge, 2002.

Baskes, Jeremy. *Indians, Merchants, and Markets: A Reinterpretation of the Repartimiento and Spanish-Indian Economic Relations in Colonial Oaxaca, 1750–1821*. Stanford, CA: Stanford University Press, 2000.

Beezley, William, Cheryl Martin, and William E. French, eds. *Rituals of Rule, Rituals of Resistance: Public Celebrations and Popular Culture in Mexico*. Wilmington, DE: Scholarly Resources, 1994.

Bell, Rudolph. *How To Do It: Guides to Good Living for Renaissance Italians*. Chicago: University of Chicago Press, 1999.

Benhabib, Seyla. "Models of Public Space: Hannah Arendt, the Liberal Tradition, and Jürgen Habermas." In *Habermas and the Public Sphere*, ed. Craig Calhoun. Cambridge, MA: MIT Press, 1992.

Bensaude-Vincent, Bernadette, and Christine Blondel, eds. *Science and Spectacle in the European Enlightenment*. Burlington, VT: Ashgate Publishing Co., 2008.

Benzaquén, Adriana S. "Childhood, Identity and Human Science in the Enlightenment." *History Workshop Journal* 57 (2004): 35–57.

Bleichmar, Daniela. *Visible Empire: Botanical Expeditions and Visual Culture in the Hispanic Enlightenment*. Chicago: University of Chicago Press, 2012.

———. "A Visible and Useful Empire: Visual Culture and Colonial Natural History in the Eighteenth-Century Spanish World." In *Science in the Spanish and*

Portuguese Empires, 1500–1800, ed. Daniela Bleichmar et al. Stanford, CA: Stanford University Press, 2009.

Bleichmar, Daniela, et al., eds. *Science in the Spanish and Portuguese Empires, 1500–1800*. Stanford, CA: Stanford University Press, 2009.

Bliss, Katherine. "The Science of Redemption: Syphilis, Sexual Promiscuity, and Reformism in Revolutionary Mexico City." *HAHR* 79:1 (February 1999): 1–40.

Bliss, Michael. *The Making of Modern Medicine: Turning Points in the Treatment of Disease*. Chicago: University of Chicago Press, 2011.

Bloom, Lansing B. "Early Vaccination in New Mexico." *Historical Society of New Mexico* 27 (1924): 3–12.

Bolufer Peruga, Mónica. "De la historia de las ideas a la de las prácticas culturales: Reflexiones sobre la historiografía de la Ilustración." In *La ilustración y las ciencias: Para una historia de la objetividad*, ed. Josep Lluís Barona, Javier Moscoso, and Juan Pimentel. Valencia, Spain: Universitat de València, 2003.

Booth, Christopher. *John Haygarth, FRS (1740–1827): Physician of the Enlightenment*. Philadelphia: American Philosophical Society, 2005.

Borah, Woodrow. "Alguna luz sobre el autor de las *Enfermedades políticas*." *Estudios de historia novohispana* 8:8 (1985): 51–79.

Bourdieu, Pierre. *Language and Symbolic Power*, trans. Gino Raymond and Matthew Adamson. Cambridge, MA: Harvard University Press, 1991.

Brading, David A. *The First America: The Spanish Monarchy, Creole Patriots, and the Liberal State, 1492–1867*. Cambridge: Cambridge University Press, 1991.

———. *Mexican Phoenix: Our Lady of Guadalupe: Image and Tradition across Five Centuries*. Cambridge: Cambridge University Press, 2001.

———. *Miners and Merchants in Bourbon Mexico, 1763–1810*. New York: Cambridge University Press, 1971.

———. "Power and Justice in Catorce, 1779–1805." *Ibero-amerikanisches Archiv* 20:3–4 (January 1994): 357–380.

Braudel, Fernand. *The Structures of Everyday Life*. Vol. 1, trans. Sian Reynolds. New York: Harper & Row Publishers, 1981.

Braun, Theodore, and John Radner, eds. *The Lisbon Earthquake of 1755: Representations and Reactions*. Oxford: Voltaire Foundation, 2005.

Brown, Anna, and David Hall. "Family Strategies and Religious Practice: Baptism and the Lord's Supper in Early New England." In *Lived Religion in America: Toward a History of Practice*, ed. David Hall. Princeton, NJ: Princeton University Press, 1997.

Burdette, Derek. "*Caritas* and the Christ of the Seven Veils: The Cult Statue as Confraternal Charity during Mexico City's Smallpox Outbreak of 1779." Paper delivered at the Congress of the Latin American Studies Association, Toronto, 2010.

———. "Miraculous Crucifixes and Colonial Mexican Society: The Artistic, Devotional, and Political Lives of Mexico City's Early-Colonial Cristos." Ph.D diss., Tulane University, 2012.

Burke, Michael E. *The Royal College of San Carlos: Surgery and Spanish Medical Reform in the Late Eighteenth Century*. Durham, NC: Duke University Press, 1977.

Bynum, W. F., Stephen Lock, and Roy Porter, eds. *Medical Journals and Medical Knowledge: Historical Essays*. New York: Routledge, 1992.

Calhoun, Craig, ed. *Habermas and the Public Sphere*. Cambridge, MA: MIT Press, 1992.

Calvo, Hortensia. "The Politics of Print: The Historiography of the Book in Early Spanish America." *Book History* 6 (2003): 277–305.

Camacho Alberto, Neibeth. "Guanajuato y Valladolid de Michoacán durante la epidemia de viruela." In In *El impacto demográfico de la viruela en México de la época colonial al siglo XX*. Vol. 1, ed. Chantal Cramaussel. Zamora, Michoacán: El Colegio de Michoacán, 2010.

Cañeque, Alejandro. *The King's Living Image: The Culture and Politics of Viceregal Power in Colonial Mexico*. New York: Routledge, 2004.

Cañizares-Esguerra, Jorge. *How To Write the History of the New World: Histories, Epistemologies, and Identities in the Eighteenth-Century Atlantic World*. Stanford, CA: Stanford University Press, 2001.

———. Introduction to *Science in the Spanish and Portuguese Empires*, ed. Bleichmar et al.

———. "Nation and Nature: Natural History and the Fashioning of Creole National Identity in Late Colonial Spanish America." Paper delivered at the Latin American Studies Association Meeting, Guadalajara, Mexico, 1997.

———. *Nature, Empire, and Nation: Explorations of the History of Science in the Iberian World*. Stanford, CA: Stanford University Press, 2006.

Carbajal López, David. "La epidemia de viruela de 1830–1831 en el obispado de Guadalajara." In *El impacto demográfico de la viruela en México de la época colonial al siglo XX*. Vol. 2, ed. Chantal Cramaussel and Mario Alberto Magaña Mancillas. Zamora, Michoacán: El Colegio de Michoacán, 2010.

———. *La población en Bolaños, 1740–1848: Dinámica demográfica, familiar y mestizaje*. Zamora, Michoacán: El Colegio de Michoacán, 2008.

Carmagnani, Marcello. *El regreso de los dioses: El proceso de reconstitución de la identidad étnica en Oaxaca, siglos XVII y XVIII*. Mexico City: Fondo de Cultura Económica, 1988.

Carmichael, Ann. *Plague and the Poor in Renaissance Florence*. Cambridge: Cambridge University Press, 1986.

Carreón Nieto, María del Carmen. *Epidemias y desastres en el Obispado de Michoacán, 1737–1804*. Morelia, Michoacán: Morevallado Editores, 2015.

Carrillo, Anna María. "Por voluntad o por fuerza: La lucha contra la viruela en el porfirismo." In *El impacto demográfico de la viruela en México de la época colonial al siglo XX*. Vol. 2, ed. Cramaussel et al.

Cavallo, Sandra. *Charity and Power in Early Modern Italy: Benefactors and Their Motives in Turin, 1541–1789*. Cambridge: Cambridge University Press, 1995.

Certeau, Michel de. *The Practice of Everyday Life*, trans. Steven Rendall. Berkeley: University of California Press, 1984.

———. *The Writing of History*, trans. Tom Conley. New York: Columbia University Press, 1988.

Cervantes Bello, Francisco Javier, et al., eds. *Poder civil y catolicismo en México: Siglos XVI al XIX*. Puebla, Mexico: Benemérita Universidad Autónoma de Puebla, UNAM, 2008.

Chalhoub, Sidney. *Cidade febril: Cortiços e epidemias na corte imperial.* São Paulo: Companhia das Letras, 1996.

———. "The Politics of Disease Control: Yellow Fever and Race in Nineteenth-Century Rio de Janeiro." *Journal of Latin American Studies* 25:5 (1993): 441–463.

Chalhoub, Sidney, et al., eds. *Artes e ofícios de curar no Brasil: Capítulos de história social.* Campinas, Brazil: Universidad Estadual de Campinas, 2003.

Chance, John. *Conquest of the Sierra: Spaniards and Indians in Colonial Oaxaca.* Norman: University of Oklahoma Press, 1989.

———. *Race and Class in Colonial Oaxaca.* Stanford, CA: Stanford University Press, 1978.

Chassen-Lopez, Francie. *From Liberal to Revolutionary Oaxaca: The View from the South.* University Park: Pennsylvania State University Press, 2005.

Chaves de Resende, Maria Leônia. "Entre a cura e a cruz: Jesuítas e pajés nas missões do novo mundo." In *Artes e ofícios de curar no Brasil,* ed. Chalhoub et al.

Chowning, Margaret. "Convent Reform, Catholic Reform, and Bourbon Reform: The View from the Nunnery." *HAHR* 85:1 (February 2005): 1–37.

———. *Rebellious Nuns: The Troubled History of a Mexican Convent, 1752–1863.* New York: Oxford University Press, 2005.

Christian, William A. *Apparitions in Late Medieval and Renaissance Spain.* Princeton, NJ: Princeton University Press, 1981.

———. *Local Religion in Sixteenth Century Spain.* Princeton, NJ: Princeton University Press, 1981.

Cipolla, Carlo. *Faith, Reason, and the Plague in Seventeenth-Century Tuscany,* trans. Muriel Kittel. New York: Norton, 1979.

———. *Public Health and the Medical Profession in the Renaissance.* Cambridge: Cambridge University Press, 1976.

Clark, Fiona. "The *Gazeta de Literatura de México* (1788–1795): The Formation of a Literary-Scientific Periodical in Late-Viceregal Mexico." *Dieciocho* 28:1 (Spring 2005): 7–30.

———. "'Read All About It': Science, Translation, Adaptation, and Confrontation in the Gazeta de Literatura de México, 1788–1795." In *Science in the Spanish and Portuguese Empires, 1500–1800,* ed. Bleichmar et al.

Clark, William, Jan Golinski, and Simon Schaffer, eds. *The Sciences in Enlightened Europe.* Chicago: University of Chicago Press, 1999.

Clendinnen, Inga. "Ways to the Sacred: Reconstructing 'Religion' in Sixteenth-Century Mexico." *History and Anthropology* 5 (1990): 105–141.

Coatsworth, John. "Obstacles to Economic Growth in Nineteenth-Century Mexico." *AHR* 83 (1978): 80–100.

Cody, W. F. "An Index to the Periodicals Published by José Antonio Alzate y Ramírez." *HAHR* 33:3 (August 1953): 442–475.

Conis, Elena. *Vaccine Nation: America's Changing Relationship with Immunizations.* Chicago: University of Chicago Press, 2015.

Connaughton, Brian. *Clerical Ideology in a Revolutionary Age: The Guadalajara Church and the Idea of the Mexican Nation, 1788–1853,* trans. Mark Healey. Boulder: University Press of Colorado, 2003.

———. "Los curas y la feligresía ciudadana en México, siglo XIX." In *Las nuevas naciones: España y México, 1800–1850*, ed. Jaime E. Rodríguez. Madrid: Fundación MAPFRE, 2008.
———. "A Most Delicate Balance: Representative Government, Public Opinion, and Priests in Mexico, 1821–1834." *Mexican Studies/Estudios Mexicanos* 17:1 (2001): 41–69.
———. "Transiciones en la cultura político-religiosa mexicana, siglo XVII–1860: El aguijón de la economía política." In *Poder civil y catolicismo en México, Siglos XVI al XIX*, ed. Cervantes Bello et al.
Cook, Noble David. *Born To Die: Disease and New World Conquest, 1492–1650*. Cambridge: Cambridge University Press, 1998.
Cook, Noble David, and W. George Lovell, eds. *"Secret Judgments of God": Old World Disease in Colonial Spanish America*. Norman: University of Oklahoma Press, 1991.
Cook, Sherburne F. "Francisco Xavier Balmis and the Introduction of Vaccination in Latin America." *BHM* 12:5 (1942): 543–560.
———. "Francisco Xavier Balmis and the Introduction of Vaccination in Latin America." *BHM* 12:6 (1942): 70–101.
———. "The Smallpox Epidemic of 1797 in Mexico." *BHM* 7:1 (1939): 937–969.
———. "Smallpox in Spanish and Mexican California, 1770–1845." *BHM* 7:2 (1939): 153–191.
Cooper, Donald. *Epidemic Disease in Mexico City, 1761–1813: An Administrative, Social, and Medical Study*. Austin: University of Texas Press, 1965.
Cooper, Frederick. "Conflict and Connection: Rethinking Colonial African History." *AHR* 99:5 (December 1994): 1516–1545.
Cope, Douglas R. *The Limits of Racial Domination: Plebeian Society in Colonial Mexico City, 1660–1720*. Madison, WI: University of Wisconsin Press, 1994.
Corbin, Alain. *The Foul and the Fragrant: Odor and the French Social Imagination*. Cambridge, MA: Harvard University Press, 1986.
———. *Village Bells: Sound and Meaning in the 19th-Century French Countryside*, trans. Martin Thom. New York: Columbia University Press, 1998.
Coronil, Fernando. "Smelling Like a Market." *AHR* 106:1 (February 2001): 119–129.
Cramaussel, Chantal, et al., eds. *El impacto demográfico de la viruela en México de la época colonial al siglo XX*. 3 vols. Zamora, Michoacán: El Colegio de Michoacán, 2010.
———. "Epidemias y endemias: La viruela en Chihuahua del siglo XVIII al XX." In *El impacto demográfico de la viruela en México de la época colonial al siglo XX*. Vol. 3, ed. Cramaussel and David Carbajal López.
———. "La lucha contra la viruela en Chihuahua durante el siglo XIX." *Relaciones* 114 (Spring 2008): 101–132.
Cruz Soto, Rosalba. "El nacionalismo de José Antonio de Alzate en el periódico científico *Gaceta de literatura*." In *Periodísmo científico en el siglo XVIII*, ed. Aceves Pastrana.
Cuenya Mateos, Miguel Ángel. *Puebla de los Ángeles en tiempos de una peste colonial*. Zamora, Michoacán: El Colegio de Michoacán, 1999.

Cunningham, Andrew, and Bridie Andrews, eds. *Western Medicine as Contested Knowledge*. New York: Manchester University Press, 1997.
Cunningham, Andrew, and Roger French, eds. *The Medical Enlightenment of the Eighteenth Century*. Cambridge: Cambridge University Press, 1990.
Darnton, Robert. "The High Enlightenment and the Low-Life of Literature in Pre-Revolutionary France." *Past and Present* 51 (1971): 81–115.
Daston, Lorraine, and Peter Galison. "The Image of Objectivity." *Representations* 40 (Autumn 1992): 81–128.
———. *Objectivity*. New York: Zone Books, 2007.
Dávalos, Marcela. *De basuras, inmundicias y movimiento: De cómo se limpiaba la ciudad de México a finales del siglo XIII*. Mexico City: Cien Fuegos, 1989.
de Vos, Paula. "The Art of Pharmacy in Seventeenth- and Eighteenth-Century Mexico." Ph.D. diss., University of California, Berkeley, 2001.
———. "Natural History and the Pursuit of Empire in Eighteenth-Century Spain." *Eighteenth-Century Studies* 40:2 (2007): 209–239.
———. "The Rare, the Singular, and the Extraordinary: Natural History and the Collection of Curiosities in the Spanish Empire." In *Science in the Spanish and Portuguese Empires, 1500–1800*, ed. Bleichmar et al.
———. "Research, Development, and Empire: State Support of Science in the Later Spanish Empire." *Colonial Latin American Review* 15:1 (2006): 55–79.
Decorme, Gerard, S.J. *La obra de los jesuitas mexicanos durante la época colonial, 1572–1767*. Vol. 1. Mexico City: Antigua Libreria Robredo de J. Porrúa e Hijos, 1941.
Delgado Carranco, Susana María. "Un acercamiento a la segunda época del *Diario de México* (1812–1817)." In *Historia de la prensa en Iberoamérica*, ed. Celia del Palacio Montiel. Mexico City: ALTEXTO, 2000.
Desjarlais, Robert. "Presence." In *The Performance of Healing*, ed. Carol Laderman and Marina Roseman. New York: Routledge, 1996.
Donahue-Wallace, Kelly. "Picturing Prints in Early Modern New Spain." *The Americas* 64:3 (January 2008): 325–349.
Ducey, Michael T. "Village, Nation, and Constitution: Insurgent Politics in Papantla, Veracruz, 1810–1821." *HAHR* 79:3 (August 1999): 463–493.
Durbach, Nadja. *Bodily Matters: The Anti-Vaccination Movement in England, 1853–1907*. Durham, NC: Duke University Press, 2005.
Durkheim, Emile. *The Elementary Forms of Religious Life*, trans. Karen E. Fields. New York: The Free Press, 1995 [1912].
Dutcher Mann, Kristin. "Opus Dei, 'The Work of God': Franciscan and Jesuit Music." In *Religion in New Spain*, ed. Susan Schroeder and Stafford Poole. Albuquerque: University of New Mexico Press, 2007.
Earle, Rebecca. *The Body of the Conquistador: Food, Race, and the Colonial Experience in Spanish America, 1492–1700*. Cambridge: Cambridge University Press, 2012.
———. "The Role of Print in the Spanish American Wars of Independence." In *The Political Power of the Word: Press and Oratory in Nineteenth-Century Latin America*, ed. Iván Jaksic. London: Institute of Latin American Studies, 2002.

Early, James. *The Colonial Architecture of Mexico*. Albuquerque: University of New Mexico Press, 1994.
Eire, Carlos. *From Madrid to Purgatory: The Art and Craft of Dying in Sixteenth-Century Spain*. Cambridge: Cambridge University Press, 1995.
Eisenstein, Elizabeth. *The Printing Press as an Agent of Change: Communications and Cultural Transformations in Early Modern Europe*. 2 vols. New York: Cambridge University Press, 1979.
Eley, Geoff. "Nations, Publics, and Political Cultures: Placing Habermas in the Nineteenth Century." In *Habermas and the Public Sphere*, ed. Calhoun.
Emch-Dériaz, Antoinette. *Tissot: Physician of the Enlightenment*. New York: Peter Lang International Academic Publishers, 1992.
Espinosa Cortés, Luz María, and Raúl Miranda Ocampo. "La epidemia de viruela de 1796–1798: De Teotitlán del Valle, Oax., a la Ciudad de México." In *El impacto demográfico de la viruela en México de la época colonial al siglo XX*. Vol. 1, ed. Cramaussel.
Espinosa, Mariola. *Epidemic Invasions: Yellow Fever and the Limits of Cuban Independence, 1870–1930*. Chicago: University of Chicago Press, 2009.
Etlin, Richard. *The Architecture of Death: The Transformation of the Cemetery in Eighteenth-Century Paris*. Cambridge, MA: MIT Press, 1984.
Farge, Arlette. *Subversive Words: Public Opinion in Eighteenth-Century France*, trans. Rosemary Morris. University Park: Pennsylvania State University Press, 1995.
Farge, Arlette, and Jacque Revel. *The Vanishing Children of Paris: Rumor and Politics before the French Revolution*, trans. Claudia Miéville. Cambridge, MA: Harvard University Press, 1991.
Farriss, Nancy. *Maya Society under Colonial Rule: The Colonial Enterprise of Survival*. Princeton, NJ: Princeton University Press, 1984.
Fenn, Elizabeth A. *Pox Americana: The Great Smallpox Epidemic of 1775–82*. New York: Hill and Wang, 2001.
Fernández del Castillo, Francisco. *Los viajes de don Francisco Xavier de Balmis*. Mexico City: Sociedad Médica Hispano Mexicana, 1985 [1960].
Few, Martha. *For All of Humanity: Mesoamerican and Colonial Medicine in Enlightenment Guatemala*. Tucson: University of Arizona Press, 2015.
———. "Medical Mestizaje and the Politics of Pregnancy in Colonial Guatemala, 1660–1730." In *Science in the Spanish and Portuguese Empires, 1500–1800*, ed. Bleichmar et al.
Fields, Sherry. *Pestilence and Headcolds: Encountering Illness in Colonial Mexico*. New York: Columbia University Press, 2008.
Findlen, Paula. *Possessing Nature: Museums, Collecting, and Scientific Culture in Early Modern Italy*. Berkeley: University of California Press, 1994.
Fissell, Mary. "Making a Masterpiece: The Aristotle Texts in Vernacular Medicine Culture." In *Right Living: Anglo-American Tradition of Self-Help Medicine and Hygiene*, ed. Charles Rosenberg. Baltimore: The Johns Hopkins University Press, 2003.
———. "Readers, Texts, and Contexts: Vernacular Medical Works in Early Modern England." In *The Popularization of Medicine, 1650–1850*, ed. Roy Porter. New York: Routledge, 1992.

Florescano, Enrique. *Precios de maíz y crisis agrícolas en México, 1708–1810.* Mexico City: Ediciones Era, 1986.

Florescano, Enrique, and Elsa Malvino, eds. *Ensayos sobre la historia de las epidemias en México.* 2 vols. Mexico City: Instituto Mexicano del Seguro Social, 1982.

Foster, George M. "Hippocrates' Latin American Legacy: 'Hot' and 'Cold' in Contemporary Folk Medicine." In *Colloquia in Anthropology*, ed. R. K. Wetherington, vol. 2. Taos, NM: Fort Burgwin Research Center, 1978.

Fox, Christopher, Roy Porter, and Robert Wokler, eds. *Inventing Human Science: Eighteenth-Century Domains.* Berkeley: University of California Press, 1995.

Foucault, Michel. *Discipline and Punish: The Birth of the Prison*, trans. Alan Sheridan. New York: Vintage Books, 1977.

———. "The Politics of Health in the Eighteenth Century." In *Power/Knowledge: Selected Interviews and Other Writing, 1972–1977*, ed. Colin Gordon. New York: Pantheon Books, 1980.

Franco, Jean. *Plotting Women: Gender and Representation in Mexico.* New York: Columbia University Press, 1989.

Fraser, Nancy. "Rethinking the Public Sphere: A Contribution to the Critique of Actually Existing Democracy." In *Habermas and the Public Sphere*, ed. Calhoun.

Frías Núñez, Marcelo. *Enfermedad y sociedad en la crisis colonial del Antiguo Régimen: Nueva Granada en el tránsito del siglo XVIII al XIX, las epidemias de viruelas.* Madrid: Consejo Superior de Investigaciones Científicas, 1992.

Furdell, Elizabeth Lane. *Publishing and Medicine in Early Modern England.* Rochester, NY: University of Rochester Press, 2002.

García Flores, Raúl. "Morbilidad y vulnerabilidad en una epidemia de viruela: Nuevo Reino de León, 1798." *Relaciones* 114 (Spring 2008): 45–75.

Garner, Richard. "Price Trends in Eighteenth-Century Mexico." *HAHR* 65 (1985): 279–325.

Geertz, Clifford. *The Interpretation of Cultures.* New York: Basic Books, 1973.

Gibson, Charles. *The Aztecs under Spanish Rule: A History of the Indians of the Valley of Mexico, 1519–1810.* Stanford, CA: Stanford University Press, 1964.

Gilman, Sander. *Difference and Pathology: Stereotypes of Sexuality, Race, and Madness.* Ithaca, NY: Cornell University Press, 1985.

Gluckman, Max. "Gossip and Scandal." *Current Anthropology* 4:3 (1963): 307–316.

Golinski, Jan. *British Weather and the Climate of Enlightenment.* Chicago: University of Chicago Press, 2007.

———. *Science as Public Culture: Chemistry and Enlightenment in Britain, 1760–1820.* Cambridge: Cambridge University Press, 1992.

Goodman, Dena. *The Republic of Letters: A Cultural History of the French Enlightenment.* Ithaca, NY: Cornell University Press, 1994.

Granados Salinas, Rosario Inés. "Mexico City's Symbolic Geography: The Processions of Our Lady of Remedios." *Journal of Latin American Geography* 11 (2012): 145–173.

Grandin, Greg. *The Blood of Guatemala: A History of Race and Nation.* Durham, NC: Duke University Press, 2000.

Granjel, Luis. *Anatomía española de la ilustración*. Salamanca, Spain: Universidad de Salamanca, 1963.

Greer, Alan, and Jodi Bilinkoff, eds. *Colonial Saints: Discovering the Holy in the Americas, 1500–1800*. New York: Routledge, 2003.

Grell, Ole Peter, et al., eds. *Religio Medici: Medicine and Religion in Seventeenth-Century England*. Aldershot, England: Scolar Press, 1996.

Gruzinski, Serge. "Las cenizas del deseo: Homosexuales novohispanos a mediados del siglo XVII." In *De la santidad a la perversión: O de por qué no se cumplía la ley de Dios en la sociedad novohispana*, ed. Sergio Ortega. Mexico City: INAH, 1986.

———. *The Conquest of Mexico*, trans. Eileen Corrigan. Cambridge, UK: Polity Press, 1993.

Guardino, Peter. *The Time of Liberty: Popular Political Culture in Oaxaca, 1750–1850*. Durham, NC: Duke University Press, 2005.

Guarisco, Claudia. *Los indios del valle de México y la construcción de una nueva sociabilidad política, 1770–1835*. Zinacantepec, Mexico: Colegio Mexiquense, 2003.

Guedea, Virginia. "La medicina en las gacetas de México." *Mexican Studies/Estudios Mexicanos* 5:2 (Summer 1989): 175–199.

Guerra, Francisco, ed. *El tesoro de medicinas de Gregorio López, 1542–1596: Estudio, texto, y versión*. Madrid: Ediciones Cultura Hispánica del Instituto de Cooperación Iberoamericana, 1982.

Guerra, François-Xavier. *Modernidad e independencias: Ensayos sobre las revoluciones hispánicas*. Madrid: Editorial MAPFRE, 1992.

———. "The Spanish-American Tradition of Representation and Its European Roots." *Journal of Latin American Studies* 26:1 (February 1994): 1–35.

Guerra, François-Xavier, and Annick Lempérière, eds. *Los espacios públicos en Iberoamerica: Ambigüedades y problemas, siglos XVIII–XIX*. Mexico City: Centro Francés de Estudios Mexicanos y Centroamericanos, Fondo de Cultura Económica, 1998.

———. Introduction to *Los espacios públicos en Iberoamerica*, ed. Guerra and Lempérière.

Guerrini, Anita. "Newtonianism, Medicine and Religion." In *Religio Medici*, ed. Grell et al.

Guha, Ranajit. "On Some Aspects of the Historiography of Colonial India." In *Selected Subaltern Studies*, ed. Ranajit Guha and Chakravorty Spivak. New York: Oxford University Press, 1988.

———. "The Prose of Counter-Insurgency." In *Selected Subaltern Studies*, ed. Guha and Spivak.

Guha, Ranajit, and Gayatri Chakravorty Spivak, eds. *Selected Subaltern Studies*. New York: Oxford University Press, 1988.

Gunn, J.A.W. *Queen of the World: Opinion in the Public Life of France from the Renaissance to the Revolution*. Oxford: Voltaire Foundation, 1995.

Gurevich, Aron. *Medieval Popular Culture: Problems of Belief and Perception*, trans. Janos M. Bak and Paul A. Hollingworth. Cambridge: Cambridge University Press, 1988.

Hall, David, ed. *Lived Religion in America: Toward a History of Practice*. Princeton, NJ: Princeton University Press, 1997.

Hanks, William F. "Discourse Genres in a Theory of Practice." *American Ethnologist* 14:4 (1987): 64–88.

———. *Intertexts: Writings on Language, Utterance, and Context*. New York: Rowman & Littlefield Publishers, 2000.

Harris, Olivia. "The Coming of the White People: Reflections on the Mythologization of History in Latin America." *Bulletin of Latin American Research* 14:1 (1995): 9–24.

Headrick, Daniel. *When Information Came of Age: Technologies of Knowledge in the Age of Reason and Revolution, 1700–1850*. New York: Oxford University Press, 2000.

Hernández Palomo, José Jesús, ed. *Enfermedad y muerte en América y Andalucía (Siglos XVI–XX)*. Seville, Spain: Escuela de Estudios Hispano-Americanos, 2004.

Hernández Sáenz, Luz María. *Learning To Heal: The Medical Profession in Colonial Mexico, 1767–1831*. New York: Peter Lang Publishers, 1997.

Herrejón Peredo, Carlos. *Del sermón al discurso cívico, México, 1760–1834*. Zamora, Michoacán: El Colegio de Michoacán, El Colegio de México, 2003.

Hopkins, Donald. *Princes and Peasants: Smallpox in History*. Chicago: University of Chicago Press, 1983.

Houdaille, Jacques. "Frenchmen and Francophiles in New Spain from 1760 to 1810." *The Americas* 13:1 (July 1956): 1–29.

Howard, David A. *The Royal Indian Hospital of Mexico City*. Tempe: Center for Latin American Studies, Arizona State University, 1990.

Huguet-Termes, Teresa. "New World Materia Medica in Spanish Renaissance Medicine: From Scholarly Reception to Practical Input." *Medical History* 45 (2001): 358–376.

Ibarra, Ana Carolina. "De tareas ingratas y épocas difíciles: Francisco Xavier de Lizana y Beaumont, Arzobispo de México, 1802–1811." In *Poder civil y catolicismo en México*, ed. Cervantes Bello et al.

Jacobs, Margaret C., and Larry Stewart. *Practical Matter: Newton's Science in the Service of Industry and Empire, 1687–1751*. Cambridge, MA: Harvard University Press, 2004.

Jaffary, Nora E. *False Mystics: Deviant Orthodoxy in Colonial Mexico*. Lincoln: University of Nebraska Press, 2004.

Jaksic, Iván, ed. *The Political Power of the Word: Press and Oratory in Nineteenth-Century Latin America*. London: Institute of Latin American Studies, 2002.

Jones, David. *Rationalizing Epidemics: Meanings and Uses of American Indian Mortality since 1600*. Cambridge, MA: Harvard University Press, 2004.

Jones, Oakah. *Los Paisanos: Spanish Settlers on the Northern Frontier of New Spain*. Norman: University of Oklahoma Press, 1979.

Kellogg, Susan. *Weaving the Past: A History of Latin America's Indigenous Women from the Prehispanic Period to the Present*. New York: Oxford University Press, 2005.

Kuethe, Allan J., and Lowell Blaisdell. "French Influence and the Origins of Bourbon Colonial Reorganization." *HAHR* 71:3 (August 1991): 579–608.

Laderman, Carol, and Marina Roseman, eds. *The Performance of Healing*. New York: Routledge, 1996.

Lafuente, Antonio. "Institucionalización metropolitana de la ciencia española en el siglo XVIII." In *Ciencia colonial en América*, ed. Lafuente and Sala Catalá.

Lafuente, Antonio, and José Sala Catalá, eds. *Ciencia colonial en América*. Madrid: Alianza Editorial, S.A., 1992.

Lafuente, Antonio, and Leoncio López-Ocón. "Tradiciones científicas y expediciones ilustradas en la América hispana del siglo XVIII." In *Historia social de las ciencias en América Latina*, ed. Juan José Saldaña. Mexico City: UNAM, 1996.

Lafuente, Antonio, and Nuria Valverde. "Linnaean Botany and Spanish Imperial Biopolitics." In *Colonial Botany: Science, Commerce, and Politics in the Early Modern World*, ed. Londa Schiebinger and Claudia Swan. Philadelphia: University of Pennsylvania Press, 2005.

Lambert, Helen. "Plural Traditions? Folk Therapeutics and 'English' Medicine in Rajasthan." In *Western Medicine as Contested Knowledge*, ed. Cunningham and Andrews.

Landes, Joan. *Women and the Public Sphere in the Age of the French Revolution*. Ithaca, NY: Cornell University Press, 1988.

Lanning, John Tate. *The Royal Protomedicato: The Regulation of the Medical Professions in the Spanish Empire*. Durham, NC: Duke University Press, 1985.

Larkin, Brian. *The Very Nature of God: Baroque Catholicism and Religious Reform in Bourbon Mexico City*. Albuquerque: University of New Mexico Press, 2010.

Lawrence, Christopher. "Medical Minds, Surgical Bodies: Corporeality and the Doctors." In *Science Incarnate: Historical Embodiments of Natural Knowledge*, ed. Christopher Lawrence and Steven Shapin. Chicago: University of Chicago Press, 1998.

Lawrence, Christopher, and Steven Shapin, eds. *Science Incarnate: Historical Embodiments of Natural Knowledge*. Chicago: University of Chicago Press, 1998.

León García, María del Carmen. "Espacio, olor y salubridad en Toluca al final del siglo XVIII." *Historia Mexicana* 52:1 (2002): 163–199.

León Sanz, Pilar, and Dolores Barettino Coloma. *Vicente Ferrer Gorraiz Beaumont y Montesa (1718–1792), un polemista navarro de la Ilustración*. Pamplona: Fondo de Publicaciones del Gobierno de Navarra, 2007.

Lévi-Strauss, Claude. *The Raw and the Cooked*, trans. John and Doreen Weightman. Chicago: University of Chicago Press, 1969.

———. *The Savage Mind*, trans. George Weidenfield and Nicholson Ltd. Chicago: University of Chicago Press, 1966.

Levitt, Marcus C. *Visual Dominant in Eighteenth-Century Russia*. DeKalb: Northern Illinois University Press, 2012.

Lipsett-Rivera, Sonya. *Gender and the Negotiation of Daily Life in Mexico, 1750–1856*. Lincoln: University of Nebraska Press, 2012.

Lomnitz, Claudio. *Deep Mexico, Silent Mexico: An Anthropology of Nationalism*. Minneapolis: University of Minnesota Press, 2001.

López Austin, Alfredo. *The Human Body and Ideology: Concepts of the Ancient*

Nahuas. Vol. 1, trans. Thelma Ortiz de Montellano et al. Salt Lake City: University of Utah Press, 1988.

Lynch, Kevin. *The Image of the City*. Cambridge, MA: MIT Press, 1960.

Machuca Gallegos, Laura. *Comercio de sal y redes de poder en Tehuantepec durante la época colonial*. Mexico City: Centro de Investigaciones y Estudios Superiores en Antropología Social, 2007.

———. "La viruela de 1795–1797 en Tehuantepec, Oaxaca." In *El impacto demográfico de la viruela en México de la época colonial al siglo XX*. Vol. 1, ed. Cramaussel.

MacLeod, Roy. Introduction to *Disease, Medicine, and Empire: Perspectives on Western Medicine and the Experience of European Expansion*, ed. Roy MacLeod and Milton Lewis. New York: Routledge, 1988.

MacLeod, Roy, and Milton Lewis, eds. *Disease, Medicine, and Empire: Perspectives on Western Medicine and the Experience of European Expansion*. New York: Routledge, 1988.

Magaña Mancillas, Mario Alberto, ed. *Epidemias y rutas de propagación en la Nueva España y México (siglos XVIII–XIX)*. Mexicali, Baja California, Mexico: Universidad Autónoma de Baja California, 2013.

Manning, Susan, and Francis Cogliano, eds. *The Atlantic Enlightenment*. Burlington, VT: Ashgate Publishing Company, 2008.

Maravall, José Antonio. *Culture of the Baroque: Analysis of a Historical Structure*. Minneapolis: University of Minnesota Press, 1986.

Mark, Catherine, and José G. Rigau-Pérez. "The World's First Immunization Campaign: The Spanish Smallpox Vaccine Expedition, 1803–1813." *BHM* 83:1 (2009): 63–94.

Marcuse, Edgar. "Prudent Personal Belief Exemption Policies." *Archives of Pediatrics and Adolescent Medicine* 166:12 (December 2012): 1093–1094. .

Márquez Morfín, Lourdes. *La desigualdad ante la muerte en la Ciudad de México: El tifo y el cólera, 1813 y 1833*. Mexico City: Siglo XXI, 1994.

Marten, James, ed. *Children in Colonial America*. New York: New York University, 2007

Martínez, María Elena. *Genealogical Fictions: Limpieza de Sangre, Religion, and Gender in Colonial Mexico*. Stanford, CA: Stanford University Press, 2009.

Martínez Duran, Carlos. *Las ciencias médicas en Guatemala*. 3rd edition. Guatemala City, Guatemala: Editorial Universitaria, 1964.

Mauss, Marcel. *The Gift: The Form and Reason for Exchange in Archaic Societies*, trans. W. D. Halls. 1950; reprint, New York: W.W. Norton, 1990.

Mazín Gómez, Oscar. *Entre dos majestades: El obispo y la iglesia del gran Michoacán ante las reformas borbónicas (1758–1772)*. Zamora, Michoacán: El Colegio de Michoacán, 1987.

———. "Reorganización del clero secular novohispano en la segunda mitad del siglo XVIII." *Relaciones* 39 (1989): 69–86.

McCaa, Robert. "Inoculation: An Easy Means of Protecting People or Propagating Smallpox?" *Boletín Mexicano de Historia y Filosofía de la Medicina* 1:2 (1998): 4–11.

———. "Revisioning Smallpox in Mexico City-Tenochtitlán, 1520–1950: What Difference Did Charity, Quarantine, Inoculation, and Vaccination Make?" In

Living in the City, 14th–20th Centuries, ed. Eugenio Sonnino. Rome: Casa Editrice, 2004.
McClellan III, James. *Colonialism and Science: Saint Domingue in the Old Regime*, 2nd ed. 1992; reprint, Chicago: University of Chicago Press, 2010.
McCrea, Heather. *Diseased Relations: Epidemics, Public Health, and State Building in Yucatán, Mexico, 1847–1924*. Albuquerque: University of New Mexico Press, 2011.
Meade, Teresa. *"Civilizing" Rio: Reform and Resistance in a Brazilian City, 1889–1930*. University Park: Penn State University Press, 1997.
Melton, James van Horn. *The Rise of the Public in Enlightenment Europe*. New York: Cambridge University Press, 2001.
Molina del Villar, América. *La Nueva España y el matlazahuatl, 1736–1739*. Mexico City: Centro de Investigaciones y Estudios Superiores en Antropología Social, 2001.
———. *Por voluntad divina: Escasez, epidemias y otras calamidades en la Ciudad de México, 1700–1762*. Mexico City: Centro de Investigaciones y Estudios Superiores en Antropología Social, 1996.
Moravia, Sergio. "The Enlightenment and the Sciences of Man." *History of Science* 18 (1990): 247–268.
Moreno, Roberto. *Ensayos de historia de la ciencia y la tecnología en México*. Mexico City: UNAM, 1986.
Murphy, Kathleen. "Translating the Vernacular: Indigenous and African Knowledge in the Eighteenth-Century British Atlantic." *Atlantic Studies* 8:1 (March 2011): 29–48.
Nachman, Robert. "Positivism and Revolution in Brazil's First Republic: The 1904 Revolt." *The Americas* 24:1 (1977): 20–39.
Navarro García, Ramón. "Análisis de los documentos esenciales sobre la Real Expedición de Balmis-Salvany." In *La Real Expedición Filantrópica de la Vacuna: Doscientos años de lucha contra la viruela*, ed. Susana María Ramírez Martín, Luís Valenciano, Rafael Nájera, and Luis Enjuanes. Madrid: Consejo Superior de Investigaciones Científicas, 2004.
Needell, Jeffrey. "The *Revolta Contra Vacina* of 1904: The Revolt Against 'Modernization' in Belle-Époque Rio de Janeiro." *HAHR* 67:2 (May 1987): 233–269.
Nelson, Cary, and Lawrence Grossberg, eds. *Marxism and the Interpretation of Culture*. London: Macmillan, 1988.
Newson, Linda A. *Life and Death in Early Colonial Ecuador*. Norman: University of Oklahoma Press, 1995.
Norman, Donald. *The Design of Everyday Things*. New York: Basic Books, 1988.
Norton, Mary. *Sacred Gifts, Profane Pleasures: A History of Tobacco and Chocolate in the Atlantic World*. Ithaca, NY: Cornell University Press, 2008.
Numbers, Ronald, ed. *Medicine in the New World: New Spain, New France, and New England*. Knoxville: University of Tennessee Press, 1987.
O'Gorman, Edmundo. "Reflexiones sobre la distribución urbana colonial de la ciudad de México." In *Seis estudios históricos de tema mexicano*, ed. Edmundo O'Gorman. Xalapa, Mexico: Universidad Veracruzana, 1960.
O'Hara, Matthew. *A Flock Divided: Race, Religion, and Politics in Mexico, 1749–1857*. Durham, NC: Duke University Press, 2009.

Osores y Sotomayor, Félix. *Colegios de la ciudad de México*. Mexico City: Talleres Gráficos de la Nación, 1929.
Osowski, Edward. *Indigenous Miracles: Nahua Authority in Colonial Mexico*. Tucson: University of Arizona Press, 2010.
Owensby, Brian. *Empire of Law and Indian Justice in Colonial Mexico*. Stanford, CA: Stanford University Press, 2008.
Pani, Erika, and Alicia Salmerón, eds. *Conceptualizar lo que se ve: François-Xavier Guerra, historiador, homenaje*. Mexico City: Instituto Mora, 2004.
Paquette, Gabriel, ed. *Enlightened Reform in Southern Europe and Its Atlantic Colonies, c. 1750–1830*. Burlington, VT: Ashgate Publishing Co., 2009.
———. *Enlightenment, Governance, and Reform in Spain and Its Empire, 1759–1808*. New York: Palgrave Macmillan, 2008.
Pardo-Tomás, José. "'Antiguamente vivían más sanos que ahora': Explanations of Native Mortality in the Relaciones Geográficas de Indias." In *Medical Cultures of the Early Modern Spanish Empire*, ed. John Slater, Maríaluz López-Terrada, and José Pardo-Tomás. Burlington, VT: Ashgate Publishing Company, 2014.
Parrish, Susan Scott. *American Curiosity: Cultures of Natural History in the Colonial British Atlantic World*. Chapel Hill: University of North Carolina Press, 2006.
Pastor, Rodolfo. *Campesinos y reformas: La mixteca, 1700–1865*. Mexico City: Colegio de México, Centro de Estudios Históricos, 1985.
Perdiguero, Enrique. "Popularizando la ciencia: El caso de la medicina doméstica en la España de la Ilustración." In *La Ilustración y las ciencias*, ed. Barona et al.
———. "The Popularization of Medicine during the Spanish Enlightenment." In *The Popularization of Medicine, 1650–1850*, ed. Roy Porter. New York: Routledge, 1992.
Pérez Toledo, Sonia. *Trabajadores, espacio urbano y sociabilidad en la Ciudad de México, 1790–1867*. Mexico City: UAM, Miguel Ángel Porrúa, 2011.
Peset, José Luis. "Símbolos e ideas en torno al concepto de naturaleza." In *Periodismo científico en el siglo XVIII*, ed. Aceves Pastrana.
Phelan, John Leddy. *The People and the King: The Comunero Revolution in Colombia, 1781*. Madison: University of Wisconsin Press, 1978.
Piccato, Pablo. "Public Sphere in Latin America: A Map of the Historiography." *Social History* 35:2 (May 2010): 165–192.
Pierce, Donna, Rogelio Ruiz Gomar, and Clara Bargellini, eds. *Painting a New World: Mexican Art and Life, 1521–1821*. Denver, CO: Denver Art Museum, 2004.
Pizzigoni, Caterina. *The Life Within: Local Indigenous Society in Mexico's Toluca Valley, 1650–1800*. Stanford, CA: Stanford University Press, 2012.
Pino Díaz, Fermín del, ed. *Ciencia y contexto histórico nacional en las expediciones ilustradas a América*. Madrid: Consejo Superior de Investigaciones Científicas, 1988.
Plotkin, Susan, and Stanley Plotkin. "A Short History of Vaccination." In *Vaccines*, 4th edition, ed. Stanley Plotkin and Walter Orenstein. Philadelphia: Saunders, 2004.
Porter, Dorothy. *Health, Civilization, and the State: A History of Public Health from Ancient to Modern Times*. New York: Routledge, 1999.

Porter, Roy. *Bodies Politic: Disease, Death, and Doctors in Britain, 1650–1900*. Ithaca, NY: Cornell University Press, 2001.

———. *The Greatest Benefit to Mankind: A Medical History of Humanity*. New York: W.W. Norton & Company, 1997.

———. "Laymen, Doctors, and Medical Knowledge in the Eighteenth Century: The Evidence of the *Gentleman's Magazine*." In *Patients and Practitioners: Lay Perceptions of Medicine in Pre-Industrial Society*, ed. Roy Porter. Cambridge: Cambridge University Press, 1985.

———. "Medical Science and Human Science in the Enlightenment." In *Inventing Human Science*, ed. Fox et al.

———. "The Rise of Medical Journalism in Britain to 1800." In *Medical Journals and Medical Knowledge*, ed. Bynum et al.

———, ed. *Patients and Practitioners: Lay Perceptions of Medicine in Pre-Industrial Society*. Cambridge: Cambridge University Press, 1985.

———, ed. *The Popularization of Medicine, 1650–1850*. New York: Routledge, 1992.

Porter, Roy, and Dorothy Porter. *Patient's Progress: Doctors and Doctoring in Eighteenth-Century England, 1650–1850*. Stanford, CA: Stanford University Press, 1989.

———. *In Sickness and in Health: The British Experience, 1650–1850*. London: Fourth Estate, 1988.

Price, Robin. "State, Church, Charity, and Smallpox: An Epidemic Crisis in the City of Mexico, 1797–98." *Journal of the Royal Society of Medicine* 75 (May 1982): 356–367.

Prieto, Andrés. *Missionary Scientists: Jesuit Science in Spanish South America, 1570–1810*. Nashville, TN: Vanderbilt University Press, 2011.

Puerto Sarmiento, Francisco Javier. *La ilusión quebrada: Botánica, sanidad y política científica en la España Ilustrada*. Madrid: Consejo Superior de Investigaciones Científicas, 1988.

Pullan, Brian. "Plague and Perceptions of the Poor in Early Modern Italy." In *Epidemics and Ideas*, ed. Ranger and Slack.

———. *Rich and Poor in Renaissance Venice: The Social Institutions of a Catholic State, to 1620*. Cambridge, MA: Harvard University Press, 1971.

Quezada, Noemí. *Enfermedad y maleficio: El curandero en el México colonial*. Mexico City: UNAM, 1989.

Rama, Angel. *The Lettered City*, trans. John Charles Chasteen. Durham, NC: Duke University Press, 1996.

Radding, Cynthia. *Wandering Peoples: Colonialism, Ethnic Spaces, and Ecological Frontiers in Northwestern Mexico, 1700–1850*. Durham, NC: Duke University Press, 1997.

Ramírez, Paul, and William B. Taylor. "Out of Tlatelolco's Ruins: Patronage, Devotion, and Natural Disaster at the Shrine of Our Lady of the Angels, 1745–1781." *HAHR* 93:1 (February 2013): 33–65.

Ramírez Martín, Susana María. "Fuentes bibliográficas para el estudio de la inoculación y la vacunación en la Nueva España." In *El impacto demográfico de la viruela en México de la época colonial al siglo XX*. Vol. 1, ed. Cramaussel.

———. *La mayor hazaña médica de la colonia: La Real Expedición Filantrópica de la Vacuna en la Real Audiencia de Quito*. Quito: ABYA–YALA, 1999.
———. *La salud del Imperio: La Real Expedición Filantrópica de la Vacuna*. Aranjuez, Spain: Ediciones Doce Calles, 2001.
Ramírez Martín, Susana María, Luís Valenciano, Rafael Nájera, and Luis Enjuanes, eds. *La Real Expedición Filantrópica de la Vacuna: Doscientos años de lucha contra la viruela*. Madrid: Consejo Superior de Investigaciones Científicas, 2004.
Ramsey, Matthew. *Professional and Popular Medicine in France, 1770–1830: The Social World of Medical Practice*. Cambridge: Cambridge University Press, 1988.
Ranger, Terence, and Paul Slack, eds. *Epidemics and Ideas: Essays on the Historical Perception of Pestilence*. Cambridge: Cambridge University Press, 1992.
Razzell, Peter. *The Conquest of Smallpox: The Impact of Inoculation on Smallpox Mortality in Eighteenth-Century Britain*. Firle, UK: Caliban Books, 1977.
Reff, Daniel T. *Disease, Depopulation, and Culture Change in Northwestern New Spain, 1518–1764*. Salt Lake City: University of Utah Press, 1991.
Ricard, Robert. *The Spiritual Conquest of Mexico*, trans. Lesley Byrd Simpson. Berkeley: University of California Press, 1966.
Riera, Juan, and Juan Granda-Juesas, eds. *La inoculación de la viruela en la España ilustrada*. Valladolid: Universidad de Valladolid, Secretariado de Publicaciones, 1987.
Rigau-Pérez, José. "The Introduction of Smallpox Vaccine in 1803 and the Adoption of Immunization as a Government Function in Puerto Rico." *HAHR* 69:3 (August 1989): 393–423.
———. "Surgery at the Service of Theology: Postmortem Cesarean Sections in Puerto Rico and the Royal Cedula of 1804." *HAHR* 75:3 (August 1995): 377–404.
Riskin, Jessica. *Science in the Age of Sensibility: The Sentimental Empiricists of the French Enlightenment*. Chicago: University of Chicago Press, 2002.
Rodríguez, Martha Eugenia. *Contaminación e insalubridad en la ciudad de México en el siglo XVIII*. Mexico City: Facultad de Medicina, UNAM, 2000.
———. "El doctor José Felipe Flores, primer Protomédico de Guatemala." *Boletín Mexicano de Historia y Filosofía de la Medicina* 13 (1990): 111–123.
Rosen, George. *A History of Public Health*. Baltimore, MD: Johns Hopkins University Press, 1993.
Rosenberg, Charles. *Explaining Epidemics, and Other Studies in the History of Medicine*. Cambridge: Cambridge University Press, 1992.
———. "Medical Text and Social Context: Explaining William Buchan's Domestic Medicine." *BHM* 57:1 (Spring 1983): 22–42.
———. "What Is an Epidemic? AIDS in Historical Perspective." *Daedalus* 118:2 (1989): 1–17.
———, ed. *Right Living: An Anglo-American Tradition of Self-Help Medicine and Hygiene*. Baltimore: The Johns Hopkins University Press, 2003.
Ross, Paul. "Mexico's Superior Health Council and the American Public Health Association: The Transnational Archive of Porfirian Public Health, 1887–1910." *HAHR* 89:4 (2009): 573–602.

Ruiz Castañeda, María del Carmen. "La tercera gaceta de la Nueva España: *Gazeta de México* (1784–1809)." *Boletín del Instituto de Investigaciones Bibliográficas* (July–December 1971): 137–150.

Rusnock, Andrea. "Biopolitics: Political Arithmetic in the Enlightenment." In *The Sciences in Enlightened Europe*, ed. Clark et al.

———. *Vital Accounts: Quantifying Health and Population in Eighteenth-Century England and France.* Cambridge: Cambridge University Press, 2002.

Ryan, Mary P. "Gender and Public Access: Women's Politics in Nineteenth-Century America." In *Habermas and the Public Sphere*, ed. Craig Calhoun. Cambridge, MA: MIT Press, 1992.

Sahlins, Marshall. *Islands of History*. Chicago: University of Chicago Press, 1985.

Saladino García, Alberto. *Ciencia y prensa durante la ilustración latinoamericana.* Mexico City: UNAM, 1992.

———. *Dos científicos de la Ilustración hispanoamericana: J. A. Alzate y F. J. de Caldas*. Mexico City: UNAM, Universidad Autónoma del Estado de México, 1990.

———. "José Antonio de Alzate y Ramírez: Figura de la cultura novohispana del siglo XVIII." In *Periodismo científico en el siglo XVIII*, ed. Aceves Pastrana.

Saldaña, Juan José. "Ciencia y felicidad pública en la Ilustración americana." In *Historia social de las ciencias en América Latina*, ed. Saldaña.

———, ed. *Historia social de las ciencias en América Latina*. Mexico City: UNAM, 1996.

———. "Introducción: Teatro científico americano." In *Historia social de las ciencias en América Latina*, ed. Saldaña.

Salgado Pimenta, Tânia. "Barbeiros-sangradores e curandeiros no Brasil (1808–28)." *História, ciências, saúde-manguinhos* 5:2 (July–October 1998): 349–72.

Schaffer, Simon. "Measuring Virtue: Eudiometry, Enlightenment and Pneumatic Medicine." In *The Medical Enlightenment of the Eighteenth Century*, ed. Cunningham and French.

Scheper-Hughes, Nancy, and Margaret Lock. "The Mindful Body: A Prolegomenon to Future Work in Medical Anthropology." *Medical Anthropology Quarterly* 1:1 (1987): 6–41.

Schiebinger, Londa. "The Anatomy of Difference: Race and Sex in Eighteenth-Century Science." *Eighteenth-Century Studies* 23:4 (Summer 1990): 387–405.

———. *The Mind Has No Sex? Women in the Origins of Modern Science*. Cambridge, MA: Harvard University Press, 1989.

———. *Plants and Empire: Colonial Bioprospecting in the Atlantic World*. Cambridge, MA: Harvard University Press, 2004.

———. *Secret Cures of Slaves: People, Plants, and Medicine in the Eighteenth-Century Atlantic World*. Stanford, CA: Stanford University Press, 2017.

Schiebinger, Londa, and Claudia Swan, eds. *Colonial Botany: Science, Commerce, and Politics in the Early Modern World*. Philadelphia: University of Pennsylvania Press, 2005.

Schifter Aceves, Liliana. *Medicina, minería e inquisición en la Nueva España: Esteban Morel, 1744–1795*. Mexico City: UAM–Xochimilco, 2002.

Schroeder, Susan. "Jesuits, Nahuas, and the Good Death Society in Mexico City, 1718–1767." *HAHR* 80:1 (February 2000): 43–76.

Schroeder, Susan and Stafford Poole, eds. *Religion in New Spain*. Albuquerque: University of New Mexico Press, 2007.

Scott, James. *Seeing Like a State: How Certain Schemes to Improve the Human Condition Have Failed*. New Haven, CT: Yale University Press, 1998.

Scott, Robert A. *Miracle Cures: Saints, Pilgrimage, and the Healing Powers of Belief*. Berkeley: University of California Press, 2010.

Sennhauser, Rolf Widmer. "Política sanitaria y lucha social en tiempos de viruelas: Corona, comercio y comunidades indígenas en Tehuantepec, 1795–96." *Relaciones* 44 (Winter 1991): 33–74.

Serrano, Sol, and Iván Jaksic. "Church and Liberal State Strategies on the Dissemination of Print in Nineteenth-Century Chile." In *The Political Power of the Word*, ed. Jaksic.

Shapin, Steven. "The Philosopher and the Chicken: On the Dietetics of Disembodied Knowledge." In *Science Incarnate*, ed. Lawrence and Shapin.

———. *A Social History of Truth: Civility and Science in Seventeenth-Century England*. Chicago: University of Chicago Press, 1995.

———. "Trusting George Cheyne: Scientific Expertise, Common Sense, and Moral Authority in Early Eighteenth-Century Dietetic Medicine." *BHM* 77:2 (2003): 263–97.

Shapin, Steven and Simon Schaffer. *Leviathan and the Air Pump: Hobbes, Boyle, and the Experimental Life*. Princeton, NJ: Princeton University Press, 1985.

Sheehan, Jonathan. "Enlightenment, Religion, and the Enigma of Secularization: A Review Essay." *AHR* 108:4 (October 2003): 1061–1080.

Silva, Renán. "Prácticas de lectura, ámbitos privados y formación de un espacio público moderno." In *Los espacios públicos en Iberoamerica*, ed. Guerra and Lempérière.

Silva Prada, Natalia. "El uso de los baños temascales en la visión de dos médicos novohispanos." *Historia Mexicana* 52:1 (2002): 5–56.

Simmons, Marc. *Spanish Pathways: Readings in the History of Hispanic New Mexico*. Albuquerque: University of New Mexico Press, 2001.

Slack, Paul. *The Impact of Plague in Tudor and Stuart England*. Boston: Routledge, 1985.

———. Introduction to *Epidemics and Ideas: Essays on the Historical Perception of Pestilence*, ed. Terence Ranger and Paul Slack. Cambridge: Cambridge University Press, 1992.

———. "Mirrors of Health and Treasures of Poor Men: The Uses of the Vernacular Medical Literature of Tudor England." In *Health, Medicine and Mortality in the Sixteenth Century*, ed. Charles Webster. New York: Cambridge University Press, 1979.

Slater, John, Maríaluz López-Terrada, and José Pardo-Tomás, eds. *Medical Cultures of the Early Modern Spanish Empire*. Burlington, VT: Ashgate Publishing Company, 2014.

Smith, Michael. "Balmis en la Nueva España." In *La Real Expedición Filantrópica de la Vacuna*, ed. Ramírez Martín et al.

———. *The "Real Expedición Marítima de la Vacuna" in New Spain and Guatemala*. Philadelphia: American Philosophical Society, 1974.

Smith, Pamela H., and Paula Findlen. Introduction to *Merchants and Marvels:*

Commerce, Science, and Art in Early Modern Europe, ed. Smith and Findlen. New York: Routledge, 2002.

———, eds. *Merchants and Marvels: Commerce, Science, and Art in Early Modern Europe*. New York: Routledge, 2002.

Sousa, Lisa. "Women and Crime in Colonial Oaxaca: Evidence of Complementary Gender Roles in Mixtec and Zapotec Societies." In *Indian Women of Early Mexico*, ed. Susan Schroeder, Stephanie Wood, and Robert Haskett. Norman: University of Oklahoma Press, 1997.

Spivak, Gayatri Chakravorty. "Can the Subaltern Speak?" In *Marxism and the Interpretation of Culture*, ed. Nelson and Grossberg.

Starn, Randolph. Foreword to Giulia Calvi, *Histories of a Plague Year: The Social and the Imaginary in Baroque Florence*, trans. Diario Biocca and Bryant T. Ragan, Jr. Berkeley: University of California Press, 1989.

Stein, Stanley, and Barbara Stein. *Apogee of Empire: Spain and New Spain in the Age of Charles III, 1759–1789*. Baltimore, MD: Johns Hopkins University Press, 2003.

Stepan, Nancy. *"The Hour of Eugenics": Race, Gender, and Nation in Latin America*. Ithaca, NY: Cornell University Press, 1996.

———. "Race and Gender: The Role of Analogy in Science." *Isis* 77 (1986): 261–277.

Stern, Steve. *The Secret History of Gender: Women, Men, and Power in Late Colonial Mexico*. Chapel Hill: University of North Carolina Press, 1995.

Stewart, Larry. *The Rise of Public Science: Rhetoric, Technology, and Natural Philosophy in Newtonian Britain, 1660–1750*. Cambridge: Cambridge University Press, 1992.

Sullivan, Lawrence E. "Religious Foundations of Health and Medical Power in South America." In *Healing and Restoring: Health and Medicine in the World's Religious Traditions*, ed. Sullivan. New York: Macmillan Publishing Company, 1989.

Sutphen, Mary Preston. "Rumoured Power: Hong Kong, 1894 and Cape Town, 1901." In *Western Medicine as Contested Knowledge*, ed. Cunningham and Andrews.

Sutphen, Mary, and Bridie Andrews, eds. *Medicine and Colonial Identity*. New York: Routledge, 2003.

Tackett, Timothy. "Conspiracy Obsession in a Time of Revolution: French Elites and the Origins of the Terror, 1789-1792." *AHR* 105:3 (June 2000): 691–713.

Tanck de Estrada, Dorothy. *Atlas ilustrado de los pueblos de indios: Nueva España, 1800*. Mexico City: El Colegio de México, 2005.

———. "Indian Children in Early Mexico." In *Children in Colonial America*, ed. Marten.

———. *Pueblos de indios y educación en el México colonial, 1750–1821*. Mexico City: El Colegio de México, 1999.

Tarantola, Arnaud. "Four Thousand Years of Concepts Relating to Rabies in Animals and Humans, Its Prevention and Its Cure." *Tropical Medicine and Infectious Diseases* 2:5 (2017): 1–21.

Taylor, William B. "Between Global Process and Local Knowledge: An Inquiry into Early Latin American Social History, 1500–1900." In *Reliving the Past:*

The Worlds of Social History, ed. Olivier Zunz. Chapel Hill: University of North Carolina Press, 1985.
———. "'. . . de corazón pequeño y ánimo apocado': Conceptos de los curas párrocos sobre los indios en la Nueva España del siglo XVIII." *Relaciones* 39 (Summer 1989): 5–67.
———. *Drinking, Homicide, and Rebellion in Colonial Mexican Villages*. Stanford, CA: Stanford University Press, 1979.
———. *Landlord and Peasant in Colonial Oaxaca*. Stanford, CA: Stanford University Press, 1972.
———. *Magistrates of the Sacred: Priests and Parishioners in Eighteenth-Century Mexico*. Stanford, CA: Stanford University Press, 1996.
———. "Mexico's Virgin of Guadalupe in the Seventeenth Century: Hagiography and Beyond." In *Colonial Saints*, ed. Greer and Bilinkoff.
———. *Shrines and Miraculous Images: Religious Life in Mexico before the Reforma*. Albuquerque: University of New Mexico Press, 2010.
———. *Theater of a Thousand Wonders: A History of Miraculous Images and Shrines in New Spain*. New York: Cambridge University Press, 2016.
———. "Two Shrines of the Cristo Renovado: Religion and Peasant Politics in Late Colonial Mexico." *AHR* 110:4 (2005): 945–974.
———. "The Virgin of Guadalupe in New Spain: An Inquiry into the Social History of Marian Devotion." *American Ethnologist* 14 (1987): 9–33.
Terraciano, Kevin. "Crime and Culture in Colonial Mexico: The Case of the Mixtec Murder Note." *Ethnohistory* 45:4 (Autumn 1998): 709–745.
Thompson, Angela T. "To Save the Children: Smallpox Inoculation, Vaccination, and Public Health in Guanajuato, Mexico, 1797–1840." *The Americas* 49:4 (April 1993): 431–455.
Thompson, E. P. *Customs in Common: Studies in Traditional Popular Culture*. New York: The New Press, 1993.
———. "The Moral Economy of the English Crowd in the Eighteenth Century." *Past and Present* 50 (1971): 76–136.
Tilley, Helen. *Africa as a Living Laboratory: Empire, Development, and the Problem of Scientific Knowledge, 1870–1950*. Chicago: University of Chicago Press, 2011.
Tomaselli, Sylvana. "Reflections on the History of the Science of Women." *History of Science* 29 (1991): 185–205.
Tortorici, Zeb. "'Heran Todos Putos': Sodomitical Subcultures and Disordered Desire in Early Colonial Mexico." *Ethnohistory* 54:1 (Winter 2007): 35–67.
Trennert, Robert A. *White Man's Medicine: Government Doctors and the Navajo, 1863–1955*. Albuquerque: University of New Mexico Press, 1998.
Trexler, Richard. *Religion in Social Context in Europe and America, 1200–1700*. Tempe: Arizona Center for Medieval and Renaissance Studies, 2002.
Uribe-Uran, Victor. "The Birth of a Public Sphere in Latin America during the Age of Revolution." *Comparative Studies in Society and History* 42:2 (April 2000): 425–457.
Valdez Garza, Dalia. *Libros y lectores en la* Gazeta de literatura de México *(1788–1795) de José Antonio Alzate*. Mexico City: Bonilla Artigas Editores, Instituto Tecnológico y de Estudios Superiores, 2014.

Valverde, Mariana. *Law's Dream of a Common Knowledge*. Princeton, NJ: Princeton University Press, 2003.

Van Young, Eric. *The Other Rebellion: Popular Violence, Ideology, and the Mexican Struggle for Independence, 1810–1821*. Stanford, CA: Stanford University Press, 2001.

Verdi Webster, Susan. *Art and Ritual in Golden-Age Spain*. Princeton, NJ: Princeton University Press, 1998.

Viesca Treviño, Carlos, and José Sanfilippo. "La medicina en las *Gacetas de Literatura*." In *Periodismo científico en el siglo XVIII*, ed. Aceves Pastrana.

Villaseñor Cabral, Patricia. "La epidemia de viruelas en Nueva España (1796–97) y sus repercusiones sociales, políticas, y económicas." Master's thesis, Universidad Iberoamericana, 1977.

Viqueira Albán, Juan Pedro. *Propriety and Permissiveness in Bourbon Mexico*, trans. Sonya Lipsett-Rivera and Sergio Rivera Ayala. Wilmington, DE: Scholarly Resources Inc., 1999.

Voekel, Pamela. *Alone before God: The Religious Origins of Modernity in Mexico*. Durham, NC: Duke University Press, 2002.

———. "Peeing on the Palace: Bodily Resistance to Bourbon Reforms in Mexico City." *Journal of Historical Sociology* 5:2 (June 1992): 183–208.

Wain, Harry. *A History of Preventive Medicine*. Springfield, IL: Charles C. Thomas, 1970.

Walton, Charles. *Policing Public Opinion in the French Revolution: The Culture of Calumny and the Problem of Free Speech*. New York: Oxford University Press, 2009.

Warner, Michael. *The Letters of the Republic: Publication and the Public Sphere in Eighteenth-Century America*. Cambridge, MA: Harvard University Press, 1992.

Warren, Adam. *Medicine and Politics in Colonial Peru: Population Growth and the Bourbon Reforms*. Pittsburgh: University of Pittsburgh Press, 2010.

———. "An Operation for Evangelization: Father Francisco González Laguna, the Cesarean Section, and Fetal Baptism in Late Colonial Peru." *BHM* 83:4 (Winter 2009): 647–675.

———. "Piety and Danger: Popular Ritual, Epidemics, and Medical Reforms in Lima, 1750–1860." Ph.D diss., University of California, San Diego, 2004.

Wear, Andrew. "The Popularization of Medicine in Early Modern England." In *The Popularization of Medicine, 1650–1850*, ed. Porter.

Weber, David. *Bárbaros: Spaniards and Their Savages in the Age of Enlightenment*. New Haven, CT: Yale University Press, 2005.

Webster, Charles, ed. *Health, Medicine and Mortality in the Sixteenth Century*. New York: Cambridge University Press, 1979.

Weismann, Elizabeth. *Art and Time in Mexico: From the Conquest to the Revolution*. New York: Harper & Row, 1985.

White, Luise. *Speaking with Vampires: Rumor and History in Colonial Africa*. Berkeley: University of California Press, 2000.

Yannakakis, Yanna. *The Art of Being In-between: Native Intermediaries, Indian Identity, and Local Rule in Colonial Oaxaca*. Durham, NC: Duke University Press, 2008.

———. "Hablar para distintos públicos: Testigos zapotecos y resistencia a la reforma parroquial en Oaxaca en el siglo XVIII." *Historia Mexicana* 55:3 (2006): 833–893.

Zarzoso, Alfonso. "¿Obligación moral o responsabilidad política? Las autoridades Borbónicas en tiempo de epidemias en la Cataluña del siglo XVIII." *Revista de Historia Moderna* 17 (1998–1999): 73–94.

Zunz, Olivier, ed. *Reliving the Past: The Worlds of Social History*. Chapel Hill: University of North Carolina Press, 1985.

Index

Lightning Source UK Ltd.
Milton Keynes UK
UKHW01n0820090818
326989UK00007B/244/P

9 781503 604339